Joy,

As always my gratitude and thanks for converting my awful handwriting into a typewritten script.

My very warmest good wishes to my good friend.

John

PS Don't attempt to read the book – just dip in.

People, Politics & Health

A Traveller's View

Dr John Stephen

People, Politics & Health

A Traveller's View

Dr John Stephen

ISBN 978-0-9931272-1-2

Published by W J Stephen in conjunction with Writersworld

Copy edited by Sue Croft

Cover design by Jag Lall

www.writersworld.co.uk

WRITERSWORLD
2 Bear Close Flats
Bear Close
Woodstock
Oxfordshire
OX20 1JX
United Kingdom
☎01993 812500 ☎0044 1993 812500

The text pages of this book are produced via an independent certification process that ensures the trees from which the paper is produced come from well managed sources that exclude the risk of using illegally logged timber while leaving options to use post-consumer recycled paper as well.

To the memory of Rachel who wanted me
to write this book and to whom
I owe so much

Acknowledgements

It is impossible to mention all the individuals involved in my travels; I hope they will accept my apologies.

However, I would like to mention a number of people involved in the writing of this book. Joy Peach started the initial transcription and Helen Noble continued with the task until I made the decision to undertake publication with Writersworld. Sue Croft became my editor and I would particularly like to thank her, not only for miraculously converting my illegible scrawl into orderly typescript, but also for overcoming the difficulty in working with someone without a computer. Without her professionalism, experience regarding publishing, diplomacy in correcting my text, ability to know what needed deleting or changing, and attention to detail, nothing would have been achieved.

CONTENTS

1

BACKGROUND

'This book will have no scientific value. Those who have studied birds will not find in it anything they do not already know; those who do not care for birds will not be interested in the subject. The writing of the book, and still more the publishing of it, requires some explanation.'

Thus wrote Viscount Grey of Fallodon in the Preface to *The Charm of Birds* 1927. As Sir Edward Grey, he had been Foreign Secretary at the beginning of the First World War, and is still the longest serving Foreign Secretary. On the afternoon of Monday 3 August, 1914, he spoke to the House of Commons concerning the impending war with Germany. Later, as he looked out from the Foreign Office and watched the lamps being lit in St James's Park, he turned to a friend and spoke the words for which he is always remembered: 'The lamps are going out all over Europe; we shall not see them again in our lifetime'.

Likewise, *People, Politics & Health (PPH)* will be of no value to the majority of practising physicians and politicians and of little interest to the plethora of travel writers. Nor to the now endless crowds thronging airports throughout the world.

PPH is going to be difficult to place in a particular section of a modern bookshop or library. As far as I know, except in the small number of independent bookshops which still survive, no quiet corner exists for books of general interest.

PPH is neither seriously political nor a straightforward travel book; its genesis is based on a study of medical and health matters[1] and not on high-tech medicine, which invariably catches the public's attention and is a favourite subject for TV hospital dramas and documentaries.

---

1 *An analysis of Primary Medical Care: an International Study* (Cambridge University Press 1979).
Primary Health Care in the Arab World (Somerset House 1992).
Reports and articles over a period of 30 years.

Primary medical/health care encompasses all health care taking place outside of hospitals and includes both general practice and public health. In a worldwide context the best definition was given by Dr Roger Cohen, Department of Community Medicine at Stony Brook, New York State, who in the early 1970s wrote: 'Primary care is what everybody needs and wants and can't get.'

So, why write this book and why publish it? I believe the British still have a soft spot for the amateur, a liking for the outsider. Interestingly, over the last twenty years or so, a lack of trust in the expert or scientist has come about: of course to the scientist or academic or professional I am a good example of a sciolist. But who knows, the jack of all trades may make a comeback.

PPH is a miscellany of observations, thoughts and impressions within a shared theme, and taking place in a wide variety of contexts with different political, religious, social and economic backgrounds.[2]

Since the middle of the 19th century, perhaps earlier, politics and medicine became inextricably linked, though were rarely comfortable bedfellows. Life from birth to death is the common thread which joins these uneasy companions. Politics was clearly not the prime purpose of my studies, yet it affected almost every encounter with patients, health professionals and politicians. Within Ministries of Health, local departments of public health, universities and medical schools, politics and medicine could not be disentangled, and certainly not separated.

Travel was different, unconnected with either politics or medicine; it provided a fascinating background, whilst my fortuitous brushes with serendipity enabled me to get a more hands-on feel for the diverse lives of people and the practical difficulties they experienced with their own particular health service.

Today few places in the world, even the most remote and inaccessible, are protected or remain untouched by the effects, both good and bad, of the apparently unstoppable tourist industry. Everyone wants to find their own Shangri La before it is spoilt by the

2 A number of omissions are obvious, but were not planned. East Germany, Saudi Arabia and Oman all refused visas. This was surprising in regard to Saudi and Oman as both countries are the UK's closest allies in the region. East Germany remains a puzzle, while my failure with Albania was lack of time.

hoi-polloi, often overlooking the fact that we are all part of this tide of people which is flooding the world. It was my great good fortune to journey to places which at the time were seldom visited, even urban areas and capital cities where foreigners were unusual. As recently as November 2008 the very-much-travelled John Simpson, the BBC's World Affairs' editor, wrote quite unashamedly in a British Airways *High Life* magazine:

> *'Things have much moved on here. Belgrade is cheap and pleasant and easy to visit. My advice is to come and see its weirdly interesting sights before the hordes catch on.'*

I wonder if in all his travels he has ever considered himself to be part of the hoi-polloi.

I have always been against jumping into print but, as the origins of *PPH* go back nearly fifty years, and *Analysis of Primary Medical Care* was published over twenty years ago, I can hardly be accused of that. On the other hand, if I delay any longer, I am in danger of forgetting much of what I want to include or, even worse, memory in old age being not only fickle and unreliable, it can also lie. Re-reading part of a review in *The Lancet* 7 July , 1979, has given me the confidence before it is too late:

> *'There are three ways of analysing primary care. First, by examination of primary care as it exists today: there have been a multitude of those over the past ten years. Second, by historical research because you cannot know where you are unless you know where you came from, and this approach has largely been neglected. Third, by comparing systems of primary approach in different countries: a few short studies have been published but none as comprehensive or as important as a new book which examines systems of primary care in Western Europe, Scandinavia, East Europe, the USSR, Canada, Australia, New Zealand, the USA, Japan, Chile and Cuba.*
>
> *It is the kind of book that might have been produced by a number of authors from different countries, or by a working party, or a committee from the United Nations or some other multi-national organisation. In fact it has single-handedly been written by a general practitioner in Wells, Somerset – and it is all the better for that.*[3] *For many years Dr Stephen has been interested in patterns of primary care in other countries and, with remarkably little outside help, he has travelled from one country to another like some intrepid Victorian*

---

[3] *'Single authorship'* is not strictly true as help was received from a colleague who wrote the chapters on Canada, Australia and New Zealand.

explorer, armed with a sharp eye and a notebook. All the virtues of single authorship are here . . . Some of the author's statements are highly personal and provocative; and there shines through the book a humanely sympathetic approach to the needs of patients, combined with a balanced and realistic appreciation of general practice based on first-hand experience. It is these qualities that give the book authority . . .

At another level it is an excellent work of reference which could be described as the hitch-hikers' guide to general practice.

The greatest value of the book may be that it will stimulate everyone concerned with planning to take a much less insular view of primary care . . . There is an urgency in the need to develop and improve primary care in most countries. Sometimes it seems today that books on primary care of any size or importance can be undertaken only by 'teams' of authors. This book splendidly demonstrates that the best size for a team is often one!'

Some people, after reading these generous comments, will feel uncomfortable and believe I am indulging in self-publicity of the worst kind. They may be right, but will be relieved to learn that the book was virtually ignored in the United Kingdom.

In retrospect I realise it is rarely a good idea to be ahead of your time, and neither is it advisable for an outsider to enter the academic world. At the time my book was published I did not understand or have experience in the ways of academia; I was an amateur in the sense of having neither an academic background nor training, nor an attachment to any university or medical school. Nor was I involved with any international organisation such as the WHO or UNICEF, and in the eyes of many I was writing with no authority. Looking back I now realise that quite a number of my colleagues found this unacceptable, whilst others were mystified or irritated by the support given by the Cambridge University Press to an author with no bona fide track record to his name.

Working and researching as an individual rather than as one of a team gives you complete freedom of action and planning with no need to consult colleagues and no decisions to be made by a committee or majority vote. As I am a hopeless team player this suited me perfectly. However, these advantages must be measured against a number of disadvantages.

First, I had no secretary or research assistant; everything that needed to be done I had to do myself – travel arrangements, visa applications, writing to Ministers and Ministries of Health, searching through libraries and organising contacts and advisers. Second, the reciprocal benefits and arrangements between universities, academic institutions, international government agencies and media contacts, were not available. Such contacts are taken for granted by those who benefit from them. Often a familiar face and always a network of people are there to help with on-the-spot research, enquiries or guidance, and if they should run into potentially serious trouble of a political nature, then ready support would be at hand. I often look or listen with some amusement, and sometimes with a little irritation, as correspondents or travel writers tell their tales with hardly a mention of the back-up teams of photographers and colleagues and those who are organising food and drink and accommodation. A strong impression is given that they are travelling on their own.

But, initially unrecognised by me, was the problem my presence would pose for most of the countries I visited. It is one thing to invite an expert in a particular field to your country to share his or her expertise, but quite another to give permission to an unknown individual such as myself to come and study – or as some might say, poke my nose into the workings of their health service and then write a report on my findings.

It says a great deal about these countries, in particular those which had poor diplomatic relations with the UK and two countries in which diplomatic relations had been broken off. Almost everywhere I received cooperation and remarkable freedom to see what I wanted, although not before, I must add, much hard work and preparation had gone into the planning of my visits. But I was determined not to be fobbed off. In addition, each country provided transport, a driver and an interpreter, usually a fellow physician, all without cost to me. Nothing could have been achieved without such help.

People, Politics & Health covers the time of the Cold War, the fall of the Berlin Wall and the collapse of the Soviet Union (USSR). It had been in existence since 1922 until its disintegration at midnight on 31 December, 1991, followed quickly by Yeltsin's inspired formation of the unlikely-sounding Commonwealth of Independent States. Throughout the Soviet period the republics and a number of autonomous regions had remained dormant, suppressed and hidden within the USSR, but by the middle to late '80s most of them wanted independence, each having separate cultures as well as different religions and customs. The majority viewed themselves as independent nations within this vast landmass. It was difficult to believe that over a hundred different non-Slav dialects were spoken in the old Soviet Union.

The changes in Europe following the fall of the Berlin Wall have not been easy to take in. Albania, Bulgaria, Czechoslovakia, East Germany, Hungary, Poland and Romania all eventually rid themselves of their communist regimes. The Republics of Latvia, Lithuania, Estonia, Ukraine and Moldova all declared themselves independent of the USSR. In 1990 East and West Germany became one nation as they had been before the Second World War. In 1993 Czechoslovakia split into the Czech Republic and the Republic of Slovakia as they had been before the Versailles arrangement (Treaty of Trianon) just after the First World War. During the early 1990s Yugoslavia broke up during the Civil War, and four of the constituent republics – Slovenia, Croatia, Bosnia-Herzegovina and Macedonia – seceded to become independent countries. In 1992/3 Serbia and Montenegro declared themselves to be the new Republic of Yugoslavia, but subsequently separated in 2006 to become two separate nations. The independence of Kosovo remains unsolved, and hostility between the Serbs and the Albanians living in the new Republic of Serbia continues unabated.

With the break-up of the Soviet Union and Yugoslavia, eleven new countries in Europe became part of the United Nations, and to complicate matters further, two countries, East and West Germany, have become one, while Czechoslovakia has become two.

Kazakhstan and Mongolia are both geographically part of Asia but only Kazakhstan was a republic within the old Soviet Union; they decided against independence and joined the Commonwealth of Independent States in 1991.

For two hundred years at least, both historically and politically, Kazakhstan has been connected with or been part of, first the old Tsarist Empire and then the Soviet Union. Mongolia on the other hand has had a completely different history, being famous for having been the centre and origin of one of the largest and greatest Empires ever to exist: Genghis Khan and the Golden Hordes and all that. After the demise of the Empire in the middle of the 14th century, Mongolia then became a province of China and did not gain independence until 1911. In 1924 it became a communist state based on the Soviet model, marooned first between the Soviet Union and Chiang Kai-shek's Nationalist right-wing government, and then the first communist government of China led by Mao Tse-tung. Throughout the 60s, 70s and 80s Mongolia endeavoured whenever possible to play off its powerful neighbours one against the other. It was not until 1992, following the fall of the Berlin Wall, that a democratic-style constitution was introduced.

In the years between my two visits in 1972 and 1994, Japan had become a great economic power. To a superficial observer like myself, the country gave an impression of sound finances, a strong economy, political stability, safety in the streets and an increasingly positive influence throughout the world. Japan was certainly not a threat to her close neighbours or anyone else. Yet within a few months of my wife and I returning from Japan in 1994 the country had suffered the sarin nerve gas attack on the Tokyo underground, a severe earthquake in and around Osaka, and the start of the collapse of the banking system with the ensuing decline in its economy which persists to the present time. Of course nobody could have foreseen the earthquake and tsunami of 2011 and the devastation that has followed.

Chile and Cuba in 1974 were in the midst of the Cold War with both the United States and the Soviet Union striving to increase their power and influence in the ideological struggle at the time. Both major powers were always happy to see small countries promoting their propaganda, or fighting their cause by proxy, or interfering clandestinely in their internal politics at every opportunity.

The background to my travels in the Arab world between 1981 and 1988 was the never-ending Arab-Israeli conflict, the never-ending question of the Palestine State, the Iran-Iraq war, the Israeli invasion of Lebanon and the US bombing of Libya. It was a different world and more complicated. Certainly religion has been more significant, with Judaism (and over the last 100 years Zionism), Christianity and Islam being responsible for much of the unrest and misery in the

Middle East, whilst since the end of the Second World War the different sects of Islam have increasingly created enmity within Islam itself – and not only in the Arab world.

Politically the Arabs have had many reasons to be suspicious of the West, particularly Britain and France following the end of the First World War, and the United States at the end of the Second World War; their lack of trust is understandable. However, the Arabs have not helped themselves, and until the poisonous entanglement between religion and politics is resolved, conflict will remain. The future of the State of Israel and the land of Palestine continues to be a seemingly insurmountable problem, with all participants at fault. Finally, and most important of all, while dictatorship is the only form of government, whether it be an oligarchy, a theocracy, or the absolute authority of the military or a family, little progress can be made.

Ideally I would have liked to visit Israel, in part because it is the only country in the region (except Turkey) with a democratically elected government. However, a visit proved to be impossible as no Arab country would allow entry if your passport had been stamped by the Israelis, and I was not prepared to get a second passport in order to deceive the countries I was intending to visit.

Do I remember comments on and even opposition to my visits? Yes, I do. Nearly thirty years after the Second World War a generation gap, not surprisingly, still divided the country concerning Japan and the Japanese; an unforgiving hatred persisted amongst those who had been POWs and had seen and experienced their barbarism and cruelty at first hand.

I remember and was surprised by the anger of a good Polish friend, even forty-five years after the end of the war, when she discovered I was going to Kazakhstan. How could I possibly contemplate such a visit after everything Stalin had done? How he had uprooted millions of people before, during and after the war, and had transported them to Kazakhstan for a life of imprisonment, slavery, poverty and isolation.

Among my colleagues I was considered left-wing and to have been seduced by communist propaganda. I accepted this as almost inevitable – in the medical profession it is not difficult to be labelled in this way. Nonetheless, on occasions it did get under my skin. 'One only has to see where he's been . . .' was a typical reaction whilst conveniently forgetting my visits to Western Europe, Scandinavia, the USA, Japan, and of course Chile. No credit for deciding not to include South Africa or for being honest with regard to Israel.

I would have been quite content with labels such as 'non-conformist' or 'a bit anti-establishment' . . . never mind, it's of no consequence.

2

CENTRAL EUROPE

Throughout the Cold War, Czechoslovakia, Hungary and Poland were always considered to be part of Eastern Europe. This was accurate in a geographical sense and certainly politically and economically as the three countries had fallen behind the 'Iron Curtain' – a designation that was quickly incorporated into the English language after a speech by Churchill. It is interesting to look back at Churchill's speech, delivered in Fulton, Missouri in 1946, as he had recognised the difference between Central and Eastern Europe:

> '*From Stettin in the Baltic to Trieste in the Adriatic an Iron Curtain has descended across the Continent. Behind that line lie all the capitals of the ancient states of Central and Eastern Europe . . .*'

Sadly Churchill the historian was not listened to by the great majority of fellow politicians and certainly by none of the press, radio or television. It was therefore a great surprise to discover that the citizens of these three countries were irritated and amazed at our ignorance. These intensely individualistic and talented peoples, each with their own language, culture and traditions, had been grouped together as East European, part of that amorphous mass – the communist bloc.

No, these countries were not like Bulgaria, Romania and Yugoslavia which to a large extent had been occupied by the Ottoman Empire off and on for hundreds of years. But neither should they be included with the West. *Central* Europe was where they belonged, at the centre of European civilisation and culture. Didn't we understand history? Didn't we recognise the enormous pride these people felt for their music, literature, art and architecture?

Our apparent lack of understanding of the complexity of their history, and a seeming indifference to the geographical misfortune of their homelands, which had been a convenient battleground over the centuries with the consequent frequent alterations of their national frontiers, was an additional resentment. In contrast we British, more than any other European nation, have been so blessed by our geography and our history, that we can barely begin to understand their misfortunes. Certainly this view was confirmed by Neville Chamberlain speaking in 1938 about these 'faraway places'.

Of course included in the hundred million Europeans who lived on the wrong side of the Iron Curtain were the Bulgarians, the Romanians and Yugoslavs, who were equally irritated, even despairing about the West, but for different reasons.

I soon realised that the visits I hoped to arrange to various parts of the communist world would produce their own particular headaches. I had chosen the communist world before any other country as I felt their health services would be easier to describe and analyse since all were based on the Soviet Union, although minor differences were permitted or developed according to the culture and history of each country.

For many years there had been debate about the Soviet model – in a sense just a luxury for academics as there could be no prospect of change. In fact the USSR was in a good position to advise on the building up and organisation of medical services from nothing, following the chaos and destruction at the end of the Second World War. The Soviets had had their own experience after revolution and civil war when they had identified essential priorities – maternity services and child care, the control of infections and communicable diseases, preventive medicine and, later on, industrial health services. However, this is not to say the Soviet Union were able to implement their own priorities as they had hoped.

Little help came from the Department of Health, the British Medical Association or the Royal College of General Practitioners, but individuals provided support and guidance which proved invaluable. It would have been easier if I had been a member of the Socialist Medical Association or a trade union as both had direct contacts on the other side of the Iron Curtain.

Surprisingly, help was at hand within the European Economic Union (EEC) where the International Society of General Practice had been set up in the late '50s in West Germany; its General Secretary, Dr K Engelmeier, from Oelde, Westphalia, provided contacts in Hungary, Poland and Romania.

Living as we do today in a world of emails, texting, twittering et al and rarely putting pen to paper, it will be hard for readers to understand the difficulties of corresponding and making contact through the Iron Curtain into the communist world. A reply in six weeks was rare, three months more likely. It was not unusual to get no response at all.

3

PEOPLE'S REPUBLIC OF HUNGARY

My travels began on 7 May, 1966. It had been a perfect spring day, a cloudless azure blue sky with the first signs of real heat in the midday sun. In Paris by early evening, it was still just warm enough to eat at a pavement table on the Rue Dante – a small, narrow street at the junction of Rue St Jacques and the Boulevard St Germain leading quickly down to the Seine and a dramatic view of Notre Dame.

I remember repeatedly looking at the Zug-Begleiter, Die Deutsche Bundesbahn with its timetable for the F S Orient Express. I knew perfectly well the train left the Gare de l'Est at 9.45pm for Budapest. Being unfamiliar with the modern 24 hour clock, as well as fidgeting with my passport and ticket and travellers cheques, I was constantly double-checking my watch to make certain that 21.45 was indeed 9.45pm and not 8.45pm or indeed 10.45pm. And of course the time difference in France had to come into the calculation. It all seems utterly pathetic but I'm much the same, even today.

The train left exactly on time. The journey was expected to take just over twenty-two hours. I was filled with nervous excitement. The Cold War was at its height – John le Carré and all that – although the actual danger of a Soviet attack had lessened. President Kennedy's successful strategy over the Cuban Missile Crisis in 1962 could largely take the credit for this.

But this was a Western perspective. What would the Hungarians and the Czechs think of the West? The dramatic crackling voice of one of the students supporting the uprising, who had occupied Hungarian State Radio, will never be forgotten by those who heard his message. On the morning of 4 November, 1956, as the Soviet tanks lumbered into Budapest, the early success of the uprising was in critical danger and the patriotic voice of this young man could be heard pleading with the outside world for help against the Soviet invasion. Britain and France were still immersed in the sordid deceit of the Suez fiasco, whilst the United States was busy opposing Britain and France at the United Nations. No other countries in Western Europe were prepared or able to support the Hungarians, who were left to their fate. The West shed crocodile tears. The Hungarians rapidly learnt that sympathy did not extend into action. This depressing reality was accepted by all the People's Republics over the next forty years.

So, ten years after the fated uprising I was wondering how much bitterness against the West remained. How fresh in the minds of the Hungarians I was to meet would be the memory of the hopeless street fighting and the final shutdown of Hungarian State Radio.

The journey across Europe was uneventful, although I was surprised by the meandering route between Strasburg and Ülm, stopping at places I'd never heard of. As always one wakes when the train is stationary, and in the middle of the night uncertainty took over as I caught sight of unfamiliar names on ill-lit platforms – was I on the right train? Eventually we reached Vienna. Alas, there was none of the glamour associated with the days between 1883 and 1961 when the Orient Express ran between Paris and Istanbul via Vienna and through the Balkans. I missed it by five years. Since then the name had been used by a number of transport companies, all covering different parts of the old route and developing routes of their own.

Vienna to Budapest by train is just 165 miles and the journey took five hours. It was my first experience of these border hold-ups between the capitalist and the communist world. On the Austrian side the passport and customs officials came on board, stamped what needed to be stamped, decided whose luggage they wanted to inspect, and we were quickly on our way.

On the Hungarian side it was a different matter; just a mile or so across the border was Hegyeshalen with barbed-wire watch towers and Alsatian dogs straining at the leash. As we drew alongside the platform, armed soldiers immediately took up their positions, one standing at the end of each coach guarding the doors, which had now been locked. Soldiers were on both sides of the train and on the roofs of the carriages. No one was allowed to get out or even look out of the windows without much shouting and threatening gestures. The passport and customs officials, both men and women, then proceeded through each carriage without any sense of urgency. As they flicked through them it was as if our passports held secret information and, before returning them, all passengers had to move into the corridor whilst the officials searched every corner of the apartment – under the seats and in the overflowing luggage racks. I had no trouble. It was the Hungarians returning from the West who were subjected to the most aggressive searching. Cigarettes, spirits, and any kind of luxury item were confiscated, though foreign currency seemed to be their main target. The whole palaver must have taken a good hour and a half.

I had corresponded briefly with Dr Engelmeier's Hungarian contacts but nothing more. Dr and Mrs Rado Sandor – Sonyi and Suzie – were on the platform. I forget how we were to recognise each other, but after a quick, rather formal handshake we found their clapped-out Lada and I was driven home to meet their three children – Gabor, about 16 years, Ester 13 or 14, Judit who was 11 – and one of their grandmothers, Suzie's mother, who lived in Vienna and was on holiday.

Their flat, at 11 Kükülo, was in the woody, hilly area of the city. Buda was the original medieval city on the right bank of the Danube, which in the nineteenth century became fashionable for anyone who wasn't working-class. It has remained 'an attractive and desirable residential area' (as estate agents would say). The largest and most elegant houses were of course no longer occupied by the aristocracy or nouveau-riche but by a different elite – top government ministers, the crème de la crème of the Party and, it seemed, senior members of the University.

On the flat land surrounding the town of Pest on the opposite side of the river, factories and industry were easy to see, and it was here the workers were housed in the grey, soulless blocks of flats so typical of Soviet planning. Certainly twenty years of communist egalitarianism hadn't altered the fact that Pest was for the workers and Buda for the rest.

Sonyi and Suzie were both doctors and considered themselves to be general practitioners. Suzie worked part-time in Buda and a number of her patients were members of the government and senior members of the Party. Sonyi worked in Pest full-time; all his patients were workers, or retired, or peasants from neighbouring villages which had been swallowed up by industry. Suzie and her mother were charming, cultured people, coming as it were from another time and place. Sonyi was more a man from the Hungarian plains, a large good-looking fellow of great enthusiasm and energy and endless stories to tell, but having experienced little of the pre-war sophistication of Vienna and Budapest. He was completely at home with his working-class patients and was clearly liked by them. Both Sonyi and Suzie understood English.

I didn't meet any of Suzie's patients or see where she worked. There were a number of reasons for this. First, she wasn't happy about being involved with government and Party members as it compromised her strong anti-communist beliefs. Second, she was embarrassed about having to admit to me that this was the situation. Third, she did not want any of her patients to know that someone from the West was staying with her.

Arrangements had been made for me to stay close by in the ground floor of a house which could have been from a Turgenev or Tolstoy novel. It was surrounded by a small orchard of apples, plums and pears and a couple of large fig trees that stood against the wall of this early-nineteenth century house with its air of faded gentility and everything in need of repair and a splash of paint – the only thing missing on the wooden veranda was a samovar.

Inside, the furnishings seemed to date from the latter days of the Austro-Hungarian Empire, the antiquated lamps and fireplaces adding to its charm. It would have done credit to a Bristol Old Vic production of *The Cherry Orchard*, or *The Three Sisters*. The bathroom consisted of two old brass taps, two stone washbasins supported on bricks, and the oldest geyser I had ever seen. In winter it must have been perishingly cold.

I was sharing the place with two young Russian students. I spoke no Russian, they spoke no English, yet we chatted happily as we washed and shaved. They used open razors and were intrigued by my Gillette blade, having never seen one before.

In the morning I walked round to have breakfast with the Rado family, but before setting off with Sonyi for work we needed to visit the local police station as every foreigner and non-resident Hungarian had to 'sign on' within thirty-six hours of arrival. How officials do love to stare at documents and then stare at the owner of the documents. The policeman studied my visa and passport quite impassively for some minutes and then rather dramatically leapt into action as though he had just found what he was looking for. Having filled in the required form which confirmed where and with whom I was staying, the final flourish involved repeated stamping of the precious documents. As far as I was concerned, the whole procedure took place in silence; Sonyi had told me not to speak, he would do all the talking.

Hungary was divided into around 3,300 health districts each with a population of between 3,000 - 3,500. As in the Soviet Union, Hungary was committed to the principle that the doctor of first contact restricted her work (doctors in primary care were predominantly female) to a particular age and sex and to those who were able to work. In rural areas this was not possible and local physicians then acted as general practitioners. In urban areas a health centre was the primary care facility, but over the years the polyclinics took over.

Although both Sonyi and Suzie considered themselves to be general practitioners, in fact they were district/community doctors looking after the elderly, the chronically sick, the retired and the unemployed (this latter was never an official category as unemployment was not acceptable in the communist world). Women and children were not their responsibility, whilst workers were cared for by the Industrial Health Service at a polyclinic as close to their work as possible. Small enterprises combined together to provide a small health centre staffed by a factory doctor.

Sonyi worked at just such a health centre; it was staffed by two district doctors and a dentist, along with appropriate nurses. Not even the simplest laboratory test was carried out. No paediatric care was provided, the Soviet Union and Hungary being unique within the communist bloc in that they provided separate paediatric polyclinics.

The session would last about two and a half hours after which we would set off in his car on home visits. In no other country I visited did I find community doctors using their own cars. Sonyi received an allowance from the Ministry of Health; in other countries transport was provided by the state if it was required. The elderly and housebound had much the same problems and complaints as I encountered at home, but the great difference was that almost all the patients were elderly, although I noticed Sonyi would give unofficial advice to young mothers about their children.

Over a couple of days we did six visits. Everyone was pleased to see Sonyi, both patients and their families. His examination always included taking the blood pressure – almost obligatory in the view of any society – and often listening to the heart and chest. However, most of his time was spent listening to their social and medical difficulties. The area was poor and the houses we visited bore this out; furniture was sparse, people were wearing threadbare jackets, old faded frocks, ancient pinnies and worn shoes and slippers. Invariably they had tired, careworn faces and without exception all the men and some women smoked heavily. Simple gifts were offered – a slice of cake or a biscuit, cheap coffee or tea, a glass of homemade wine, or plum or peach *palinka*, and fruit in season: but never money. Sonyi and Suzie both assured me they had never accepted money and never would, and I believed them – bribery was part and parcel of the health service in every country I visited, and was openly admitted. My lasting impression of these home visits was that the household was reassured and felt secure, knowing that someone was keeping an eye on them. Certainly high-tech medicine didn't enter into it.

On the first day driving back to 11 Kükülo I asked Sonyi if it would be possible to spend a day with Suzie. No, was the uncompromising answer. This was a disappointment as I would have liked to compare and contrast. Undoubtedly Sonyi was happier in his work than Suzie, as he didn't feel a traitor to the principles both held dear. Still, a fascinating day lay ahead, visiting a doctor, a friend of the Rados, who worked in the rural health service.

He worked in Pannonhalma, a small village about three hours drive from Budapest. First we travelled north-west to Estergom on the banks of the Danube, the historic and spiritual home of the nation and the residence of the Primate, and then west along the river to Gyor, after which we turned south. After half an hour along narrow country roads and scattered hamlets a three-peaked hill suddenly rose out of the flat countryside. At the bottom of this hill their friend lived and worked. It was a traditional village house, slightly larger than the average and with a modern extension, thus a combined home and health centre.

It reminded me of many surgeries I had worked in after graduating in 1956 – the same wooden examination couch, a not-so-grand desk, a sphygmomanometer, kidney dishes, a small bunsen burner, simple surgical instruments and a separate area for boiling syringes and needles before storing them in surgical spirit. Pre-sterilised syringes and needles, which we now use and discard with gay abandon, were unheard of. The waiting room provided a couple of wooden benches rather than chairs, and apart from the brilliant white of the kidney dishes there was a general feeling of drabness and varying shades of brown paint.

We had arrived about midday and there were still patients waiting to be seen – middle-aged and elderly, men and women with lined, weather-beaten faces, and one mother and child. Knowing instinctively that country folk would not be happy with a complete stranger at a consultation, I declined the offer to sit in with the doctor.

During lunch I was able to question him about the patients he had seen that morning. There were about twenty-five, with much the same problems a GP in the UK would be presented with. In addition we talked about his life, his professional isolation and his work. We also talked openly about communism, which was a never-ending topic of discussion throughout Hungary, and provided Sonyi with an opportunity to argue.

As we came to the end of my questions Sonyi asked whether I would like to visit the monastery, to which I replied with an enthusiastic affirmative. I had glimpsed on arrival impressive-looking buildings at the top of one of the peaks, but at the time I had no idea it was a monastery, or of its importance. The Abbot and the doctor were good friends and an invitation had been pre-arranged, so we there and then took the car up to see him.

The original church and the Benedictine monastery had been built in 996 AD. Founded by the father of St Stephen (King of Hungary) it contained many relics, notably the coronation mantle of King Stephen as well as a large library. Over the next thousand years the village of Pannonhalma became an increasingly significant part of Hungarian culture. I was permitted to see both relics without quite realising what a privilege this was.

After formal introductions Abbot Nobert Legangi began to ask me questions – where was I from? what was the purpose of my visit? Having responded to these questions I then told him I came from a small town in the south-west of England that he would not have heard of. He pressed me for more details and at the mention of Wells a broad grin spread across his face. He said:

"I know it well – you see, I visited Downside Abbey before the war."

It transpired that the links between Pannonhalma and Downside had, surprisingly, remained. In 1935 the Abbey church of Downside was consecrated and dedicated by a legate representing Pope Pius XI – George Justin Seredi, monk of Pannonhalma, Archbishop and Prince Primate of Hungary. With the communist takeover in 1948, the government initially rounded up all catholic priests into the monastery at Pannonhalma in the hope of reducing the influence of the church. This failed, due to the legendary Cardinal Joseph Mindszenty who feared neither the Nazis nor the communists. In 1949 he was charged with treason and imprisoned, only to be released six years later on condition he did not leave the country. In the chaos at the end of the 1956 uprising and the Soviet invasion, he found refuge in the American Embassy in Budapest. He was granted asylum and remained a voluntary prisoner until 1971 when he was permitted to go abroad; he spent his final years in a religious community in Vienna.

The monastery had thus managed to remain open and was used as a house for retired priests. In addition, a boys' boarding school had been opened and was still functioning. One of the paradoxes of life in Hungary under communism was the number of catholic schools, in addition to Pannonhalma, which were allowed to survive, and even flourish. It seemed the government did not relish serious confrontation with the church.

As we left the monastery, situated like a fortress, we lingered for a moment to take in the commanding views of the flat plains laid out before us. Then we drove on to Lake Balaton and a visit to one of the many wine cellars built into the sides of the gentle hills of this region.

In 2008 I paid a visit to Downside Abbey. The Abbot, the Rt Rev Dominic Aideen Vellenger, told me he had visited Pannonhalma a few years before and could confirm that both the monastery and the school were flourishing. The house for retired priests was also still in existence and he had spoken to two of the elderly residents, both well into their nineties and able to recall life under the Nazis and communists. The Abbot was also able to look up the record of the consecration and dedication and validate the presence of the Hungarian legate from Pannonhalma representing the Pope.

My hosts were recognisably professional and I was interested to observe how strict they were with their children – it had a sort of non-conformist Lutheran feel. One evening we went to the opera to see Kodaly's 'Háry János' – my introduction to Kodaly. There was no question of Gabor coming with us:

'He's too young'.

None of the children were allowed to drink even diluted coffee – again, 'too young', and all treated their grandmother with respect. Another evening I joined Suzie, Sonyi and Grandma at the local school for a concert in which Ester and Judit were playing the piano. At the end, the usual pride amongst the parents and the excitement of all the children was no different from at home in Wells. The Rados and their friends, whilst chatting before going home, said to me:

"People are people, we're all the same as you. If only governments could understand this."

On getting home from the concert, despite all the excitement the bedtime routine was unchanged.

Throughout the communist world political jokes were a feature of life, and Sonyi was a master of the Hungarian variety. Some were at the expense of Marxism and its absurd bureaucracy, and in fact were often not jokes but simply amusing comments against his own government or that of the Soviet Union. I suppose they took the place of satire and political cartoons for which one could end up in prison. The political joke was a safety valve for frustration and anger, and now, fifty years later in the UK, endless phone-in programmes (very cheap for broadcasters) have given the public the illusion of serious participation in day to day issues, and of being able to influence politicians and society at large. I suspect phone-ins have as much effect as political jokes.

*

Snobbery and feelings of superiority were alive and well in Hungary. A couple of days before leaving for Prague, Sonyi started to talk about Czechoslovakia:

"Why do you need to go and see these Czechens? They're hopeless – you stay with us."

I just listened.

"We Hungarians are direct descendants of the Austro-Hungarian Empire, the Hapsburgs as well. We had an aristocracy, which the Czechens never had."

Again I listened. But the views of Sonyi and Suzie were clear, and Grandma Gully was in no doubt either, the only difference being her certainty that Vienna was more cultured than Budapest.

My Cold War anxieties disappeared very quickly and never once did it occur to me that I might be followed by the secret police, or that conversations I had in Sonyi's health centre might be reported on.

The main reason for the Rados' very warm welcome soon became clear; it was their desperate need to make contact with the West. The whole family would never be given permission to travel abroad; a child could go if the parents remained at home, or vice versa. It was referred to as 'hostage travel'. Furthermore, foreign travel was not possible without an invitation. Within a year of my visit I received a letter from Grandma Gully in Vienna explaining about the required invitation. By using her as an intermediary, Suzie and Sonyi felt that direct correspondence to Hungary could be kept to a minimum.

A year later they made Wells their base while they travelled round the south-east of England – they had come in their old Lada. Gabor followed in 1968, charming both young and old, although Ester didn't make it until 1973.

In 1971, on my way to the Soviet Union, I briefly stopped off in Budapest, and in 1973 my wife Rachel and I came over soon after Ester's visit to us. Our final meeting was a complete surprise. It was 1979 and we knew Gabor was staying behind as hostage (at the time he was training to be an ophthalmologist) and the rest of the family were coming over to the UK. Unfortunately their dates coincided with our family holiday in the north-west of Scotland, but they knew where to get the keys of our house, which they could use as a base, and we thought no more about it. On the final evening of our holiday, the Rado family were spotted climbing up the track to the house!

4

PEOPLE'S REPUBLIC of CZECHOSLOVAKIA

The night train to Prague left on time with Suzie and Sonyi waving from the platform while I clutched Suzie's food for the journey. I realised I had only managed to get a superficial understanding of the health services behind the Iron Curtain, and so much more needed to be explored. I also realised that arranging my visit privately had obvious limitations.

Now what about Czechoslovakia? In the end my visit had been arranged through the Ministry of Health in Prague – would this make a difference? And what would people think about the West, Great Britain in particular, a country in which they had mistakenly placed their trust?

Munich had been a great let-down for the Czech people. No wonder, as Chamberlain returned to London after his meeting with Hitler and Mussolini, thousands were on the streets of Prague, not only because of the Nazi occupation of the Sudetenland, but also because the occupation had been acceded to by a supposedly genuine ally. What a betrayal.

Both Tomas Masaryk, the first President of Czechoslovakia following the end of the First World War, and Edward Beneš, the first Foreign Secretary, who later became President following Masaryk's retirement in 1935, were strong Democrats and very pro-western, particularly towards Great Britain.

Although not directly involved, many people in post-war Britain had a feeling of guilt following the tragic death of Jan Masaryk, son of Tomas, who had returned as Foreign Secretary along with President Beneš to their homeland in 1945. On that fateful day 10 March, 1948, when his body was found beneath the open window of the Foreign Ministry in Prague, the question was – did he commit suicide or was he pushed? Debate was still raging when I was here in 1966, but today it is felt he took his own life in protest against the Stalinisation of his beloved country.

Dr John Horder, a London GP, had enabled me to correspond with the International Relations Department of the Ministry of Public Health in Prague; by chance he had met František Ošanéc, a senior member of the International Relations Department, at a meeting in London. My letter explaining the purpose of my visit received a business-like reply almost by return of post – a programme would be organised for my arrival. Hungary had been unofficial and relaxed, almost amateur, whilst Czechoslovakia looked as though it would be official and well-organised. Ošanéc had managed to find out where I was staying in Budapest through John Horder, who had contacted my wife in Wells, to let me know which hotel I would be staying at in Prague. In fact it was this cable that had fuelled Sonyi's comments about 'these Czechens'. I had requested cheap but hopefully clean accommodation; nevertheless I was slightly anxious as my funds were limited, and trying to arrange for additional money/travellers cheques from the UK would have been impossible.

František, known to us as Frank, and Katya his wife, both knew the UK well and spoke English with ease and fluency, Katya in particular. They came from entirely different backgrounds – he was a country boy from a poor background. In 1938 he had been the first pupil from his village school some forty miles from Prague to study at Charles University.

Katya was born into a rich, Jewish banking family and as a child had lived in a flat on the prosperous and secure Napiikopé street at the bottom of Wenceslas Square. In 1937 she was awarded a British Council scholarship to study biochemistry at Cambridge. In July/August 1939 she made the very difficult decision not to return to her homeland.

Frank escaped from Prague soon after the declaration of war in September 1939 and travelled to Britain via Romania, Bulgaria, the Middle East, North Africa, Spain and Portugal, arriving in Britain in the summer of 1940. He joined the Free Czech forces and was posted to their Armoured Brigade stationed close to Cambridge. It was here he met Katya. Within a couple of years they married, spending their brief honeymoon in Edinburgh having found a cheap room in either the YMCA or YWCA – they couldn't remember which!

Soon after D-Day Frank returned to the mainland of Europe; the

Czech Armoured Brigade was part of the advancing Allied forces as they fought their way across Europe. Katya meanwhile had left Cambridge in early 1945 with a D. Phil; travelling via the Middle East and the Balkans she found herself in Prague around the time of the May 5 uprising against the remaining German garrison. Soviet troops were nearing Prague from the east, while American forces including the Czech Armoured Brigade were rapidly advancing from the west. It all ended on May 8 with both Katya and Frank in Prague, though of course unknown to each other at the time.

Their home-comings were tragically different. Frank was to find his mother and younger brother still alive (his father had died before the war) and their village unscathed. For Katya every member of her family had perished in the death camps – mother, father, sisters, four grandparents, aunts, uncles and cousins, all had gone. Nobody had been spared. It was a common story for so many Jewish families.

Some years later Frank was talking to Rachel:

"It took me a little time to realise I was not only Katya's husband but for her I was everybody else too."

He could never get over the feeling he was the luckiest man alive; not only had he survived the war but most of all this wonderful woman had chosen him, a peasant boy from the countryside. They remained devoted to each other.

Katya worked as a nutritionist and quickly gained an international reputation as a researcher, epidemiologist and speaker. She was genuinely modest and felt she didn't deserve to be thought of as a scientist. She was refreshingly non-pc and as she got older became convinced there was a lot of nonsense talked about food wrapped up as science. As a nutritionist she would always say, 'It's just a matter of moderation in everything and to call that science is ridiculous. Nutritionists and doctors and even epidemiologists are endlessly pontificating about what is good or bad to eat and drink. Then a month later they are changing their minds so inevitably people just switch off.'

What mattered to Katya far more than international recognition, which genuinely irritated her, were her children, grandchildren and friends. For as long as we knew her she was up about 5am, and having left breakfast for Frank and any visitors there might be, would walk to her daughter's and give her grandchildren their breakfast while Vera left for work. Then she would go to nursery or school and when necessary pick up the children at the end of the afternoon. Her son-in-law worked for a long time at the Atomic Energy Commission in Vienna, which was not easy for Vera. Vladya and Renata, her son and daughter-in-law, also had two children and lived in a neighbouring flat, so they were not forgotten either. Auschwitz, Dachau, Buchenwald and the rest had given Katya a special view of life and a devotion to her precious family.

Frank finished his law studies at Charles university and after an unlikely eighteen months as a sports journalist applied for a job at the Ministry of Health. He was accepted in the early 1950s and joined the Department of Primary Care before being transferred to the International Relations Department in the early '60s. His ability with English must have helped his progress as was the fact he spoke German well, and he could also manage Russian. Like Katya he too developed an international reputation with his encyclopedic knowledge related to the organisation of health services on both sides of the Iron Curtain. He had a forensic mind that enabled him to disentangle facts from the statistics and propaganda coming from both right and left of the political spectrum.

Naturally when I first met him I knew nothing of this. Both had returned home as committed socialists which led to their support of the new communist government in 1948. I never knew if they had been members of the Party, but it was Katya who first began to have doubts about the lies and false propaganda of the government. Perhaps this change coincided with the infamous Stalin purges in the early fifties.

Katya reminded me of Heda Margolius Kovaly and her book *Prague Farewell* in which she writes about her efforts to try and persuade her husband that the government, of which he was an important member, was not as he saw it. She led an ordinary life, shopping and experiencing the empty shops, struggling with the children to see the doctor, climbing aboard overcrowded buses and trams, arguing with officials over almost everything, and much beside. Her husband was protected from reality by all the trappings of government and sadly he wouldn't listen until it was too late; he was arrested and became one of the victims of the Slansky Trials. At the time he was Secretary General of the Czech Communist Party. After a brief trial he was executed along with ten other Jews.

I'm not suggesting for one moment that Frank led a protected, privileged life, far from it, but he was not as 'hands-on' as Katya. Undoubtedly an idealist, it was not until the Prague Spring of 1968 and the subsequent Warsaw Pact invasion that he finally admitted the government was dishonest and could not be trusted.

Hotel Flora made me uneasy and I was surprised how readily I succumbed to Cold War propaganda. Was my rather bleak room bugged? Should I inspect it to see if there were any hidden cameras? As it was unlikely I would be speaking to anyone in my room I decided that any bugs or hidden cameras could remain in situ.

Within an hour three regular features of the communist world became apparent: no lavatory paper apart from a few pages of a daily newspaper; no soap; and no plugs for either the basin or bath. For the next twenty years, wherever I was going, soap, lavatory paper and a variety of plugs were top of my packing list.

Indifference and consciously unhelpful advice was just part of the service at the Flora, and the ever-present floor managers illustrated this behaviour to perfection. On each floor they sat at the end of the corridor to keep an eye on the lifts and stairs, making sure no unauthorised person entered her territory. Seemingly always large (like the women sweeping the streets or working on the railways), usually grim and unsmiling but ever vigilant, she handed out room keys and collected them in again with a stare and a grunt. In the majority of hotels tea and hot water and sugar could be purchased from her – in the Soviet Union there was always a samovar. If one had any complaints or problems she was the person you turned to – at least that was what the receptionists always instructed.

Fellow guests seemed suspicious of me, or was I imagining it? I never received a smile or acknowledgement or any sign of recognition. For a couple of days I was aware that every time I came out of my room the same middle-aged couple were standing in the corridor. Were they there to keep an eye on me or was I paranoid and they were just there by chance?

Frank arrived in a chauffeur-driven ministry car; he was formal and straightforward and looked much as I thought a Czech would look. He showed me the programme he had arranged – no mention of hospitals, which I thought was a good sign, and he explained carefully about the facilities to be visited. It was clear he must have read my letter to the Ministry and I now moved from the unstructured, relaxed ways of Sonyi to an official, organised study of primary medical care.

Over the next few days as we travelled around he was keen to point out to me the number of young black people in the streets:

"As you can see, we are having to educate Africans from your old empire."

It was such an absurd remark as very few Africans were to be seen and I had just come from the streets of Bristol and London, though at this time it was mostly West Indians in Bristol. The Czechs were copying the Soviet Union, who had built the Patrice Lumumba (briefly Prime Minister of the Congo after Independence) university in Moscow, which undoubtedly increased Soviet influence in post-colonial Africa. The Czechs were not building a new university but were trying to encourage as many 'blacks' as possible to Charles University. I'm afraid I didn't challenge Frank because I felt an unresolvable argument was pointless. More important, an excellent programme had been arranged for me; any questions I asked were willingly answered and I did not want to alienate him.

Looking back I have since wondered to what extent our chauffeur may have been responsible for Frank's attitude. Was he from the Ministry of the Interior? Was he in fact monitoring our relationship? Was he assessing whether Frank was safe to mix with foreigners? Was he a reliable Party member? Could he be trusted? Was it wise to allow him to travel abroad, attend conferences, give lectures and make contacts outside the communist bloc?

I remember one day in particular when we visited a number of polyclinics, two maternity units and two small factories that had cooperated to provide a joint industrial health centre. I'm certain it was not by chance that Frank chose a circuitous route that took us through the small village of Lidice, about fifteen miles out of Prague. This detour enabled him to give me a detailed account of the consequences of the assassination of Reinhard Heydrich on 27 May 1942. Heydrich had been sent to assist the Gestapo leader Hermann

Frank in his attempt to liquidate anti-Nazi resistance by encouraging quislings and informers. This strategy had failed and thousands were sent to their death on June 9/10 in revenge for the assassination. Gestapo and SS units surrounded Lidice. Women were separated from the men and children from their mothers. The women ended up in concentration camps while the children, if they did not conform to the ideal of the pure Aryan race, were sent to the gas chambers. Out of 109 children 89 were murdered. The 192 males, including boys from the age of fifteen, were shot. The village was then looted, bulldozed and set on fire.

After the war Lidice was completely rebuilt and the terror of '42 was remembered by the Rose Garden of Friendship which separated the new village from the site of the old. The initiative for this memorial garden came from a British committee 'Lidice Shall Live'. To the chauffeur it appeared Frank was explaining to a Westerner the difficulty the Germans forces had in controlling an occupied country, but to me he was pointing out the brutality of the Nazis. What the chauffeur was thinking I have no idea, but he was certainly listening. In the course of general conversation Frank often gave the impression of being a local Party bureaucrat and would endeavour to persuade me of the benefits of living in a People's Democracy! I still cannot decide on the role of that chauffeur . . .

Czechoslovakia faithfully followed the organisational pattern of the Soviet Health Service at provincial, district and community levels. The central planning by the Ministry of Health was more rigid than in Hungary, or so it seemed to me.

Polyclinics were the main primary care facility with community therapists, paediatricians, gynaecologists and dentists working alongside many different specialists. The provision of specialists was in theory excellent, the idea being to try and integrate primary and secondary care more closely. But the actual use of specialists was puzzling and unsatisfactory with much duplication of work and an enormous misuse of manpower. The specialist had no direct contact or access to the local hospital (no beds or outpatient clinics) and no responsibility for patients seen in the polyclinic. In reality, a patient who was referred to one of the specialists by a community physician was in the great majority of cases referred to the hospital without any further action being taken. The specialist merely acted as a signpost and was actually an obstacle to quick referral where specialists could take immediate clinical responsibility for the patient.

Frank was well aware of the problem and the need for urgent reform and never hesitated to point out to me the stupidity of the situation. In order to fill in the day with some clinical work, ophthalmologists would spend a lot of time doing simple eye tests (routinely carried out in the UK by opticians). An experienced surgeon might spend most of the day treating simple cuts, bruises and sprains which could have been dealt with by a trained nurse; the occasional inspection of haemorrhoids or varicose veins might be the highlight of the day. Frank was adamant that such a surgeon would have been placed in this position for political and not professional reasons – for criticising the system or the Party, for example – but how different he was when the chauffeur was not within hearing distance.

The inappropriate use of manpower, both doctors and nurses, was a sort of madness and was one of the main criticisms of the non-communist world concerning polyclinics. Over-staffing on the other hand was a different matter and was directly related to the proud boast of socialist economics that unemployment had been defeated and did not exist.

Another proud boast at the time of the communist takeover in 1948 had been that all health services would be free and accessible to the whole population. In Czechoslovakia a fully comprehensive service was not introduced by law until 1966 and in reality was not implemented for many years. Private practice continued but had been restricted to retired physicians.

Contraception was a problem as the oral contraceptive pill was not in widespread use. It appeared to be only available for those with money or in the upper echelons of the Party. Abortion on demand was easily available and was the commonest method of birth control – I suppose it was preferable to the backstreet abortions so common in many parts of the world.

To my great surprise, the night before I returned to the UK, Frank invited me to his home for supper. It was only on my next visit that I discovered that Bubenečská 33 was directly opposite the Ministry of the Interior (secret police), an impressive mid-nineteenth century neo-classical mansion with a grand portico and enclosed by elegant iron railings. Apart from the Czech flag, there was nothing to indicate the building was connected to the government.

No. 33 was part of a large late-nineteenth century residential building. The Ošanécs lived on the first floor. There was a large central area, always cold, round which a stone staircase made its way up to the fourth floor. On every subsequent visit, on my own as well as with Rachel, we were asked to keep a low profile, so if we were dropped by taxi or a friend's car we got out a block away and walked. If there was any luggage, the Ošanécs dealt with it. Certainly in the '60s and '70s they risked a lot by having foreigners to stay, but by the early '80s everything was more relaxed.

I now met Katya, and their children Vladya and Vera, for the first time. Apart from providing the meal Katya kept in the background all evening except when she asked if I had any children. Two friends of Frank's joined us. One of them was Dr Bartos who had been sent to work in Algeria and was home on leave – at that time young doctors, nurses and teachers from all Eastern Bloc countries spent some time working in Africa and the Middle East. I forget the background of the other friend except that he was medically qualified. The conversation started tentatively but confidence soon developed and we were able to discuss a wide variety of topics associated with medicine. I was questioned closely about the NHS and Western Europe and there was much interest in the position of private medicine. I didn't mention the politics of Czechoslovakia as I didn't want to embarrass Frank or make things awkward for him or his guests. On my next visit I realised I needn't have worried – the Ministry chauffeur wasn't with us! I remained in contact with Dr Bartos for a number of years. I noted he always wrote from Algeria and never from his home address in Prague.

In the summer of 1967 Frank wrote asking if he could come to Wells whilst he was on an official visit to the Department of Health in London where he was staying with Dr Horder and his wife. I remember saying to Rachel that I didn't think she would like him but that we would have to have him if only for a few days. I had previously explained that Frank had generally seemed a rather hard-line supporter of his government. When he arrived Rachel was mystified by my description, and certainly he was now unrecognisable – relaxed, amusing, and great fun with our kids, particularly our daughter Anna who reminded him of Vera at a similar age. We took him to see *Blyth Spirit* at the Bristol Old Vic, which he understood and which genuinely made him laugh, although we felt that Coward didn't quite live up to Mozart and Dvořák. According to Rachel's diary Frank was '. . . surprisingly nice and talked solidly . . . easy and amusing . . . have really enjoyed his visit.'

The next year at the time of the 'Prague Spring' and the subsequent invasion by Warsaw Pact troops, his son Vladya came to the UK for his summer holidays, staying first with the Horders in London and then intending to come down to Wells. On the day Soviet tanks entered Prague I phoned the Horders to see if Vladya was with them and to see if we could help in any way. They passed the phone to him and he politely said 'No, thank you' as he was returning to Prague as soon as he could. This he did by train within a couple of days. Katya and Frank had passed on to him their love of their country.

In November '68 Frank had been on a brief lecture tour in the States and had been given permission to stop over in the UK for a few days, having persuaded the Czech authorities he had further meetings at the Department of Health in London. In reality it was to stay with the Horders and then visit us in Wells. He was a broken man, much like a Catholic who had lost his faith. He spoke slowly in a sad, thoughtful way:

> "As I looked at the Soviet tanks in the street I couldn't believe it, Rachel, it was like your country being invaded by the United States, it just couldn't be happening."

We sat up into the early hours listening to him, occasionally asking questions. It was clear he had no intention of staying in the UK and attempting to get his family out – no, he must return to support Alexander Dubček.

It was my great good fortune and my wife's to have been introduced to Prague by someone with such knowledge and enthusiasm for his beloved city. He never tired of acting as guide, explaining its history and describing the architecture of almost every church and building of interest – each church was prefaced with 'still working' or 'not working'. Bubenečská 33 was close to the castle area and the cathedral of St Vitus and he never tired of looking down to the Lesser Town and the Old Town separated by the Vltava and joined by the magnificent Charles Bridge. In the '60s and '70s and even early '80s we were lucky as there were few tourists, mainly busloads of East Germans. It was quiet, there wasn't much to buy, and the cafés were simple and traditional, but the city itself became more and more in need of cleaning and restoration.

After the fall of the Berlin Wall everything changed and not all for the good, according to Katya and Frank and most of their friends. It was probably a generation thing, but they were disappointed by much of the influence of western culture with the sudden appearance of sex shops and the obsession with drugs and consumerism plus the quite shameless behaviour of drunken tourists. Now, twenty-five years later, the seedy side of Prague has become seedier with young women openly entertaining men in the many brothels, whilst the police and ambulance services spend much of their time clearing up after intoxicated tourists.

Friendship can be unexpected and so it was with Katya and Frank; the next thirty years saw them and two of their grandchildren Honsa and Madlenka coming to this country, and Rachel and I visiting them. We took secret pride in encouraging Madlenka and her boyfriend to take a romantic few days in south Devon. Initially they planned to stay in youth hostels but we managed to persuade them to camp, and I dropped them off on the edge of the Salcombe Estuary and saw them get on the ferry to East Portlemouth. A wedding was the result.

The climax of our friendship was in September 1993 when Vera and Alesch, their son-in-law, brought them to the UK in their car – Frank and Katya never owned a car themselves – as a celebration of fifty years of marriage. They found us with two of our sons, a daughter-in-law and baby granddaughter in our usual holiday cottage on the north-west coast of Scotland. They stayed for two or three days after eventually finding a B & B, and we celebrated the actual anniversary with a splendid meal at the traditional Sheildaig Lodge Hotel, Badachro. How unbelievable for them to be in Scotland again exactly fifty years after the YMCA/YWCA honeymoon in Edinburgh.

But perhaps the real mark of friendship was in 1996 when they came to spend a night with us barely a month before Rachel died.

5

PEOPLE'S REPUBLIC of POLAND

Over two years were to pass before my study of Central Europe was completed. The reasons as usual were time and money and the additional difficulty of coordinating the visit to Poland with Bulgaria and Romania. Looking back through old correspondence and realising the time it took to get replies to my letters it was small wonder it took so long. However, regarding Poland, I received no reply whatsoever form the Ministry of Health in Warsaw. I realised Poland was going to be similar to Hungary: this private visit would be unstructured and superficial.

Dr Engelmeier again tried to come to the rescue with the names of contacts, and I received helpful advice from Dr John Hunt, past President of the Royal College of General Practitioners, and Dr John Fry, a GP working in Beckenham, Kent, who was fast becoming the UK's answer to František Ošanec as a recognised authority on primary care throughout the industrialised world. Interestingly he was of Polish extraction; his father had been a practising GP in Krakow but had fled to Britain with his family in the summer of 1939.

After a few months I had received only one reply from the six letters I had written to Dr Engelmeier's contacts. Romnald Gutt from Bielsko-Biala, a small town in the foothills of the Carpathians close to the Czech border, replied in October 1966. He explained he only worked part-time as a GP, that he was hoping to become a full-time haematologist, and was intending to leave Bielsko-Biala at the first opportunity so as to settle eventually in a university town. He promised he would inform his colleagues of my enquiry, but nothing happened – all very discouraging.

Just as I was about to give up on Poland a letter arrived from the wife of Dr Gutt's oldest friend. Irena Bochenska was keen to make contacts in the West. She explained that neither she nor her husband were in any way connected with the medical profession but they had many 'doctor friends' and she was confident she would be able to organise a programme with their help. In addition she would act as a first-class interpreter – she taught English privately to both adults and children and also did translating for a small private publishing company. Subsequently, on one of her visits to Wells, she met John le Carré and agreed to try and get one of his books translated and published in Poland. This project was short-circuited when the publishing company told her there was an acute shortage of paper – of course the real reason was that the authorities would not permit publication. She was not surprised by such an absurd excuse and in fact wasn't even embarrassed; as she said, 'it's just one of those things'.

Similar to my experience with Hungary, it seemed I must visit privately and unofficially. This was far from what I had been hoping for but I had no alternative but to accept Irena's offer. Or would such a visit be a complete waste of time and money and should I just forget Poland? Rightly or wrongly I decided to go ahead. As it turned out it was a mistake and proved to be one of the least successful of my visits; data was sparse, information was poor, and most of the discussion with the medical profession was little more than anecdotal.

From this inauspicious beginning a long happy friendship with Irena and her daughter Mariola, aged 15 at the time, began – both were eager to travel. Staszek her husband was a lawyer. He and Romnald Gutt had been friends since their school days. He spoke no English but was interested in Britain and its history. And its football. He didn't want to visit Britain at the time and wouldn't do so until he could pay his own way and 'travel as a gentleman, not a pauper'. Permission to travel to the West was only granted provided the host agreed to accept all financial responsibility plus the ridiculous limit to the money that could be taken abroad – at the time, twenty US dollars! A proud man, he came from a minor aristocratic background – his great grandfather had owned Pieskowa Skala, an impressive Renaissance castle some twenty miles south of Krakow.

Dr Gutt and I remained in irregular contact and we didn't finally meet until September '78 in Szczecin when he, Rachel and I, spent a pleasant afternoon together over coffee, cakes, vodka and a cigar. Like Staszek he had never wanted to travel to Britain, or anywhere else for that matter, and had only once been abroad – he proudly showed us a photograph of the private audience he had had with Pope John Paul II in the Vatican: indeed he sent us a copy of it.

My journey to Poland started in Bucharest on the evening of 3 October 1968. The Trans-Caucasian Express was waiting at the platform and, as with everything given the title Express within the communist world, every traveller must accept the reality. Timetables are so arranged that the Express departs on time and arrives on time and there is never any reason to get up speed. Just a gentle measured rate of progress is all that is needed.

I was relieved to be leaving Romania for a number of reasons. Departure from Bucharest was 9.30pm and arrival time in Krakow 7.30pm the next day. I had no food or drink for the journey and no money should there be a restaurant car (there was not). What could I do? It didn't take me long to decide, as I had been vaguely watching people eating and chatting at a small café in the station concourse. Service was slow, but finally the travellers left and the café closed, leaving the remnants of food on the tables. I chose my moment and grabbed four or five bread rolls, some tomatoes, gherkins and red peppers, and moved along the platform as quickly as I could with my luggage and the stolen goods stuffed into an already overflowing bag. Half expecting to hear shouts from the café, I was mightily relieved to find my booked seat. Almost immediately the train moved and I knew I was safe.

We travelled north, with the Carpathians on our left, and eventually came to the Soviet Socialist Republic of Ukraine. The late Ryszard Kapúscinski, the acclaimed and controversial Polish writer and journalist, has graphically described the borders surrounding the Soviet Union or dividing individual countries within the communist bloc. In his book *Imperium* he writes:

> *'The border is stress – it is fear . . . Barbed-wire. Barbed-wire barriers are what you see first . . . The walls of barbed-wire have something to say to you, have something to contribute. They are saying: Be careful, you are coming to the border, into a different world . . . Best you mind your own business. Best be silent. Best not ask any questions.*
>
> *Then came the dogs, German Shepherds, furious, trembling, frenzied; the train has barely stopped when they throw themselves under the carriages, barking and baying. But who would be riding under carriages in minus forty Celsius . . . the sight of the ferreting dogs is so absorbing that for a while one doesn't*

notice the next image . . . soldiers have sprung up as if from the earth and have instantaneously lined up on both sides of the train. They stand in such a way that the train cars are under total surveillance . . . the sentries who stand in the watch towers have their rifles aimed at the doors and windows of the train cars . . . I would like to traverse the entire Soviet Union, its fifteen republics . . . a huge area of the world. Keeping in mind that whenever it's technically possible these borders are marked with thick coils of wire (I saw such barriers on the borders of Poland, China and Iran) and that the wire quickly deteriorates and therefore must be replaced across hundreds, no, thousands of kilometers . . one can assume that a significant portion of the Soviet metallurgical industry is devoted to producing barbed-wire.

For the matter doesn't end with the wiring of borders. How many thousand kilometers of wire were used to fence the Gulag Archipelago? Those hundreds of camps, staging posts and prisons . . ?

It is easy to see why in the shops of Smolensk or Omsk one can buy neither a hoe nor a hammer, never mind a knife or spoon . . . and the vigilant concern expressed in the question "Are you all really properly wired in?" And so instead of building themselves houses and hospitals, instead of repairing the continually failing sewage and electrical systems, people (although fortunately not everybody) were for years occupied with the internal and external, local and national wiring of the Emporium!

Many travellers and writers are adamant . . . it is almost impossible to understand a country unless you cross its frontiers . . . and not by plane. The accessories of a border tell you so much.'

How true.

At the border I saw for myself what Kapúscinski described in his book, and also had my first experience of the problem caused by the different gauge of the Russian track. The whole procedure took about an hour and a half and initially was under floodlight. Each carriage was lifted by two cranes whilst new wheels/bogies were fitted to suit the wider track. Romanian passport control and customs were no problem as all the officials wanted to get back to their beds. It was not so easy on the Ukrainian side. By this time it was daylight so we could see the soldiers lined up on both sides of the train and the dogs being dragged up and down. Customs were alright with me and my fellow-travellers, but it was my transit visa which interested passport control – two officials, one an insignificant man, the other a massive woman with front teeth of steel. Both scrutinised the passport and visa with furrowed brows until the female discus thrower vigorously stamped them.

The countryside was largely flat with occasional hills which might go unnoticed in another landscape. Travelling along the edge of this huge agricultural region, the breadbasket of Europe, what a pleasure it was to travel at a steady 30 or 40 mph, allowing me to absorb the views I would never see again: small villages with single-storey whitewashed or ochre-coloured houses, mainly wooden, each invariably surrounded by wooden fencing with sunflowers, geraniums, small fruit trees and bushes, and vines everywhere providing welcome shade as well as wine and vodka all the year round. Orchards and small woods completed the scene. Hens, ducks, geese, pigs and sheep were everywhere, with a few cows and cart-horses and bullocks for work on the land.

Collectivisation was easy to see with regular, very large collections of farm machinery – tractors, trailers and harvesters – as well as cattle sheds and buildings for storage and other uses. Most villages had electricity, but judging by the numbers of women and children queuing to collect water from wells, usually at both ends of the village, piped water seemed unlikely. I think telephone wires reached most villages, but I wasn't certain. On a beautiful autumn day how easily I was seduced by such a peaceful rustic scene; I had to keep reminding myself of the horrors of World War 11, not to mention the four decades of Stalin's atrocities – murder, extermination, starvation and transportation to Siberia and Kazakhstan.

Piped music was an unexpected companion – mainly classical and Russian folk with the occasional complete surprise like the Irish winner of the European Song Contest 'A Puppet on a String', immediately followed by Elgar's Introduction and Allegro for Strings suddenly transporting me to the Malvern hills. Extraordinary.

It was a relief when we reached Lvov, as it was then called; it meant Poland was getting close and Krakow not too distant. The carriage doors were unlocked and we were allowed onto the platform for a much-needed stroll. The coaches were traditional with separate compartments. On returning to my seat I found my seven companions from Bucharest had gone, to be replaced by seven new travellers all of whom were Polish and in high spirits. One spoke a smidgeon of English and over the next couple of hours we were all entertained with non-stop political jokes told by the 'joker' amongst them. He was well fuelled with beer and vodka and kept his mates happy and asking for more. The English speaker tried his very best to explain.

On reaching the Polish border my companions' high spirits evaporated as soon as the train stopped. The change of wheels/bogies took place once again and, again, armed soldiers were lined up on both sides of the train and passport and customs officials climbed on board. There was total silence. I was virtually ignored by the officials, my luggage merely glanced at, my visa stamped and retained and my unstamped passport returned. This was the first occasion I had come across this strange practice; by retaining the stamped visa and returning my unstamped passport there is no way anyone can discover if I have visited the Soviet Union. As far as I know, the Soviet Union is the only country in which the visa is a separate document.

My companions were cross-questioned, physically searched and their luggage thoroughly checked. They were cleared, but the jovial atmosphere had gone, replaced by a feeling of anxiety. According to my interpreter a crackdown on currency was the problem. Just before we were on our way again two men were taken off the train by soldiers and marched off accompanied by the barking, snarling Alsatians dogs. The general opinion was that the men were suspected of smuggling currency, but nothing more.

Staszek and Irena were waiting on the platform. They didn't have a car but a friend gave us a lift back to their flat at Swietokrska 2/5 in a district which had seen more prosperous times and was about half an hour's walk from the city centre. As we climbed the foul-smelling stone staircase, barely lit by a single dirty 40 watt bulb and stinking of cat urine, I noticed an acrid odour, the source of which would become clear in the morning.

Once inside the flat there was an atmosphere of warmth, hospitality and faded elegance plus the smell of wonderful food – by this time I was mighty hungry. Two walls were lined with books. Old-fashioned drapes covered old chairs and a turn-of-the-century settle. A good if faded carpet covered most of the floor and might well have been laid before the First World War. In one corner a large traditional wood-burning stove was heating pipes and radiators that would have done credit to an Atlantic ocean liner. I immediately felt at home.

In the morning I could see within a quarter of a mile two factory chimneys, one belching out thick black smoke and the other a purplish-yellow cocktail of chemical waste. This made a mockery of what I was subsequently told about Poland's industrial health service and the government's commitment to controlling environmental hazards. By the end of my studies it was obvious both in Central and Eastern Europe as well as the Soviet Union that their claims about the environment were simply lies and propaganda for home and foreign consumption.

As in Hungary and Bulgaria, so here in Poland, an immediate visit to the local police station was necessary. If staying in a hotel, the registration of where and how long I was staying as well as the stamping of my passport and visa, would be carried out by the State Tourist Board. Foreigners travelling on their own interested the authorities the most.

Irena had gathered together as much basic information related to the health service as she could, plus a list of health facilities connected to primary care. Armed with this background information I went first to a meeting that had been arranged with the senior administrator of the Krakow Department of Health; I was quite surprised by the open way in which he was prepared to answer questions.

Within a day or so I realised that Poland was different. First, in spite of the much trumpeted boast of the communist world, health care was not freely available in Poland and in fact was only for the 'insured' – insurance was compulsory for state employees and was organised through their wage packet. Private citizens, who amounted to at least forty percent of the population, were not covered and had to pay for medical care. In rural areas, where seventy percent of farmers did not work in collective farms and where wages were already low, these were the families most seriously affected.

Rural health cooperatives, organised by farmers themselves, were usually staffed by a single physician carrying out a role similar to that of the GP in the UK. The rural cooperatives paid the doctor a small salary and the patients paid a small, additional fee to supplement the salary. Private practice was allowed but in reality the higher fees charged could not be afforded by the majority. As a consequence of the non-payment by poor patients, around fifty percent of practitioners had organised themselves into groups where they were allowed to work privately (the fees being regulated by the Ministry of Health) after they had completed their official seven hours per day working for the state.

It would be an understatement to say that Poles were different from the rest of Central and Eastern Europe – experimental, flexible, and in some ways disorderly, which was proudly talked about. Doctors may have been happy with this more relaxed approach but it was a very different story for the patients; for them it meant less available, less comprehensive and less accessible. Most of the physicians I spoke to about this responded with merely 'yes, it's just a muddle, but that's how it is'.

After visiting health centres, polyclinics and other facilities, Irena had arranged that every day always ended with five or six physicians being prepared to answer any questions I wanted to ask. It was a splendid idea, but soon medicine was forgotten and politics, history and culture took over and I quickly began to understand the position of the large numbers of downtrodden peasantry, and the less numerous but equally downtrodden urban poor, who for centuries had been dominated by a small but powerful aristocracy, later to be joined by an emerging professional middle-class after the end of the First World War.

The discussions centred on Poland's lost identity and failed revolutionary movements in the 19th century, this lost identity only being regained again at the end of the First World War. The final tragedy was the incorporation of Poland behind the Iron Curtain thereby falling under the power of the Soviet Union. Discussions and arguments went on and on, only interrupted by united pride concerning Chopin and other musicians, the Curies and other scientists and poets I'd never heard of. Eventually I would ask if we could return to the problems of the Health Service which, after all, was the reason Irena had arranged the meetings. Customs and culture were frequently blamed for many of the difficulties, but it was all talked about in a broad sweep and rarely were specific examples given.

The 'elephant in the room' finally surfaced and I was amazed it had hardly been mentioned up to then; this was the Catholic Church. The influence of the Church was plain to see – priests were everywhere and churches were full. The communist party had never managed to gain control over it or been able to close its churches or seminaries. At the time of my visit Cardinal Archbishop, Primate of Poland, Stefan Wyszynski, was held in highest regard and had been popular since his outspoken condemnation in 1953 of the government's campaign against the Church.

In some ways the success of the Catholic Church in Poland reminded me of Hungary following the uprising in 1956, but Poland had been the first country to challenge the ruling communist party about the rising cost of food, diminishing wages and general misery, and throughout the years Stefan Wyszynski and his Church supported the workers.

There was no shortage of young men applying to enter seminaries and I wondered if it had always been a popular calling, or if it was connected with the economic situation versus the lifelong security provided by the Church. After all, you got food and clothing and a roof over your head and, perhaps just as important, a priest was not conscripted for military service.

However, the majority of the medical profession and the general population disagreed with the Church over contraception and abortion. Over the past forty years in Poland the birth rate has remained constant at just over two children per family, so it is obvious the teaching on contraception is ignored. Abortion was and is more complicated. It was carried out free for the élite of the Party or if you had money. Otherwise you had to make do with the horrors of the back streets. To confuse matters more, many maintained that abortion was the commonest form of contraception.

Another 'elephant in the room' that was never mentioned concerned the very recent invasion of Czechoslovakia by the Warsaw Pact countries (excluding Romania) following the Prague Spring. In private conversations everyone admitted regret, embarrassment and shame in equal measure.

During the 1970s the British Medical Students Association and the

BMA organised visits for foreign students to study the NHS. The majority went to hospitals but a few chose general practice. I was part of that scheme and in September 1970 Ewa Dzidkowska arrived in Wells. Her home was in Lódz and one of my colleagues, Alan, had been a POW in Poland from September 1940 to May 1945. During these years Alan's best friend had been a Polish doctor, Leszniewiecz, who came from Lódz. After much deliberation we asked Ewa if she knew a doctor of this name: 'yes he was a senior gynaecologist at the medical school'. This of course indicated he was probably a member of the Communist party; after much thought Ewa agreed to take a letter from Alan addressed to Leszniewiecz (we insisted she must first speak to her parents before delivering the letter).

About six weeks after Ewa returned home a small parcel arrived for Alan from Poland containing a letter saying how wonderful it was to be in contact again. Included in the parcel was a small, battered, old tobacco pipe which Alan had given his friend as a memento in the last chaotic days of the war as one turned east and the other west. Alan wrote back immediately and some four weeks later received another letter from Poland saying 'please Alan never write to me again . . . ' Such was the fear in those days when all mail from the western world was opened and read.

In Poland, medicine, politics and religion were an interesting mix. Politics and religion were inextricably entwined and yet largely in opposition to each other.

One thing was indisputable and was unconnected with either politics or religion – within the medical profession, primary medical care, compared with the hospital service, was considered to be the poor relation financially, in training, and in knowledge, but most of all with regard to kudos.

6

EASTERN EUROPE

Grenville A J Cole writing from Dublin about his book *The Gypsy Road* published in 1894 gives an impression of faraway Europe:

> *'When our grandfathers crossed Europe by post chaise or a rumbling diligence they did so with some sort of gravity. Of late we have been so accustomed to step from the steamer to the sleeping-car and from this to the day-express that we have forgotten on the one hand the largeness and on the other the detail of the earth. The rich variety of continental landscapes, the airy labours of the peasants, the growth of slumbering towns, the interchange of ideas along the frontier have become nigh lost to us in our rapid passages.'*

Forty years later Hessell Tiltman in the foreword to his book *Peasant Europe* published in London in 1934 writes:

> *'Western Europe, preoccupied with the problems of international relations, industry and the future of armaments, is sometimes in danger of overlooking the fact that more than half the entire population of that Continent is composed of peasants.'*

He included Austria, Bulgaria, Czechoslovakia, Hungary, Poland, Romania and Yugoslavia and observes:

> *'. . . their tools and their farming methods belong to the time of the Old Testament'.*

How were Eastern Europe and the Balkans viewed in 1968, another forty years on? Some may have dipped into Rebecca West's *Black Lamb and Grey Falcon,* 1941, or more recently Olivia Manning's wonderfully atmospheric and vivid description of Bucharest and its inhabitants living under a fascist regime and the dreaded Iron Guard who were equal to the Nazis in every way. In addition Manning reminds us the Balkans were still feudal societies, and powerfully describes the poverty of the peasants as they struggle into the capital to sell their meagre bundles of fruit and vegetables, sleeping on the pavements or sheltering under trees and bushes in the sweltering heat of summer. At the same time she captures the idleness and luxury and boredom of the aristocracy and the families of bankers and business men in extraordinary detail. *The Great Fortune,* 1960, *The Spoilt City,* 1962, and *Friends and Heroes,* 1965, formed what came to be known as the *Balkan Trilogy.*

The most informative book in my view for an introduction to Bulgaria was published in 1961; *Bulgarian Background* enabled Bernard Newman to give a good account of life behind the Iron Curtain in 1959 during the Khrushchev era as well as refreshing his memory of his initial visit thirty years earlier in 1931. I regret not reading the book until after my return.

Most of us will have heard of Tito's heroic exploits as he led the partisans during the Second World War, and these have been graphically reported by Fitzroy Maclean in *Eastern Approaches,* 1949, as well as touching on the complicated politics of the country and giving a glimpse of the old Yugoslavia.

Inevitably the spirit and popular culture of the Sixties created an indifference and ultimately a total ignorance in the West, certainly in the UK, of Eastern Europe and the Balkans. Between the end of the Ottoman Empire and the beginning of the Cold War, these countries were just faraway places arguing over frontiers, disagreeing endlessly with each other – in fact just causing trouble. After all, wasn't there a place called Sarajevo which had something to do with the First World War? If we had paid attention during our geography lessons at school a few of us might have been able to find some of these countries on a map. What language they all spoke we had little idea, probably Balkan.

Once the Soviet Union had taken its spoils after the war, anywhere behind the Iron Curtain was just part of the communist bloc – too complicated and remote to understand or bother about. However, as I write today, forty more years have passed and three events have reduced our ignorance and increased our interest. First, the introduction of the package tour, then the fall of the Berlin Wall, and finally the Yugoslav Civil War leading to the bombardment of Sarajevo, the horror of Srebrenica and the unsolved problem of Kosovo. And of course much more besides.

7

THE PEOPLE'S REPUBLIC of BULGARIA

Dr Engelmeier of the International Society was unable to help in arranging my visit, but František Ošanéc had contacts. Professor Gargov at the Department of the Organisation of Health Services, Institute of Postgraduate Training in Sofia, had worked with Frank off and on for some years and believed him when he said I was a bona fide researcher, although not an academic associated with a university or institute. A lengthy correspondence for over a year between Professor Gargov and myself eventually produced a programme of study with which I was happy. Of the twenty-two countries included in *An Analysis of Primary Medical Care* Bulgaria was in the top three for organising and arranging what I had requested to see.

The cheapest time-friendly journey to Sofia was by air to Zagreb, a change of plane to Belgrade, and then by train to Sofia. Thus on 23 September 1968 a Caravelle plane took me to Zagreb, where after a delay in changing planes I finally arrived at Belgrade. By the time I had got through passport and customs I was more than two hours late. A taxi rather than an airport bus proved wise and I arrived with barely ten minutes to spare for the Pannonian Express interestingly advertised as the Orient Express; after the Orient Express Company had finally ceased to exist in 1961 the dishonest free market advertising of the West had a firm grip in the communist world.

The station was heaving with people and providentially I found the right platform and boarded the train with barely a minute to spare. As I sank thankfully into my seat, cheering started in the corridor and on the platform. A train had just arrived from East Berlin having passed through Prague. Czech flags and pictures of the Czech leaders – Dubček the First Secretary and Svoboda the President – were stuck on the windows of the coaches. Soon it seemed everyone was shouting "Dubček!" and "Svoboda!" This spontaneous enthusiastic public demonstration of support for the Czechs against the Warsaw Pact invasion was dramatic and emotional and only later was it explained that Svoboda has two meanings, first as a name and second, 'freedom'.

The arrival time in Sofia was 5.00 am their time. We moved gently along in the darkness, never getting up speed and passing through picturesque little stations lit by oil lamps swinging in the breeze with ducks and hens roosting while a few still scratched away on the platform.

Seven fellow travellers were in the compartment and quite quickly we all tried to settle down to sleep: I found it impossible. I was anxious because I knew there would be difficulties at the Yugoslav/Bulgarian border – it hadn't been possible to buy a ticket to travel from the border to Sofia, and to make matters more complicated it was forbidden to take in any Bulgarian currency. My intention had been to buy the ticket with Yugoslav currency but the unexpected expense of the taxi had made that impossible.

Once over the frontier we stopped at Dragoman with its charming old station from another age. Here passports and customs slowly did their job in a sleepy sort of way. So far so good. Then came the ticket inspector, an elderly man with a long drooping grey moustache and a small paraffin lamp hanging round his neck. I spoke no Bulgarian and he spoke no English and none of my companions wanted to be involved. The old chap was weary yet looked at me in a kindly way – all he wanted to do was to go back to his little cubicle at the end of the carriage and fall asleep. Waving some English £1 notes eventually produced a reaction and he disappeared to return with two customs officials. It was impossible to explain why I had no Yugoslav money and in the end I paid for the Bulgarian part of the journey with English money. I've no idea who came off best out of this nocturnal negotiation, but with one of my worries settled it enabled me to sleep.

I had been told my interpreter/guide would meet me at the station and I would recognise her as she would be carrying a rose. We arrived just after 6am, only an hour or so late. The station looked too small and provincial to serve a capital city, but even at this early hour soldiers were being marched around, peasants were struggling with all manner of baggage, women were carrying crying babies while clutching small toddlers, and protesting children were being pushed along. Elderly men were carrying chickens and ducks in metal cages and hanging on tightly to the occasional goat. Chaos reigned and I just wandered up and down looking for the lady with the rose; unfortunately she had forgotten this part of the arrangements and was accompanied by her husband, who had never been mentioned.

Lilian and Tudor Bourilkova were both doctors working in the Postgraduate Medical Institute. He was researching into chest diseases, mainly asbestosis, and she was involved in the planning of primary medical care in Professor Gargov's department. In addition she often acted as a peripatetic interpreter as she understood and spoke English well.

To my great surprise it had been arranged and approved by Professor Gargov that I would be allowed to live and sleep in their flat in the centre of Sofia, but while we were having breakfast it was explained with much embarrassment that this was no longer possible. Since the recent invasion of Czechoslovakia the activity of the secret police had increased and if I stayed with them I would have to give their address when I registered with the local police. The long and short of it was I would be 'tailed', as they put it, and so would they as well as their two sons.

The Bourilkovas did everything to help me. Two government-run tourist hotels exclusively for foreigners existed in Sofia but if you were from the wrong side of the Iron Curtain the cost would be five or six times more than if you were East German or Cuban. Clearly the government understood how to make money. Instead they managed to find me a small cheap hotel where I could stay and where the owners, whom they knew, had promised not to overcharge. It was close to their flat so I could eat with them.

An elderly uncle lived with them and their two sons aged 14 and 11. The old man had been a general in the old Royal Army of King Boris and towards the end of the war he had been imprisoned for three years between 1944 and '47 by the anti-Nazi, anti-Royalist government. When the communist takeover took place he had then been forced to work as a peasant in the countryside for another fifteen years. Looking out of the window of their third-floor flat at the busy street below, I asked how he viewed life today compared with the days of King Boris. He replied:

"For me it is much worse but for most people it is much better."

At the Postgraduate Institute I was given the programme that had been arranged and was invited to ask for changes should I want any. At first glance it seemed fine but I decided to ask Lilian for her opinion. She too thought it was fine and in any case minor alterations could be organised on a day to day basis. As Lilian's work concerned primary care I couldn't have had a more useful companion.

The provision of a 'free service' paid for by central taxation applied to both primary and secondary care, and was similar to the principles of our NHS, including similar payments for prescriptions as well as direct payments for dental and optical services. One interesting difference was the payment which could be levied from patients if doctors considered any out of hours emergency calls to be unnecessary, or could have been dealt with in normal working hours. Patients could appeal – in theory.

Bulgaria had followed the Soviet Union and was committed to the principle that the doctor of first contact should look after patients according to their age, sex or ability to work; thus the basic team working in a health centre would consist of: a physician covering the old, the chronically sick and the unemployed; a paediatrician for children of both sexes; a gynaecologist for women; and dentists for both adults and children as well as the appropriate number of nurses and midwives. All workers whether on the railways or coal mines or construction would be seen at the health centres/polyclinics connected to their place of work. The army and police had separate organisations.

Work started at 8am until 2pm and then another shift took over until 8pm. On average twenty to thirty patients would be seen per session, followed by home visits accompanied by a nurse. I was able to visit a number of patients in their homes, all for much the same reasons as in the UK – for example a middle-aged man dying of cancer of the lung, an elderly woman with congestive heart failure, and a man in his mid-forties whom I remember very well as his management was so different compared with the UK. Following an uncomplicated myocardial infarct he had been taking anticoagulant drugs for six months and had been given no advice whatsoever about exercise or getting back to work. It was now seven months since the original attack and he had become a neurotic cardiac invalid. I only managed two home visits for children, one with chicken pox and the other involving paediatric development. Great emphasis was placed on assessment of children's development, which normally took place in the local health centre.

Rural areas, as in the communist bloc, had problems, particularly with regard to recruitment. Life was lonely both for a single person and for families, schools were poor and recreational facilities virtually non-existent. Consequently, over the years, because of the recruitment difficulties, a sort of 'compulsory national service' was in operation whereby for three years after graduation young doctors had to work in the villages. According to Lilian it was those who were politically suspect or unsatisfactory in some other way who were sent to the most remote regions. In recent years a fixed percentage of places at medical schools were being kept for youngsters from rural areas in the hope they would return to the village of their origin – a project that had as yet met with only limited success.

One thing was certain and Lilian agreed with me; it was connected with *feldschers.*[4] Without doubt they were more popular and valued and trusted than the young doctors and above all they provided the continuity of care since the majority had grown up in the local village.

Lopian was a small village on the northern foothills of the Balkan mountains, which run west to east almost cutting the country in two. First we drove to Botevgrad, a small town with a population of about ten thousand, and called at the health centre attached to the rural hospital (for medical and obstetric patients). Discussion was free and easy and my questions were answered clearly.

The journey onward to Lopian continued by ambulance (attached to the rural hospital) the general opinion being it would cope better

[4] In Russia around 1700 Peter the Great introduced the *feldscher* (from the German 'field barber') into the Imperial army and slowly they became an accepted part of the medical scene, particularly in the countryside. In Sweden in 1751 Linnaeus advocated that rural clergy should be trained in medicine to provide cover for the virtually doctor-less rural population. However, it was not until 1804 in Germany that Johann Christian Reil, Professor of Medicine in Halle, had the foresight to introduce a separate shorter training for medical auxiliaries in rural areas and in the under-privileged area of cities. The title 'feldscher' remained in Russia and continued in Soviet times.

with the poor roads as we neared the town. We drove initially along the edge of the Danubian plain through undulating farmland, then turning south up into the mountains with the road getting steeper and the countryside wilder and more dramatic. Lopian was off the beaten track, with small wooden houses surrounded by pretty fenced gardens, and had – much to my surprise – electricity.

The health centre was modern, built in the late '50s, and cared for a population of around 2700 that included two smaller hamlets. It was clean, had the necessary basic medical equipment, and two beds were provided for normal deliveries. In addition a simple dispensary stored the necessary day to day drugs.

The doctor and dentist were in their early thirties and I suspected had been placed there for political reasons (Lilian later confirmed this). Discussion again was easy with Lilian encouraging everyone, including the nurses, to talk. The doctor in particular was eager to criticise things he was unhappy about and to admit to difficulties. During this discussion a most impressive story emerged; in spite of having no piped water or a piped sewage system, over the past six years there had been no outbreak of serious infectious diseases although without doubt some would have been expected.

Returning in the ambulance to Botevgrad we continued to Turnovo, many centuries ago the capital of the Second Bulgarian Kingdom. In 1968 with a population of about 26000, and 160 miles from Sofia, it had officially become part of the tourist trail for those who lived behind the Iron Curtain. I see why; the river Yantra meanders through a valley with steep hills on either side, the picturesque town perched on the left bank. On the opposite bank is Trapezitsa, a beautifully wooded hill. As we drove towards the town it looked as though it were suspended from the rocks with the houses built one above the other.

Once we were in the town and looking down at the river from spectacular rocky ridges with vertical drops through steep ravines, the view was different – the houses and the many small dwellings looked almost as though they had been sprinkled onto the gentle lower slopes, but as the ground became steeper so the houses, often terraced, seemed miraculously stuck to the earth.

The main street was about half a mile long and was a mixture of

19th and 20th century architecture with some influence from the Turks, but mostly old Russia. The town is divided into old and new, the main street being part of the old with a maze of twisting cobbled streets leading from it with lanes so narrow that the balconies and even the eaves obscured the sky. It had a fairytale feel about it.

We drove straight to the Area Hygiene Institute (Public Health Directorate) where the Director was waiting. We talked for an hour and a half about the organisational, epidemiological, environmental and preventive aspects of health. Two memories stand out. First, the lavatory and hand washbasin were encrusted with excreta and dirt and the smell to go with it – and this was the office of the Director of Public Health! I couldn't understand why he showed no sign of embarrassment – Lilian certainly did – and how he was able to talk about the importance of hygiene within both the family and society with no sense of shame given his own circumstances. Second, the Director answered everything without hesitation.

We carried on with this enjoyable mixture of primary medical care and travel although I was determined not to be side-tracked by Lilian's desire to show me as much as possible of her interesting homeland. A rural health centre at the village of Polikraistle about fifteen miles from Turnovo was our first port of call, though en passant Lilian couldn't resist taking me first to one of the ten medieval monasteries surrounding Turnovo. Preobrazenski monastery is two miles from the village and in the early morning autumn sunshine it was enchanting, surrounded by vines and nestling into the wooded hill. We saw no monks, heard only birds, and saw only ducks, chickens and geese, with sheep and goats wandering along the cobbled paths.

The health centre had been built in 1953 and was much the same as we had seen at Lopian except for two things. First, the three *feldschers* were officially included in the staff, and second, the doctor was unusual in that he had worked there since it opened fifteen years earlier. He had been born in the village and had willingly returned immediately after qualifying – so the scheme had its successes at times.

Before finally leaving Turnovo we made another detour to the village of Arbanassi, famous for its seven churches and two monasteries. The village was different in that most of the 16th and 17th century stone buildings were still standing and deliberately half hidden behind high stone walls. The churches and monasteries contained many precious frescoes which unfortunately we had no time to see. In any case many were locked away and tourists were not encouraged to see them on account of neighbouring mosques; the government didn't want to offend Muslims, at least that's what I was told.

By lunchtime primary care was forgotten and politics and travel took over. We were now travelling almost directly south to Plovdiv, Bulgaria's second city, over the Balkan mountains to the Valley of the Roses and rich agricultural land almost as far as Plovdiv. First Lilian wanted me to understand the historical relationship with their powerful neighbour, the Soviet Union. As we drove through one of the many passes on the mountains two memorials were pointed out. They commemorated famous battles between Russia and Ottoman armies during the War of Liberation 1877 - 1878; the Bulgarians have obviously never forgotten how much they owe the Russians. The first was a spectacular orthodox church with golden domes and tall spires in the village of Shipka, and then in the pass itself a massive granite monument in memory of a handful of Russians and Bulgarians who had defended the pass against the forces of Suleima Pasha, the Ottoman leader. Lilian was able to describe a further memorial, not quite visible, a hundred-foot-high monument to Liberty; it was the largest memorial connected with the Russo-Turkish war.

I remained unclear about the relationship between Bulgaria and the Soviet Union but eventually I think I began to understand what Lilian was saying. Historically Imperial Russia had always befriended Bulgaria, especially against the Ottoman Turks, so that Lilian's generation was able to dissociate Russian people from the Soviet Union, thus permitting them to believe the two peoples could remain friends even if the two governments disagreed.

In addition Bulgarians are taught from an early age that two orthodox priests, the brothers Cyril and Methodius, during the 9th century AD created the Cyrillic alphabet thus allowing Bulgaria to take credit for being the originator of the Slav-speaking language and reinforcing their relations with the Russian people. The Greeks have a different slant on this version of history.

Plovdiv was not reached until late afternoon and we were eventually sight-seeing in semi-darkness, though before the light went altogether we managed to see the old part of the town with its narrow, steep, winding streets leading to the three hills upon which the original medieval town had been built. Of further interest to me was 'Gladstone Street' close to the railway station – but no evidence of anything for Disraeli.

Three places in Sofia graphically illustrate how ignorance makes it difficult to understand what you are looking at. Why is there still a street also named after William Gladstone in Sofia as well? Why was it that in 1959, according to the writer and traveller Bernard Newman, when the name of Disraeli was mentioned people spat on the ground, but mention Gladstone's name and they raised their hats? Undoubtedly it was related to the occasion in the House of Commons when Gladstone had openly supported the Russian intervention in the War of Liberation whilst Disraeli had taken the opposing view.

Why in a communist country was a forty-foot-high statue of Tsar Alexander the Second mounted on horseback allowed to remain as 'The Liberator's Monument' standing paradoxically in front of the Naradno Subranye (National Assembly)? After all, no communist had ever considered the Tsars to be liberators.

Finally, what about the 'largest and artistically most valuable monument in the capital' (according to the official government Guide Book 1963), the Alexander Nevski Memorial Church? Since 1948 gold had been stolen from most of its domes which over the years had been replaced using government money. At the same time this massive building at the centre of the Bulgarian Orthodox Church had been in imminent danger of collapsing. Again the communist government had given the church enough money to restore and sometimes rebuild it.

According to Owen Chadwick in his book *The Christian Church in the Cold War*, the Bulgarian Academy of Science –

> *'held an enquiry into 42,644 people in 1962: no religion 65.4%; some religion 35.5% but half the babies were baptised in church; a third of brides were married in church; and four-fifths of funerals happened in church. The enquiry was gloomy about the success of the atheist campaign . . . it reached only those who were already atheists'.*

Perhaps the babushkas of the nation had more power and influence than the Central Committee, and maybe the Academy of Science had the wisdom to realise this.

Lilian and Tudor described themselves as non-believers, not aggressively, just matter of fact.

> "Would you like to go to a service in the Alexandra Nevski?"
> "Yes, I would, but please don't feel you must come."
> "No, we'd like to come."

And so we set off from their flat, a ten-minute walk. On the way they explained why they wanted to come. First, going to church was often used as a way of protesting against the government –

> "What is the protest now?"
> "The invasion by the Warsaw Pact - we're really ashamed."

Second –

> "Our lives are dreary and dull. There's little beauty unless we can get out into the countryside. Of course, we can go to concerts and art galleries but many of us want more – just you wait and see."

I was looking forward to my first Orthodox service and didn't know quite what to expect. The huge area under the central dome was packed, everyone standing, no chairs or benches. The iconostasis took my eye immediately, but it was the rich colours of the robed priests that stunned me, the Patriarch of All Bulgaria at their centre adding further grandeur to the proceeding. What amazing good fortune.

The singing was unlike anything I had ever heard; it was unaccompanied, as the use of instruments was forbidden, not even an organ or piano. The strength and depth of the bass voices of the priests was profound and deeply spiritual; it was counter-balanced by two women's choirs on the opposite sides of the church. Their voices conveyed a feeling of sorrow and anguish, almost a sense of grief and suffering. It was so different from the tradition of the Anglican Church reaching its apotheosis in the sublime purity of treble voices in cathedral or university college choirs where women were excluded (now of course girls supplement the treble voices of the boys in most church choirs). Did the Orthodox and Anglican communions view life differently? One from the ever-present experience of suffering and grief, the other from the beauty of holiness?

Although we had arrived more than an hour after the service had begun, when we left about an hour later Lilian and Tudor assured me that only about half the litany had been completed; this was my introduction to the physical stamina required to survive the whole of an Orthodox service.

"Well, what did you think? Can you see why people go even if they're not believers? Did you enjoy it?"
"Yes, I can see what you mean. I've never seen or heard anything like it. I don't think I've ever been asked if I've enjoyed a church service . . . but perhaps you didn't mean 'enjoy'?"
"Yes, we did."
"Alright, maybe it was the right word. In some ways it was like a concert, a sort of performance. The congregation is the audience."

Bulgaria had gone exceedingly well as regards my studies, and certainly way beyond what I had expected, which was largely due to Lilian. I had one regret – Professor Gargov was out of the country in Moscow so we never met.

Lilian and Tudor had introduced me to Goran Moskowski, a rheumatologist, and his wife Zdravka. The friendship between Tudor and Goran was nothing to do with medicine but through playing bridge. Goran's family had been refugees from Poland (Moskowski is not a Bulgarian name and was perhaps one of the reasons he had become an outsider) and after the war Goran had been trained at the American University in Beirut. A committed non-believer, it was extraordinary listening to him singing a wide variety of Christian hymns, especially Christmas carols, and reciting bits of English poetry, all picked from his days in Beirut. He was fiercely anti-communist and unsurprisingly against the influence of the Soviet Union in Bulgaria – one of his sisters had been in prison for six years for anti-government activities. She had been betrayed by one of her colleagues, which was the reason Goran trusted no one except his family. Curiously he was equally opposed to the United States, or more accurately to the spread of American culture, which he hated. He had one obsession and this favoured the United Kingdom; the BBC World Service represented the truth and he had listened two or three times a day since the early 1950s and had continued to do so until he died in the mid-90s. When Rachel and I were staying with them in 1989 it was fascinating to realise he had gone through the same routine for fifty years. Before turning on the wireless he made certain the door of the flat was locked, other doors were closed, and the volume was as low as possible. For him and Zdravka and Martha his daughter the World Service could be relied on to provide an honest, balanced account. During our visit we all listened to reports of the dramatic opening of a Hungarian/Austrian border post that was followed by a flood of Hungarians moving west and then thousands of Czechs and East Germans pouring into West Germany. All three Moskowskis were stunned almost speechless and hardly able to believe what they were hearing – but it was safe to believe because it was the BBC. The three of them remained nervous that something would go wrong, and listening to the fall of the Berlin Wall was beyond anything they could imagine.

Over the years Martha visited the UK many times and on one occasion came with her son, Dimitaz, to see if he could get a scholarship to study at Wells Cathedral School, one of four specialist music schools in the country. He was clearly a talented musician and been offered a place to study at the Moscow Conservatoire, but the Moskowski family was keen to get away from any Soviet influence. Eventually he went to America (not with the approval of his grandfather) and studied at the Juilliard School of Music in New York, after which he worked as a classical clarinetist for twelve years. By this time he had married and decided he couldn't stomach the American way of life any longer so he and his wife and son returned home to work in the Sofia Philharmonic (his grandfather, who by then had died, would have been extremely pleased!).

Goran and Zdravka only visited Britain once. This was in 1990 when the highlight of the trip was a visit to the BBC World Service and meeting presenters who for more than half his lifetime had been his saviour – the light that had brought hope to the Moskowskis and thousands like him.

Lilian came to Wells in the '80s and her two sons, Jordan and Danni, in the early '90s. Lilian was much more realistic and objective about the West than poor Goran whose visit to Britain had been a disappointment. Her two sons were of a different generation and enjoyed western culture, particularly the United States. Neither had had the experience of Goran's or their mother's generation.

As I left Sofia on the train to Bucharest I felt genuinely sad and more than a little apprehensive.

8

THE PEOPLE'S REPUBLIC of ROMANIA

Dr Engelmeier continued to be my first port of enquiry; he provided a few names and addresses, only one of which was in any way connected with primary care. Dr Alexandra Cuica worked at the Institute of Geriatrics in Bucharest and his reply was enthusiastic as he was hoping to improve the exchange of medical information and even take in the possibility of travel. His wife was a paediatrician also working in the capital, and they would be pleased to invite me to stay in their home. It all seemed too good to be true and five days before leaving for Bulgaria I received a letter informing me that he and his wife had been invited to Italy, Switzerland, West Germany and Sweden for two months and would not be in Bucharest for my proposed visit; my forebodings were realised.

The Royal Society of Medicine (RSM) of which I was a member had contacts with many scientific/medical societies and institutes throughout the world including a number behind the Iron Curtain. One of these was the Union des Sociétas des Sciences Médicales de la République Socialiste de Roumanie. Explaining that I was a member of the RSM I requested any help they could give in making contacts. Within six weeks Dr Caloenescu, the General Secretary, had replied advising me he could not give me official assistance but promising he would try to organise an official invitation through the Ministerul Sanătătii Prevederilor Sociale – in other words with official government approval. In the meantime the first National Conference with International Participation of the Sociétas des Sciences Médicales was being organised and I would be invited as an official guest; the conference however would not be for at least another two years! A further letter from Dr Caloenescu confirmed he had contacted the Ministerul Sanătătii Prevederilor Sociale and had put in a good word for me.

In late December 1967/early January '68 Dr Florea Duna from the Ministère de la Santé et de la Prevoyance Sociale agreed to my visit for the autumn of 1968 and requested I should send details of what I wanted to see and discuss so that a programme could be organised. Everything was now in the official hands of the State.

On 21 August '68 the invasion of Czechoslovakia commenced. I was due to reach Romania on 23 September and during that time there was much speculation about the future of Eastern Europe. The newspapers and the media in the UK floated the idea that the Soviet Union was about to invade Romania in retaliation for their provocative action in refusing to join the other Warsaw Pact countries. Soviet forces were reported to be on manoeuvres along the Romanian border.

I had been vaguely aware that Romania had pursued a sort of independent foreign policy vis-à-vis the Soviet Union and often joined China in their criticism of the USSR, perhaps endeavouring to follow the independence of Yugoslavia and President Tito.

During those four weeks I wondered if I should cancel my visit. Would an invasion take place, as so many people suggested? Even the Foreign Office considered it to be a possibility. Was I being irresponsible/stupid? Well, as the weeks went by and nothing happened I decided it was unlikely.

I was met off the train and taken to the Hotel Lido and my interpreter/guide/minder told me she would collect me at 9am the following day. She was a physician, artificially blond, over-made-up and arrogant. I immediately thought she might be in direct contact with the Securitate (secret police). Romania felt different from the other countries I had visited – there was a sense of hidden watchfulness, nobody speaking out of turn, a strict formality on meeting anyone and a wariness of each other. Certainly the streets were not full of happy smiling faces.

The staff at the reception desk were grim in every sense of the word, and after they had told me the cost per night and for meals it was obvious the Lido would be far too expensive. I had requested to be put up in a modest hotel or B & B, not realising it would never have occurred to a government official that my visit was not financed by my government or a university or institute. In addition, all foreigners from the West stayed in government-run hotels so they could be watched carefully and followed if necessary. In 1968 only two such hotels existed in Bucharest. I had to make a decision, and quickly.

The only thing I could think to do was to phone Dr Cuica's home, although thinking about it now I can't imagine how I plucked up the courage to contact someone I'd never met or spoken to and who didn't know me. But far more than this I didn't know what danger I might be putting them in. If I could stay with whoever was, I hoped, in the house looking after their daughter, I could book out of the Lido in the morning without telling my interpreter/guide. I didn't want the Cuica household to be in any trouble so I decided that each morning I would return to the Lido to be picked up. In my panic I had forgotten the hotel receptionist might contact the Ministry of Health when it was discovered my bed hadn't been slept in (and anyway I had booked out!).

I spoke to Dr Cuica's sister, who spoke French, and somehow we managed to communicate. The next day, after finishing my work, I walked to St Aviator Papa Marin No. 3, which took about forty minutes. She was a most warm, friendly lady who seemed to be enjoying looking after her ten-year-old niece Svetlana. Eventually her husband arrived home from work and was mighty surprised to find me there. He chatted with his wife and they assured me I could stay; mercifully they didn't seem too concerned. They spoke quietly to Svetlana and I gathered they were telling her not to mention to any of her friends or teachers that I was staying in her home. After returning to the hotel to collect my luggage we spent a very pleasant evening chatting as best we could. It seemed that French was the second language and English came after German. On retiring to bed I felt somewhat more relaxed and certainly very very grateful. I just hoped that nothing would go wrong – and nothing did.

My walk back to the Lido in the morning worked well and I was in plenty of time for my guide. Off we went to a meeting at the Ministry of Health and Social Maintenance with the Director-General himself, Dr Constantinescu Gheorghe. I was surprised to be talking to the 'top man' and it made me realise that my visit was under strict surveillance – there was no other way in Romania. Compared to my experience in Hungary it was almost laughable.

From my notes it is clear I was able to cover most aspects of primary care but I received only the minimum amount of information in answer to my questions – everything was strictly formal and the health workers were careful about what they said. Even whilst talking to the Director General about abortion he was cautious, as if our conversation might be bugged. In 1953 Romania had introduced abortion on demand with no restrictions – probably the freest abortion legislation in the world. In 1966, a year after Nicolae Ceausesçu became President, everything changed without any discussion or debate; abortion was restricted to women aged over forty-five, to those who already had four children, after rape and for a number of medical and psychiatric conditions. This policy remained in place until Ceausesçu was murdered on Christmas Day 1989. Women found ways around the new legislation, which mostly meant resorting to back-street practitioners with the accompanying dangers of infection and haemorrhage. Money was the answer for the minority.

No discussion on this issue or implied criticism of Ceausesçu was allowed by the Director-General. He simply stated that the changes had taken place. He was of course living in a police state and when I tried to question one or two Romanian colleagues about the reaction of society, and how health professionals dealt with controversial medical topics, the reply was 'that's government policy', and nothing more would be said.

Whenever possible urban and rural areas were organised in similar ways. The basic health centre, covering a population of between four and six thousand, was staffed by an internist (a physician looking after medical problems), a paediatrician, a midwife, and nurses, all working on a shift pattern and in pairs; one would be working in the health centre with the other doing home visits. Great emphasis was placed on preventive care in children. Up to the age of one all children were examined each month; between one and three years this was four times a year; between three and seven twice yearly. In urban areas, health centres, sometimes called dispensaries, were closely connected to a crèche (three months to three years), and a *camin* or playschool (three to seven years). In this way each child's development, at least in theory, was carefully monitored.

Care of women and maternity work in urban areas took place in polyclinics which, where possible, were attached to hospitals. In rural areas the midwife and internist were responsible for ante-natal, post-natal care and delivery. In reality most babies were delivered in hospital. The internist was also responsible for simple gynaecological problems.

I managed to visit a number of health centres, a crèche and a *camin*, a clinique de pédiatrie and the obstetric and gynaecological departments within a polyclinic as well as a visit to the Public Health Directorate of the City of Bucharest.

It was not for medical reasons that I most clearly remember polyclinic number four. Opened only two years previously, it was a facility the authorities were happy to show foreigners – but it was the meeting with Dr Nicolae Constantinescu (not related to the Director General) which was later going to have an impact on me – and subsequently Rachel – for many years and would give us an idea from a safe distance of just what living in a police state was like.

As I was walking round the polyclinic Nicolae had been looking directly at me to catch my eye as though he wanted to speak to me. At the end of the visit we were all just standing around and Nicolae quietly and quickly disappeared down a corridor and through a door on the left. Almost immediately I followed him without my interpreter or anyone else seeming to notice – perhaps they thought I was looking for a toilet. Anyway, Nicolae was there, we shook hands and I listened. He spoke rapidly in reasonably clear English and it was obvious he had much to tell; his brother was an Orthodox priest and he was a rheumatologist. He was unmarried and wanted contact with the West. He told me how professionally isolated he felt and how imprisoned politically by being unable to travel. We quickly exchanged addresses and he asked me most earnestly to keep in contact – not by letter but by postcard, which would be less likely to attract attention and cause trouble. We hadn't spoken for more than five minutes before he was urging me to get back to my interpreter and the polyclinic officials as quickly as possible. This I did; they appeared not to have missed me.

As I left Romania it was the Cuica family, however, who were in my thoughts. Without them I don't know what I would have done. Their generous welcome, their openness, the way they made me feel I wasn't a danger to them, and all for a complete stranger, was quite remarkable, and made me wonder, if the roles had been reversed, whether I would have responded in the same way: I hope so.

On my return to the UK, almost the first thing I did was to send a postcard to Nicolae. Written 27 November, his reply arrived at the beginning of December apologising for the delay and saying how glad he was to receive my postcard. He wrote:

> 'I need to be quiet to write my first letter in English. I am very exciting (sic) and want to have the free time to correct my letter . . I promise you the following letter will be better. This shortage of communication leads to the poverty of idea and to the effective isolation; on the other hand the books, the reviews, the papers are not enough to know the life and the peoples . . . I was very pleased to receive your visit but was sorry your visit was so short, very official and we had no time to talk about our medical affairs. It is very interesting to know their idea, the opinions of a man the same age, the same profession but from the other side of the country. I hope I can see you and your children. I am not yet married but it is not from my guilt. I shall be very glad if you all understand my letter. I hope to have the possibility to meet you again but until that happy occasion I send you and all your family my best wishes.'

I continued to send a postcard twice a year and would receive a short letter saying nothing once a year. I cannot begin to describe my astonishment when in 1977 I received a letter from Nicolae in West Germany. He had defected to the West with his wife Ruxandra – his marriage was unknown to us – and in May he came to stay with us for two weeks on his own. He was an academic and loved books; on a particularly miserable, cold damp windy day in May he took the bus to Oxford. I remember we were a bit anxious and very disappointed for him on account of the weather, but on his return late in the evening he was happy:

> "What more could I have asked for but to ride on a bus through the wonderful English countryside reading the Times of London and for Oxford to be my destination?"

Their story is painful to recall and relate. Ruxandra and Nicolae married in the early 1970s and soon their daughter Stanna was born.

At some stage they had decided to defect but would have to leave Stanna behind as a 'hostage' when they applied for a visa to go on holiday. Nicolae's father was dead, and they did not know how to tell his mother and Ruxandra's parents who all knew each other. They were afraid to tell them too soon before they went on their supposed 'holiday' because the two mothers were bound to be greatly upset and the authorities would inevitably very quickly find out the truth from this close-knit community. It was not until two nights before departure that the disclosure was made and their fear was justified as even in the short time the mothers were given the news their tears and anguish were plain for all to see. Throughout all the next day Nicolae and Ruxandra feared the Securitate (internal security force/secret police) might appear at any moment. Nicolae's brother, the priest, was the only other person to be told and in fact he had known for a month. On the final evening he was asked to come and pray for all concerned.

The parting next morning was too painful to bear; no embrace for the parents and barely a kiss for the two-and-a-half-year-old Stanna. As they travelled west through Yugoslavia and finally to the Swiss border, they had agreed they would only talk about their plans for the 'holiday'. The previous year acquaintances of theirs had done the same thing, but unknown to them their car had been bugged and they were arrested at the Romanian/Yugoslav border, later to be imprisoned. Nicolae told me they were so nervous they didn't speak freely until they had crossed into Switzerland.

Initially he had been able to find only temporary work in West Germany so they moved to the Netherlands; he learned Dutch, passed further exams and was able to practise as a rheumatologist. For Ruxandra the story was different. For a year she never stopped weeping; day after day she was inconsolable and news from her mother brought no relief.

By chance they read in a newspaper that Queen Juliana was to make a state visit to Romania, so Nicolae wrote to her explaining their situation and asking if there was anything she could do to influence the Romanian government and let little Stanna go free. Within two weeks a reply had come from the Queen's private secretary informing them that her representative would speak to the appropriate officials, but of course she could not promise anything. Neither Nicolae nor Ruxandra could believe this response seeing that they were not citizens of the Netherlands and did not even have Dutch passports.

Some six weeks after the Queen's return, a message came from the Dutch Foreign Ministry that Stanna had been given permission to leave Romania and would be accompanied by a Dutch children's officer on the plane to Amsterdam. A wonderful happy ending! Or so we thought.

We kept in touch and in 1984 Ruxandra, Nicolae, Stanna and Alexandru came over for three weeks (Alexandru had been born soon after Stanna's arrival). At first everything seemed fine, but soon it was clear something was amiss. Nicolae was behaving as though he had no children and his wife didn't exist. He spent most of the day in the cathedral or praying in his room (they were staying in a cottage about five minutes' walk from us). The more I got to know him the more it seemed to me that perhaps Nicolae should have become a priest like his brother, or even a monk, and should never have married. I am ashamed to say I even thought the reason for his marriage and having Stanna was to use her as a hostage.

Not surprisingly, Ruxandra spent much of the three weeks suffering from migraines or lying about exhausted before she finally unburdened herself to Rachel. Both parents seemed unwilling or unable to cope with their children. After returning home, frequent phone calls over the next nine months came from Ruxandra in Heidelberg, where they were now living, bewailing her frustration and despair. Silence and Christmas cards followed, then a letter from Cluj, Romania, where Ruxandra was living with her mother, and another from Nicolae telling us he was still working as a rheumatologist in Heidelberg. There was no mention in either letter of Stanna and Alexandru. That was the end of our friendship with the Constantinescu family.

My connection with Romania had ended rather sadly. How could I imagine that five years later on 27 November 1993 I would find myself back in Bucharest, a city I had last visited in October 1968, sitting on a bench in the concourse of the Gară de Nord waiting for a train to take me to Bacau in the north-east Province of Moldavia. This was the same concourse where I had stolen the leftover bread rolls and gherkins and tomatoes from the little restaurant all those years ago, catching the same train that took me to Poland. What a change – no restaurant, not even a café, just a ledge selling lukewarm coffee, rubbish strewn everywhere and Romany gypsies and beggars pestering travellers, most of whom looked like refugees themselves. Within an hour I had seen three amputees, two of whom were bilaterals on homemade wooden sledges with pram wheels, and a single one with an above-knee wooden stump looking like Long John Silver from *Treasure Island.* I quickly learnt that the health service had totally collapsed since the death of Ceausesçu – no diabetic clinics, no supervision, little insulin and in any case too expensive for the majority of patients. Gangrene was the most common complication and amputation the standard treatment.

The snow had come with a vengeance, piled up in the streets, and a fresh fall had nearly cancelled or diverted my flight from London. The train was delayed and a temperature of -15° added to the misery of my wait in the barely-lit station with drunks either collapsed on the floor or shouting abuse. The four-and-a-half hour journey was further delayed by continuing snow so Bacau was not reached until 2.30am.

The Relief Fund for Romania (RFFR) started working in the environs of Bacau, a clapped-out industrial town in the summer of 1991. Unlike every other charity working in Romania, all of which concentrated exclusively on children in asylums, mental hospitals, children's homes and orphanages, the Relief Fund had decided to concentrate on the elderly to be found in poverty-stricken villages without any medical care. At the end of the Ceausesçu era the newly-qualified doctors who had been forced to work in the rural health service quickly disappeared and were not replaced.

The province of Moldavia in the north-east corner of the country had been recognised for many years as the poorest region and so the RFFR organised a Mobile Health Care programme to selected villages that were without doctors and often without medical assistants (equivalent to the State Enrolled Nurses – SENs – who worked in the NHS until the mid '80s). There were sixteen such villages plus outlying communities, in total around 20,000 people. A British nurse was in charge of the small team, based in Bacau, that included a British doctor and a Romanian interpreter. Each village would be visited on either a weekly or a fortnightly basis, initially from a converted caravan. The roads were little more than rutted muddy tracks, so not surprisingly the axle finally broke – in 1993 on my watch. Village dispensaries were used and the houses of two Roman Catholic priests who also provided a cooked lunch. Sometimes a villager would allow us to use their small humble dwelling, which was amazing as by the end of the day there was as much mud in their home as in the street. The dispensaries had been poorly maintained and now the roofs were leaking, the doors were banging and the wooden stoves rarely produced enough warmth to allow patients to be examined without their layers of clothing. Not surprisingly the medical assistants were poorly-motivated, poorly paid – and sometimes never paid.

Patients had a grim time. On my first day the first patient I saw on a home visit was a woman in her mid-thirties who had recently had an unsuccessful operation for ovarian cancer and was dying. She had a small child to look after and her neighbours did their best, but her husband had disappeared. And yet this woman considered herself fortunate – at least she had paracetamol, one in the morning and one at night. I could have wept.

I made only one visit in the summer and I recall going to a man in his eighties with a malignant tumour on the right side of his face and jaw, half of which had been eaten away. He was lying on a couch in a small, dismal, dirty room with flies buzzing around and maggots wriggling about in this ghastly suppurating mess. Against his wishes, his dear wife had been forcibly taken to the hospital in Bacau two days before where she had died the next day. According to his neighbour he had pleaded for her to be brought home so he could see her for the last time, but nobody could find the money for the ambulance or hearse. Now he was pleading for someone to end his life. I'm still filled with regret that I ignored his desperate mumbling request. He died two days later. These are only two examples but there were many more occasions in the desperate poverty and neglect of those remote villages. It was sometimes difficult to remember I was in Europe and not in parts of Africa or India.

For political reasons the RFFR closed down in 1995 but continued to support the programme, which was taken over by a few hard-working and dedicated young Romanians. By 2013 this had become the Fundatia de Sprijin Comunitar (Community Support Foundation) and one of the most successful non-governmental organisations in the country.

During many visits to Romania in the late 1990s and the early years of the 21st century I was keen to find out how people remembered life when they were young. Almost all recalled a childhood of security, not well-off but not poor. They believed they lived in a good society – they were certainly told so at school. They had a home, always food on the table, went to school, had Young Communist summer camps and regular summer holidays with their parents, usually on the Black Sea. They remembered having immunisations at school. It seemed ordinary folk just accepted the propaganda of the government.

The communist regime under Ceausesçu was widely believed to be one of the most authoritarian and brutal in the former Eastern bloc. So what did older people remember about the Securitate? Almost always the answer was nothing; most of those I questioned would have had humble jobs or worked in the oil industry or were teachers. All said politics was rarely mentioned either at work or home; they simply kept their heads down as the best way not to come to the notice of the authorities.

On talking to the medical profession a different picture emerged. I remember two doctors in particular who were attached to the Medical School in Bucharest; they had been conscious of the Securitate although had not had any direct contact. They knew of colleagues who had been interrogated and imprisoned, but felt they had only themselves to blame; commonsense and caution were the essential ingredients that kept you safe and they knew how to be careful.

One further question:

"What did you resent most about living under communist rule?"

Their replies were identical and corresponded with what Nicolae had always said:

> "We resent our isolation from new ideas and meeting colleagues from abroad. We are cut off with no chance for argument or discussion, and

> professionally we are in a backwater with nothing to compare ourselves against."

It was only after the Berlin Wall came down that they realised just how successful government propaganda had been.

9

SOCIALIST FEDERAL REPUBLIC of YUGOSLAVIA

Eastern Europe would be incomplete without including Yugoslavia, yet that is how *An Analysis of Primary Medical Care* was published in 1979. It was a serious omission, but inevitable with the usual time/finance constraints and my unwillingness to ask a colleague to undertake the work, plus the deadline insisted upon by the Cambridge University Press. However, a Stanning Foundation/Royal College of General Practitioners Travelling Fellowship enabled me to visit in 1980.

The big difference between Yugoslavia and the rest of Eastern Europe was the relative ease of getting a visa and the emergence of package tours; this had given rise to a superficial familiarity with the country. People knew that Yugoslavia was right in the middle of the Balkans and had a long, beautiful Adriatic coastline. It was also common knowledge that Yugoslavia, as far as the Soviet Union and the other People's Republics were concerned, was the 'black sheep' as described by Misha Glenny in *The Balkans.* This reputation was almost entirely due to Tito (Joseph Broz) following his election as President in 1945. He remained President for the next thirty-five years until he died, four months before I arrived in Zagreb.

Phyllis Anty in *Tito: a Biography,* 1974, wrote:

> *'The news of the break between Tito and Stalin was announced to an astonished and incredulous world on June 28th 1948, by a simple statement in a Czech newspaper, that Yugoslavia has been expelled from the Cominform.'*

The Cominform was a new international organisation of communist states run along similar lines to the defunct Comintern. From then on Yugoslavia remained fiercely independent of the USSR and in the middle '50s Tito officially created the movement of non-aligned states; it spread throughout the world, enabling countries to remain separate from the two main power blocs of the United States and the USSR. Tito quickly became an honoured and much respected statesman.

The death of Tito and the end of his dictatorship began to highlight the weakness of the country's constitution, and by the time of my arrival the resulting political instability was being discussed. Nobody could have foretold the inhumanity, conflict, hatred and war crimes that lay ahead.

During my visit only a few would talk of the implications of Tito's death or hazard a guess about how successful the rotating leadership would be, or how Belgrade as the capital of Yugoslavia would work out with the other Republics. Neither would they conjecture for how long the rich north – Slovenia and Croatia – would subsidise the poverty of Montenegro, Macedonia and the Autonomous Province of Kosovo. The most anyone would say was that there were going to be many problems in the years to come, but they made no mention whatsoever of impending disaster in Bosnia-Herzegovina. The one exception was a young Muslim doctor who drove me to visit a rural hospital in Han Pijesak high in the mountains about fifty miles from Sarajevo; he was adamant that Yugoslavia would break up.

Separate languages can only reinforce differences and remind everyone of the bitter legacies of history and the poisonous embrace of religion and politics. Croats, Serbs and Montenegrins have a common language, Serbo-Croat, while Slovenians and Macedonians have their own language. Two alphabets are used, Latin and Cyrillic. Historically each Republic can be thought of as a separate nation or kingdom except Bosnia-Herzegovina which has a mixed population of Serbs, Croats and Moslems, none of which was in an absolute majority. In addition, two autonomous provinces Vojvodina and Kosovo, are part of the Republic of Serbia. Finally, religion brings its own seemingly insoluble problems with Roman Catholicism mainly in Slovenia and Croatia, Orthodox Christianity mainly in Serbia, Macedonia and Montenegro, and Islam rooted in Bosnia-Herzegovina.

All this is true, and yet Tito's communist dictatorship had enabled Bosnian Serbs, Croats and Muslims to live alongside each other in such similar villages it was impossible to tell them apart. I'm certain that this young doctor could have had no inkling of the horror and brutality that was to enfold Sarajevo and most of Herzegovina where murder and rape were carried out by all sections of society.

All was not gloom and doom, however, and on our way to the hospital he was keen to show me where the Olympic Winter games were to be held. He remarked:

"How we'll afford it I don't know, but I do know we'll have enough snow!"

The impression I had been given was that my programme of study had been organised and it was just a matter of having a meeting at the Andrija Stampar School of Public Health in Zagreb to get agreement.

Andrija Stampar in 1931 was in the Chair of Hygiene and Social Medicine at the University of Zagreb, later to become Dean of the Faculty and Rector of the University. Throughout the '30s and immediately following the end of the Second World War his national and international reputation grew, as a fighter for the reform of medical training and for the right to health and better living conditions for working people. He played a leading role in the establishment of international collaboration in health matters and the formation of the constitution of the World Health Organisation (WHO) which was accepted at the first meeting of the World Health Assembly in Geneva in 1948, presided over by Stampar himself.

My entrée into Yugoslavia had depended on two contacts, who quite independently directed me to the same person: Associate Professor Zivko Kulčar at the Andrija Stampar School of Public Health. My first contact was the ever-present, always enthusiastic and helpful Frank Ošanéc in Prague who had worked with Kulčar over a number of years, and the second, Professor Robert Kohn at the London School of Hygiene and Tropical Medicine. I forget how exactly I came to get in touch with the latter, but looking back at our correspondence, he had recently reviewed *An Analysis of Primary Medical Care* and I must have spoken to him because of what he had already written about Yugoslavia. Interestingly one of his letters should have prepared me (but didn't) for the rather disorganised last-minute measures and the confused and casual ways I was to encounter:

'There's no accounting for Zivko's ways of communicating! Why he should implicate you when he wants to communicate with me is beyond me; he had both my addresses and telephone numbers etc and in fact I had a very long letter from him to which I replied.

But thank you very much for relating the message. He really is very helpful and kind . . . '

On arriving for my first meeting with Kulčar I realised very quickly that primary care might take second place – not to hospitals but to politics and wider discussions. My diary records:

'. . . philosophical and political discussions regarding social work, care of the dying with a secular rather than a theological or medical perspective of life and death.'

My next meeting records:

'. . . a broad sweeping assessment of the crisis brought about by the success of technological medicine, and the need to change direction, followed by his explanation of Croatia's next five-year plan.'

I became extremely frustrated, however interesting his discussions with his colleagues concerning the history of Serbia as opposed to the rest of Yugoslavia might be. It was very difficult to keep to the simple basics and in fact my programme was never mentioned. Modern secular attitudes and the dangers of religious beliefs would intrude into straightforward discussions about the organisation of primary care. Again in my diary:

'Still every question is answered "Yes that is difficult" and then Zivko and his colleagues would proceed to talk about anything that interested them: awkward and difficult to combat.'

Whilst in Zagreb a WHO meeting was taking place regarding primary health care in the developing world. Without warning, at most half an hour, I was told I was to appear on Croatian TV with Dr Chien, Deputy Director of WHO.

"What are we to discuss?"
"Oh, you must talk about the ideal situation for general practice."

This was a quite impossible and absurd topic in relation to the state of primary care in the developing world.

A week later at the Institute of Public Health in Sarajevo I was asked to lecture on Chile and Cuba – no problem for me and I had been given time to decide what I wanted to say, but literally a moment before going to the meeting:

"We think it would be a good idea for you to talk about economics and primary care."

When we were discussing about how I should get from Rijeka on the Adriatic coast to Belgrade where snow had blocked the railway line, I was assured with enthusiastic certainty that there were a number of flights every day. In reality there were none at all on Sunday, the day I was due to travel!

My visit to Novi Sad, the capital of the Autonomous Province of Vojvodina, provides yet another example of the slap-happy approach to doing things.

> "Yes, it is essential to stay overnight as it will be impossible to finish everything in one day."

On arrival the next day:

> "Yes, the programme has been arranged and it will be finished in the day so there's no need for you to stay overnight."

Nobody had thought to check if there was an available bus back to Belgrade so I had to catch a train; much more expensive and requiring a taxi at the other end. It was the same assumption as in other communist countries, that the government or an institute or medical school would be paying my expenses.

And so it went on. Perhaps what annoyed me the most concerned fully-agreed and pre-arranged meetings written into everyone's diaries. But when I phoned to check the arrangements I would get:

"Yes, he is still away in Ljubljana but will be here tomorrow." (when I would have departed) Or:

> "Yes, he is expecting you today but he is away. You can come tomorrow but he will not be expecting you."

Never any embarrassment or shame, just the routine 'it's how things are'.

Following the break with the Soviet Union in 1948 it was decided that in health as in the economic, social and political spheres, the concept of decentralisation suited the independent nature of the individual republics and the general reaction against the stifling centralised bureaucracy and the inefficiency of the Marxist economy. And so decentralisation and self-management became part of the Yugoslav way of life. Interestingly agriculture was excluded from these changes until the early 1960s.

After the Second World War the health service was financed exclusively by central taxation until in the early '50s social security was introduced with payments being made by both employer and employee. Initially this was only for industrial workers and their families, but by 1969 comprehensive health insurance covered everyone (in theory). Around the same time new methods of financing the health service were being introduced, such as individual health facilities being operated on a self-financing arrangement.

The following extract appeared in an article in the *International Journal of Health Services* in 1979:

> *'The form of communism developed in Yugoslavia in the early 1950s – called workers self-management – has been of interest to many westerners concerned with the idea of participating democracy and workers self-management. It is generally said that self-management is responsible for the remarkable success that Yugoslavia has achieved. This paper suggests on the other hand that many of the successes achieved in the health care system are attributable largely to the fact that self-management is not allowed to work as freely as it does in other sectors of the economy.'*

A minority of Yugoslavs took this view, but I found it impossible to assess whether decentralisation and self-management had been a success or not. In fact it seemed possible that it could have aggravated the differences between the rich and poor republics and between the north and south. Self-management had clearly not prevented the development of special interest groups both in the medical profession and within patient groups who were pressurising for the development of high-tech medicine and tertiary care. I came across one patient group that was even advocating the building of what would be a totally superfluous hospital, and another group representing a small hospital suggesting that a renal dialysis unit should be installed. As always, whatever the society, it is those with the loudest voice who have the greatest influence, but not the necessary knowledge. Self-management kept the articulate members of the community happy but it certainly had no positive effect on the conflict between primary care and hospitals, or the antagonism between public health doctors and clinicians.

Decentralisation seemed to have been both a failure and a success. The majority of people seemed to have been aware of the danger of the principle being taken to the extreme and perhaps leading to political and social unrest. However, any return to the centralised Marxist control of the past was rejected; at least when mistakes were made the blame could no longer be laid at the door of the Federal or Republican governments. Bureaucracy didn't seem to have been much reduced, but the consensus appeared to be that at least the bureaucrats were more accessible and less remote from the people.

On my first day at the Stampar School of Public Health I had eventually been given the programme, including a note of the facilities that had been arranged for me to visit and the topics I wished to discuss. To my astonishment, where and when all this was to take place was a blank sheet of paper. Yes, Belgrade and Sarajevo were on the list but nothing had been organised. It was only by chance that Professor Smajkič from the Department of Social Medicine at the University of Sarajevo happened to be in the building and under pressure from me agreed to prepare for my visit. Similarly the colleagues in Belgrade and Novi Sad had nothing organised.

The big downside to this lack of organisation was the amount of unnecessary travelling involved – I would have to criss-cross the country and although it was only early November snow had been lying in the streets of Prague during my brief stop-over there; this should have prepared me. With road and rail links often blocked and airports closed, inevitably there were going to be problems, and yet the Yugoslavs themselves seemed no more prepared than I was. Instead of flying from Zagreb to Rijeka on the Adriatic coast I was taken with difficulty by car via Ljubljana, thus increasing the journey from 110 to 190 miles. The train journey back to Belgrade from the Adriatic coast went via Sarajevo where I had to change trains for Belgrade; a journey of only 240 miles took five minutes short of eight hours. There was no thought of stopping at Sarajevo to meet Professor Smajkič although I returned there later from Zagreb. Absolutely nothing was coordinated and there was no planning ahead nor attempt to do so. The one useful aspect of this chaos, that helped control my intense frustration, was that a number of my train journeys were undertaken at night so I didn't have to book into a hotel!

*

I had decided to visit Croatia rather than Slovenia for two reasons. First, Croatia's population was nearly three times bigger than Slovenia and second, Slovenia had the reputation of being the most westernised republic. In the south the Republics of Macedonia and Montenegro were both small – only about eight percent of the total population, and both were pretty inaccessible even without snow.

Frank Ošanéc had suggested if at all possible I should visit Kosovo and Vojvodina, both Autonomous Provinces within the Republic of Serbia yet with widely differing health statistics. Kosovo, along with Macedonia and Montenegro had the worst statistics in the country so I requested to visit Kosovo as it was the easiest to reach. The Serbian authorities stubbornly refused permission; it seemed to be a no-go area. In discussion with non-Serbian colleagues the reason soon became clear – 80% of the population were ethnic Albanians so the per capita spending on health (as well as everything else) was the lowest in Serbia and in the rest of Yugoslavia. Obviously foreigners were not allowed to see this less acceptable face of communism.

Since the early 1960s the importance of general practice as carried out in many countries in western Europe and other parts of the world had been accepted in the hope it would provide a comprehensive and accessible service along with continuity of care. One of the main obstacles to this policy was the poor education and training of general practitioners compared with their specialist colleagues. As a result GPs had a poor reputation with patients as well as within the profession and amongst medical students. Patients I spoke to told me repeatedly:

> 'GPs only sign certificates and bits of paper and refer me to a specialist.'

In practice, in urban areas the Soviet system was still followed, primary care being carried out by doctors restricting their work according to the age or sex of the patient whilst the working population was the responsibility of the industrial health service. I found it difficult to fathom how the impression had grown up both in the literature of the West and in the information coming out of Yugoslavia, that primary care was being carried out by GPs. It was simply untrue, just wishful thinking. There were of course exceptions, and in some remote rural areas the doctor of first contact worked in the same way as a GP and could be compared in a superficial way, but it would be untrue to say it was the norm.

If Yugoslavia was serious about trying to introduce general practice then success would depend on improving education and training – to my surprise this had already begun. In 1977 Experimental Centres involving courses of further education and the supervision of training were set up, leading eventually to an examination and qualification of Specialist in General Medicine.

The Experimental Centre in Sarajevo was attached to the Department of Social Medicine at the Medical School and was run by Professor Smajkič; he showed me round and was optimistic that the further qualification would bring about a change in primary care. He had set up two more Centres in Bosnia-Herzegovina at Banja Luka and Mostar. The Stampar Institute in Zagreb had been responsible for developing and supervising Centres in Croatia at Rijeka, Spit, Osijek, Varazedin and Zagreb itself. As yet Slovenia was not involved and I was never given a satisfactory answer as to why Serbia, the largest republic, had decided not to participate. Obviously Macedonia and Montenegro were never likely to be concerned with such Centres.

Refreshing my memory after so many years, I have been amazed by the number of facilities I had been able to visit despite the disorganisation already described – primary health care units in towns and villages in Croatia, villages in Vojvodina and Bosnia-Herzegovina, paediatric dispensaries in Sarajevo and Labin on the Adriatic coast, health centres in Zagreb and Novi Sad, an emergency centre in Sarajevo and a rural hospital in Han Pijesak, a village high in the mountains. I did not visit any facility in Serbia other than the Institute of Public Health in Belgrade.

Sarajevo, along with Hiroshima, are two places which have altered the history of the twentieth century in a most profound way, and in the course of my travels I have visited both. Edward Grey had been right when he said 'The lamps are going out all over Europe. We shall not see them lit again in our lifetime'.

But if anything Grey underestimated the worldwide consequences of the events in Sarajevo, the shadow it would cast and the terrible memories it would leave over the next hundred years. Many, however, foresaw the effects of the dropping of the atomic bombs on Hiroshima and Negasaki and the fear that would be generated by this most horrific weapon of war.

On my arrival in Sarajevo I took a taxi to the Hotel Nacional which had been recommended to me by a fellow traveller as not costing too much and being reasonably clean. There were no vacancies so I walked over the river to the nearby Hotel Europa where a room was available. From the outside it was a run-of-the-mill mid-nineteenth century Ottoman building, but its interior gave a wonderfully old-fashioned feel as of a bygone age with heavy solid furniture, thick carpets and a lot of brown paint. The dining room had charm and the waitresses and wine waiter were in outmoded dress with old-fashioned courtesies to match.

Reading the hotel booklet at breakfast I was informed that Archduke Franz Ferdinand, the nephew of Emperor Franz Joseph of Austria and his wife Sophie, the Duchess of Höhenburg, had slept in the hotel the night before his assassination. I couldn't believe it but immediately felt part of history and strangely excited.

A few years later I realised I shouldn't have believed that booklet or any other guide book as in fact Franz and Sophie had never stayed in Sarajevo but had spent their time in a small fashionable spa town, Ilidza, on the outskirts of the city. On that fateful Sunday morning 28 June 1914, they had proceeded to Sarajevo by train and were then driven to the official reception at the City Hall in an open car.

At a short distance from the Hotel Europa at the Princip Bridge a plaque had been set into the wall of a building to commemorate the action of Gavrilo Princip, the leader of a number of young Bosnians who were waiting to shoot the Archduke and his wife. They were members of a revolutionary group opposing the Austro-Hungarian Empire's occupation of their country. The building is now the Mlada Bosna (Young Bosnia) Museum.

It is fascinating how Gavrilo Princip has been judged over the years. At the time of the assassination, those living in Sarajevo and thus under the control of the Austro-Hungarian Empire, called him a murderer; following the end of the First World War the new royalist Yugoslavia referred to him as a messenger of freedom, whilst at the time of Tito's dictatorship he had become the hero of the people in their protest against all occupying powers.

The plaque embodies part of history yet it was difficult to take in the enormity of what it represented: disbelief that at this very spot European and in fact world history had been changed forever; that in the space of five weeks, the great powers – Germany, Russia, France, Austro-Hungary and Britain – managed to misunderstand and distrust each other to such an extent that a state of self-destruction inevitably ensued. Britain's reaction to Germany's invasion of Belgium was finally to declare war. World peace was shattered.

The anger of these young men was understandable; their land had been occupied for centuries by the Ottoman Empire and then replaced by a further occupation, the Austro-Hungarian Empire, a decision made by the Great Powers of Europe who had no interest or knowledge of the people of Bosnia. Why are we surprised that now on every continent young men and increasingly young women are reacting like Gavrilo Princip and his compatriots?

Do we never learn from history?

One evening whilst having supper in Smajkič's flat with his wife and a friend, he told me about a conference on Primary Care that he was helping to organise the following year (1981) with a small number of international participants. He invited me to be one of the speakers and to attend at the expense of the Yugoslav government. I decided not to accept his generous offer, basically because I had no time – the Arab world was now beckoning. Smajkič came to Wells instead. Unexpectedly this was to be my last contact with him and Yugoslavia; we corresponded intermittently but to my great regret I never discovered whether Arif, his wife and their friend, survived the siege of Sarajevo.

10

UNION of SOVIET SOCIALIST REPUBLICS

The Soviet Union. What would I find in this huge, fascinating and puzzling country which straddles all Asia and half Europe and covers ten time zones? At the time of my first visit in 1971 I had no thought of writing *People, Politics & Health*, but looking back now it is clear that medicine and politics were equal partners.

It was a time-consuming and complicated project, certainly *labor improbus,* yet also a labour of love. Like many of my fellow countrymen Russia had long held a spell over me – its history, music, literature, and the position of the Orthodox Church provided the framework of this mysterious country from which I've never had any desire to break free.

Professor Gargov of the Postgraduate Institute in Sofia who had successfully arranged my visit to Bulgaria in 1968, wrote on 26 December 1968:

> '. . . As to your trip to the USSR I would recommend to you to write first to Dr M Akhmeteli at the Ministry of Health, Moscow, mentioning that I have given you his name. I hope he will arrange for you to stay there in the best possible way. . .'

I duly wrote on 14 January 1969 and received a reply dated 25 March, signed Z Iakashin. It transpired that Dr Akhmeteli no longer worked at the Ministry; moving or being moved from one post or institute or ministry to another was a notable feature of the Soviet health service.

My original enquiries had begun in 1966. I wrote quite out-of-the-blue to the Department of Foreign Relations at the Ministry of Health in Moscow on 26 July 1966 and received a reply dated 8 August signed V Makarov, written not surprisingly in Russian. I was able to get it translated quite quickly and responded ten days later. I received a reply – in English – dated 8 September:

> 'In reply to your kind letter of August 20th we wish to inform you that your visit to the Soviet Union can be arranged either through the company for foreign travel (Intourist), or by certain authority

of your country in accordance with the Anglo-Soviet Cultural Agreement of 1966/67.'

M Veprintsev.

Well, two letters written and two replies received between the end of July and the beginning of September was remarkable and really surprised me. Exactly *how* remarkable became very clear as it wasn't until 21 September 1971, five years later, that I finally set foot on Russian soil.

Over a period of about three and a half years I had been in correspondence with five separate Russian colleagues without any progress being made; it was time to get off this bureaucratic roundabout – action was needed. To be involved with the Intourist company was pointless. First of all I was not a tourist; second, I didn't want to be restricted to Moscow and Leningrad (the only places foreigners were allowed to visit at that time); third, a programme for tourists would concentrate on the most prestigious medical institutions and hospitals, certainly nothing remotely connected with primary care.

The Anglo-Soviet Cultural and Scientific Agreement appeared to be the only possibility. In fact I had already been in contact with the Foreign and Commonwealth Office (FCO) in April '69. They had directed me to the British Council who explained that a small number of exchange visits were catered for in the Agreement, but only for academic and research work; that counted me out.

Mercifully a 'facultative' clause in the Agreement allowed some leeway and requests could be made for help in arranging a programme of study provided it had been accepted. I would be responsible both financially and also for organising travel within the Soviet Union. This was a formidable task as Aeroflot would only consider booking any flights if I had a visa, and the Soviet Embassy would not consider a visa application until three months before the visit. Only later did I discover that the visa department at the Embassy had no authority to issue a visa – all they could do was send my passport to Moscow for action. I must mention *en passant* that the Embassy was expensively furnished inside and was situated in one of the most pricey areas of London – Kensington Palace Gardens, surrounded by millionaires.

The British Council couldn't have been more helpful. They

contacted Mr T Garrett, the Scientific Counsellor at our embassy in Moscow, with my request under the Cultural Agreement along with the official letter from Dr Simonyan in Moscow, who had finally agreed to the visit.

After approaching Dr Simonyan, Terry Garrett wrote triumphantly to say I had been accepted under Article VII (3) and in addition Dr Simonyan had agreed to arrange accommodation as she had pointed out that accommodation directly arranged by a westerner would be extremely expensive, certainly five times more than a tourist from the Eastern Bloc. Furthermore an interpreter and a driver would be provided when needed without cost. I was surprised, as was Terry Garrett, about the interpreter, as the Russians didn't like individual travellers for the reason that all foreigners had to be 'supervised' and it was more cost-effective for an interpreter/guide to accompany a group. Both of us had expected the interpreter to have been quite an expense for me.

There can be no doubt that without the interest and determination on my behalf of Miss E M Ball, the Regional Officer for the USSR and East Europe at the Council, and Terry Garrett at the Embassy, my visit would never have taken place, or would have ended up a complete waste of time and money.

But one potentially serious problem remained outstanding; the Soviets had agreed in principle to arrange a programme, but not until my arrival. My instinct was to arrange as much as possible before leaving the UK and this was reinforced by Laurens van der Post in chapter one of his book *Journey into Russia* which describes his solo travels in the early 1960s. Seeking advice from friends and diplomats in London who were familiar with the Soviet Union, one emphatically declared:

> 'Once you've agree to a date and a travel plan with the Russians they won't vary it by a yard or a second. Take my tip and ask for all you want now.'

And so I did. I tried my luck, having already been warned by the FCO and the British Council that it was difficult, particularly as an individual, to travel widely, and to my surprise it was agreed that my study of primary care would include Moscow, Tashkent (Uzbekistan), Yerevan (Armenia), Tbilisi (Georgia), Odessa and Kiev (Ukraine). In visiting these different parts of the USSR I was hoping I might be able to assess how uniform or otherwise the Soviet Health Service would turn out to be and how they managed to plan and provide on such an enormous scale. In addition I wanted to see as much of the country as possible; would it be depressingly uniform with soulless grey concrete tower blocks, occasional views of the faded grandeur of past centuries, and the majority of people drably clad and glumly queuing up for food or soap or lavatory paper or whatever?

I had also decided to indulge myself; I would take three days off to visit the ancient cities of Bukhara and Samarkand (all anyway relatively close to Tashkent) and become an unashamed tourist. Primary care could be put on the back burner.

In my ignorance, my thoughts on the USSR were only superficially correct – I had failed to take on board how the many individual languages, the many and varied cultures, customs, traditions and religious beliefs were not only present in the separate Republics but within the Republics themselves. This produced a wonderful diversity of cuisine and fragrant aromas, an interesting mix of ethnic Russians and local folk and an explosion of rainbow colours in everyday dress.

A few months before departure I received a small pamphlet *Security Advice about Visits to Communist Countries.* I forget whether it came from the FCO or the British Council. It was a rather scary and explicit document:

> '. . . No one, however, can automatically assume that he is immune from attention . . . a visitor may still attract attention from the moment he enters the country. Reports may be obtained from nearly every person with whom he has dealings including his business contacts, the tourist guide, the maid in the hotel, the railway conductor, the bar-tender, and any apparent acquaintances he may make . . . they may be trailed before him so that their meetings appear to be entirely fortuitous . . . In the main hotels all the telephones can be tapped, and in a large number of rooms visual or photographic surveillance of the occupants can be carried out. Infra-red cameras enable photographs to be taken in the dark. In restaurants tables can be fitted with microphones connected to a central listening point where conversations are recorded. Portable miniature microphones are built into ashtrays etc and can be used on tables, in cars or at open-air meetings! Visitors are

most likely to get into trouble in one of four ways. First they may be invited to take part in some unofficial financial transaction . . . Second they may be approached by a local inhabitant and asked to take a letter or present out of the country . . . or to take messages into a communist country . . . can lead to imprisonment. Third there are dangers in taking photographs and finally irregularity of personal behaviour . . . drinking too much . . compromised sexually with a local girl . . . A homosexual affair carries the same risks . . . but to an enhanced degree. Local homosexuals are deliberately trailed before visitors who are thought to be homosexual . . .'

It is interesting there was no mention of women visitors and what awaited them, which seemed to imply that women just didn't visit the communist world on their own at that time. The only mention of women is as an enticement to men.

I set off for Moscow on 20 September via Budapest for an overnight stay at the Rados, partly to renew our friendship and partly to catch up on any changes in primary care. The next day, on a half-empty, very noisy Aeroflot flight to Moscow I sat between two Albanians. They had recently arrived on a Malev flight from Tirana along with fifteen compatriots, all part of the same group en route to China. The Sino-Soviet split at this time was occasionally mentioned in the West and Mao Tse-tung's endeavours to woo three countries in Eastern Europe – successfully in terms of Albania and Romania. Yugoslavia however had resisted and remained in the Non-Aligned group of nations, thus rebuffing the overtures of both China and the Soviet Union.

Both my companions spoke some English and almost the entire journey was filled by their explaining their mistrust of the Soviet Union and their confident friendship with China. They were a group of engineers who were to spend nine months in Peking for further training. This distrust became evident when they told me not one of them would willingly leave the airport.

"Why not?"
"We will be arrested."

As I left the aircraft I turned and waved; none of the Albanians had moved from their seats. Presumably they caught their flight to Peking without mishap.

It was late in the evening at Sheremetyevo airport and too late for airport buses to be running. After an hour's wait I shared a taxi with a couple of equally impatient fellow travellers. As we approached the National Hotel to drop them off it was possible to get a brief glimpse of the floodlit Kremlin, breathtaking with its golden domes, towers, spires and fortressed walls. We then drove through empty streets to another hotel for foreigners – the Ukraina, a thirty-storey building with a spire reaching a height of 558 feet and boasting 1000 bedrooms: a perfect example of Stalinist architecture and one of his famous 'wedding cake' buildings. Of course I had no roubles to pay for the taxi as it was forbidden to bring Russian currency into the country and the exchange bank at the airport had been closed. Confusion and delay plus an angry taxi driver were inevitable as the reception staff seemed eager not to help, but finally around 2.30am I opened the door to my room after getting the key from one of the grimmest *dezhurnayas* (floor manager) imaginable.

In the morning I found the restaurant without difficulty. It was truly enormous and ninety percent empty. Groups of waitresses in traditional pre-war style clothing were standing around talking to each other and seemingly indifferent to the few of us who wanted breakfast. After ten minutes or so a feeling of paranoia began to surface. Why was I being ignored whilst most of the other guests had been served? I walked over to the nearest group of waitresses to point out where I was sitting; they simply shrugged their shoulders and continued chatting to each other. As I was returning to my table a friendly group of Scandinavians beckoned me over to explain that I was sitting in the wrong area of the restaurant and would never get served. They suggested I sat near them and almost immediately a waitress arrived. Such deliberately unhelpful bloody-mindedness could only flourish in a country where unemployment was not allowed.

More followed. Immediately after breakfast I went to the reception desk where I found a woman who understood and spoke English. I explained I wanted to cash some travellers cheques.

"Impossible."
"Why?"
"Because the exchange bureau is closed till midday."

Her response to further enquiries was a non-committal nod and raised eyebrows. I demanded to see the hotel manager who eventually asked a receptionist to phone the bureau and it was opened.

The next evening I had been invited by Terry Garrett and his wife for dinner at their flat. I had to be there by 8pm and as it was on the other side of Moscow and I had no idea how long the Metro would take, I endeavoured to organise a taxi. It was now about 5.30pm.

"Could you please book a taxi for me."
"It may be difficult."

This was the reply from the reception desk and so it proved to be. By 6.30pm I had been back to reception three times and still a shake of the head and:

"Yes, it is very difficult."

I was genuinely mystified and quite by chance a hotel doorman heard my increasingly anxious enquiries and beckoned me over. To my surprise he spoke English:

"Why do you want to book a taxi? All you need do is stand on the street outside the hotel and hail one down."

I thanked him profusely, gave him some roubles and asked why the reception staff hadn't told me the same.

"Because you didn't ask *them* - you asked them to phone for a taxi."

I was beginning to understand what top-class bureaucracy really meant and that I would need to get to grips with the extraordinary and very unfamiliar mindset of officials and bureaucrats. On the other hand I met many individuals who were just as helpful as the doorman.

As I was taking off my coat in the Garrett's flat he asked if I had heard about the recent extraordinary events in London, to which I replied I hadn't.

A couple of days before, I think it was 21 September, the Foreign Secretary Sir Alec Douglas-Home, had expelled over a hundred Soviet diplomats from their Embassy. This was unprecedented and apparently a complete surprise to the British Embassy in Moscow. Terry Garrett and his guests were anxious about the likely Russian response and what tit-for-tat reprisals there might be. He thought I wouldn't be affected personally and he was right. None of my guides/ interpreters questioned me or asked my views and nor was it mentioned by anyone.

During the evening my fellow guests – the Swiss Chargé d'Affaires and his wife, an English businessman and his German wife, a Canadian diplomat and his wife, and an American physician doing research at one of the Cancer Institutes in Moscow – all told me how exceptionally fortunate I had been to be allowed to travel so extensively, particularly on my own. All of them had found travelling round the Soviet Union well nigh impossible and every obstacle had been put in their way. It was difficult enough to get to Leningrad or Kiev or even forty miles out of Moscow. They were truly jealous!

I had been hoping to meet Dr Simonyan, but yet again a change of personnel: Dr Eristavis was now Head of Protocol. He was sitting behind a large desk in a large room with heavy dark furniture and heavy dark curtains. At right-angles to the desk was a long table with chairs ranged along both sides and along the walls black leather armchairs and small settees. Ashtrays were everywhere. Behind Eristavis was a large portrait of Lenin surrounded on both sides by Eristavis's numerous titles, awards and diplomas. Presumably the size of the room and the desk indicated the importance of the occupant.

In fact Eristavis was a mild man despite his steely eyes and penetrating stare; he chain-smoked throughout the interview. On the desk directly in front of him was thick file marked W J STEPHEN in English. He thumbed through it asking questions about my professional life, about my close family, my parents and in-laws, noting they had been to university. He wanted to know how long I had served in the army and was particularly interested to know I had served in West Germany, close to the East German border. Why was I interested in the Soviet Union? His questioning was thorough but never aggressive.

My programme was confirmed in general terms and Eristavis explained I would have to negotiate locally what I wanted to see and discuss. He assured me he had explained to those concerned that the purpose of my visit was primary not secondary care, and already he had decided that paediatrics was to be the topic in Moscow, and which facilities were to be visited; there was certainly no room for negotiation.

*

The Paediatric Research Institute attached to the Soviet Academy of Science was as far away from primary care as you could get. Both Professor Nosov and Dr Shtyahtina were understandably proud of what they were showing me and the standard of academic research. In addition, a forty-six-bed tertiary care hospital and a specialist consultation polyclinic were attached to the Institute, both providing care for children, who would have been referred from all parts of the Soviet Union. Nosov and Shtyahtina were confident about comparisons with the United States and Western Europe and emphasised that similar Institutes could be found in the other fourteen Republics – I was later to visit one in Tashkent.

I wondered if Eristavis was saying one thing to my face – yes, primary care was my objective – but that the programme of visits wouldn't reflect this. I hoped not. Anyway I was being naive to think that in a country like the Soviet Union officials wouldn't feel duty bound to show off what they considered 'the best'. But if this were to be the case my visit would be a complete waste of time and money.

I hoped my anxiety didn't show, especially as Nosov and Shtyahtina couldn't have been more helpful in answering my queries about the paediatric service. I was asked to sign the visitors book and noticed that two days before was the signature of Madame Pompidou who was accompanying the French President on a state visit. Naturally, high-ranking dignitaries would be shown the most prestigious facilities and would respond with praise. Although I signed the book, to write an honest comment about primary care proved rather difficult!

Paediatric polyclinic 50 in industrial Kuhstevske, one of 160 such clinics in Moscow, was in an affluent area of the city. Again it was a high-quality facility perfectly safe to show to foreigners. One thing stood out: thirty-one doctors and three dentists staffed the polyclinic and were responsible for the care of between twelve and thirteen thousand children up to the age of fifteen years. In the UK the ratio would be four to five doctors for a population of that size.

As Vnukova airport disappeared beneath us it was announced that the flight time to Samarkand was about four and a half hours – yet we would only be a third of the way across the country.

Samarkand has held a romantic grip over many British people, largely due to travellers, scholars, archeologists, historians and diplomats working and living in Mesopotamia, Persia and parts of Central Asia. In addition, for hundreds of years traders had told their tales of adventures along the famous Silk Road between China and the West. James Elroy Flecker, a student of oriental languages, who after graduating entered the consular service first in Constantinople and then Beirut, died in 1915 at the early age of thirty-one, but not before writing *The Golden Journey to Samarkand*, his most famous work, which stirred the imaginations of several generations.

The Ilyushin Il-18 four-engined turbo-prop provided a noisy, vibrating but comfortable journey in what can only be described as wooden armchairs. I was woken for an unexpected breakfast of caviar and grilled meat as we flew over Baku and the Caspian Sea with its vast oil fields flickering below. Only half a dozen passengers disembarked at Samarkand and the plane almost immediately took off again for Tashkent.

It was 4.30am (6.30am Samarkand time) with nobody about. The airport building was single storey like a small bus station, with a large stone statue of Lenin and a small wooden notice board announcing Samarkand. There was no trouble with passport or customs and the officials even smiled. Neither was there any wait for a shared taxi into the centre of town where I was dropped off at the Intourist Hotel, the only one for foreigners.

Sometimes one can be disappointed by unrealistic expectations. Not so with Samarkand – neither its history, its architecture nor its people, and above all its colour, disappointed. Little remains of the earliest city. Legends abound and nobody knows its exact origins, but it is known that as far back as before Christ, the Greeks and Romans destroyed a good deal, and much later Genghis Khan renewed the destruction in the 13th century. However, another Mongol ruler, Tamerlane, started to rebuild the old part of the present city towards the end of the 14th century, which Ulugh-Beg, his son, continued.

As a conscientious tourist I set forth and slowly made my way through the unexpected gardens, tree-lined cobbled streets and unmade dirt tracks. The population was roughly fifty percent Russian and the rest a mix of Uzbeks and neighbouring Asiatic Republics.

Judging from the hotel most visitors were from the Eastern Bloc with an occasional American, Australian and West European. The locals favoured national dress, the men in turbans, lightly coloured *khalats* (originally ceremonial robes), baggy trousers and felted boots. The women also wore traditional costume – long, brightly-coloured silk dresses with scarves over their heads (some were completely veiled). The children were beautiful, with black eyes, black hair and enchanting smiles, and even though the temperature was 80°C in the mid-afternoon the babies wore woollen hats and leggings. Girls wore pretty frocks and many boys wore *tyubeteikas* (the traditional Uzbec headgear – an embroidered skull cap).

In the bazaars and narrow alleyways of the old town few Russians seemed to venture. Every fifty yards or so chestnut and plane trees shaded *chaikhanas* or tea houses occupied by middle-aged and elderly men lying on mattresses, talking, always smoking and playing chess or draughts. I don't recall seeing any women. I spoke no Russian or Uzbek and they spoke no English, but occasionally they managed a little German, and as soon as I sat down I would be surrounded as they attempted to talk to me; they would nod happily at my replies while I would smile at them. Utterly bizarre but somehow reassuring, and the hot sweet tea they insisted I drank was most welcome.

So much to see. Probably the most spectacular and impressive sight was Shah-i Zinda (Street of Tombs) along a half-hidden passageway with ascending steps to thirteen mausoleums and a mosque all dedicated to Tamerlane's family. They stretched ahead for about two hundred yards, all arranged in a haphazard way. The wealth of colour – tiles of green, white, purple and red along with the richness of Islamic decoration and the brilliant blue domes – was just breathtaking. Shah-i Zinda remains one of the holiest places in Islam, a place of homage and prayer. If you're unable to make the *Hajj* to Mecca, then some Muslims maintain that two hajjs to Shah-i Zinda would be a fitting alternative. I believe there are one or two other holy places which fulfil the same function.

The Gur-Emir Mausoleum, a building of stunning beauty, contains the bodies of Tamerlane, his two sons, and Ulugh-Beg his grandson: a dynasty. Tamerlane's tomb of dark green jade is quite separate and inscribed with the words:

'When I rise from the dead, the world will tremble.
He who opens the tomb will bring to his country
an invader even more terrible than I.'

Professor Gerasinov, a famous archeologist, anthropologist and sculptor opened the tomb in order to create the face of the great conqueror from his actual skull. Most of Gerasinov's generation (and today's for that matter) considered the ways of Islam to be ignorant and full of superstition, hence no thought was given to the inscription. But on that day in June 1941 came the news that the Soviet Union had been invaded by Nazi Germany.

The mausoleum itself has a magnificent ribbed dome of bright turquoise and tiles of many colours, which contributes to its great richness. On beholding it you are simply stopped in your tracks – small wonder it is the image most frequently used by the Soviet authorities and travel brochures to publicise Samarkand.

Having no map I just wandered around, suddenly coming upon another of Samarkand's most magnificent sights – its vast central square, the Registan. Three great *medrasas* – Islamic colleges for higher education and Islamic study – enclosed three sides of the square, the courtyards within each *medrasa* exhibiting near perfect symmetry – truly remarkable composition. In the centre of the Registan was a large flower bed fitted out with that most English of flowers, the rose. The colours were stunning, of every conceivable shade. How could this flower survive the summer heat of Central Asia when it had recently contributed to the granite city of Aberdeen, famous for its cold northerly winds and haars, being awarded the coveted title 'City of Flowers UK'? The wonders of nature.

There was much more of historical interest to be seen but time was against me. And, although I was on holiday from primary care, I had deliberately meandered around some of the poorer areas where to my surprise the foul smell of human excrement rising from the drains was almost absent, and there was little evidence of rat-infested rubbish lying in the streets. Presumably the public health service must have been functioning even 2500 miles from Moscow.

Even though the traditional Soviet-style flats and buildings along tarmacked roads now surrounded the old city, and drably-dressed Russians glumly going about their daily life had affected the overall feel of the place, Samarkand was unforgettable. The old quarter readily made up for the modernisation and I was pleased to have been on my own without an Intourist guide telling me what she thought I should hear. My lasting memory would be the explosion of colour against a clear blue sky.

Bukhara, about 140 miles west of Samarkand, is surrounded to the north by the vast sandy, rocky desert of Kyzyl-Kum and to the west by the equally vast desert of Kara-Kum. The Zeravshan river runs between Samarkand and Bukhara, eventually reaching the river Amu Darya which finally flows into the Aral Sea, a 1500-mile journey from the Pamir mountains in Tadzhikistan. As we left Samarkand it was easy to see the Zeravshan about five mile away with irrigation canals leaving the river.

The flight was in a small propeller-driven bi-plane – Biggles would happily have been the pilot! The journey took about an hour and a half and as we flew low it was easy to see the effects of irrigation – a large green belt on both sides of the river stretching five to ten miles into the desert. The irrigation had been accomplished by reversing the flow of both the Amu Darya and the Zeravshan and had been done to increase the production of cotton.

Few in the Soviet Union appeared to have anticipated the environmental disaster that would ensue, and few in the West were aware of what was happening. By 2015 the Aral Sea has almost disappeared with most of the agriculture and all the fishing in the area lost. The lives of well over thirty million people in the region are estimated to have been affected by this catastrophe. The obsession with cotton started with Stalin, continued with his successors and has never been explained. Since the collapse of the USSR it has become clear that local people and some scientists tried in vain to warn the authorities. During my brief stay in Bukhara and Samarkand, and later in Tashkent, I was informed on a number of occasions about the progress and success in increasing cotton production; this was not surprising because it would take the fall of the Berlin Wall before the truth came out.

The Syr Darya rises from two headwaters in the Tien Shan mountains of eastern Uzbekistan and flows some 1400 miles north past Tashkent into the Aral Sea; its flow too had been reversed.

Bukhara airport was very small with no tarmac, just grass, so it was even more rustic than Samarkand, but had the same obligatory statue of Lenin. Again no problem with customs or passports and again – smiles. I told myself not to expect this to become routine. Eight passengers were on board and we shared two taxis into the centre of town. Along with a Canadian couple I was dropped off at the only Intourist Hotel, the other passengers being local Uzbeks. Breakfast was brought at great speed and I decided to take a short Intourist tour of the old town. Again no maps, so I hoped I might get some idea of the layout of the place. The guide was a young married teacher with a six-month-old baby. He was keen to tell me he had five brothers and sisters and was genuinely surprised and quite impressed to learn I had four children myself.

The origins of Bukhara are shrouded in mystery and it was not until after the death of Muhammad in 632 AD that there was broad agreement as to its beginnings. First it was conquered by the Arabs, then attacked by the Turks, fell under the influence of Persia and was finally occupied by the Mongols. At the height of its power in the 16th century the population was about 450,000 – London at the time roughly 150,000 – with four hundred or more *medrases* and mosques. Under Uzbek rule it became known as Bukhara the Holy and was the core of Islamic culture in Central Asia. Bukhara and Samarkand have always been rivals, and very much later during the Russian Revolution after the First World War, Bukhara became one of the centres of refuge for anti-Bolshevik forces and was renamed Bukhara the Bold by the followers of the Tsar.

After the initial guided introduction by the Intourist school teacher I decided to proceed on my own. From everyone I had spoken to and books I had glanced at I was well aware that it was going to be difficult without a guide or a map. The narrow winding alleyways and streets and the higgledy-piggledy richness of the old town would mean many hidden treasures would remain unseen.

I had been left in the centre of town at the thousand-year-old Citadel which dominated the square. Part of the original massive forty-foot-high crenellated defence wall that used to surround the city still remains, but it is now crumbling away leaving large gaps although the crenellated battlements remain intact in places. Amazingly, individual original mud bricks of varying shades of brown, red and grey were easy to see. I now understand what people mean when they say that Samarkand is green and Bukhara brown.

I embarked on the maze of criss-cross lanes lined with flat-roofed, single-storey, sun-baked mud brick dwellings, a few white-washed, the majority dusty brown with high windowless walls. Again vaguely thinking about the Soviet Health Service, I was amazed to find that most homes had piped water or if not, had easy access to the frequent street pumps. By chance I came across one of the infamous small ponds or reservoirs (*khanz*) which used to supply the town with water. A canal (*Shakhrud*) brought the water from the Zeravshan river and it ran through the entire town in narrow water gutters (*Aryks*) supplying about a hundred *khanz*. Not surprisingly they provided a perfect supply of stagnant polluted water so that over the centuries Bukhara gained a reputation for poor health and frequent widespread epidemics of every kind. Whatever we may think of the Soviets, one of the first things they did for Bukhara, the stronghold of the Tsarist cause, was, in 1924 at the end of the Revolution, to supply its citizens with clean drinking water.

As in Samarkand, *chaikhana* were everywhere but I had no need of one; close to a *khanz*, one of three which had been carefully preserved and used for recreation, a park had been built and was full of people of all ages, mostly sitting on white-painted, wooden double-beds covered with carpets and mats; on small wooden tables food was piled. Eventually I plucked up courage and sat down with five Uzbeks who insisted I ate and drank with them – soup and kebabs, which had been cooked on a nearby communal brazier. We communicated somehow, ate the food and drank vodka for an hour and a half. On departing we toasted eternal friendship, smiled and shook hands.

Again as in Samarkand, a profusion of fruits and vegetables, particularly water melons, lined the streets; I should think the majority of the population had better food than in many western parts of the Soviet Union, despite poorer wages.

How much of this historic city did I manage to see on my 'American-style' visit and was it different from Samarkand? Yes, it was, mainly due to the Old Town being more compact and the bazaars still in use. They operated through a system of roofed streets with small cupolas marking the crossing points. Of the original five only three remained, the Dome of the Shroffs (money lenders and dealers), the Dome of the Milliners and the Dome of the Jewellers. I only ventured into the Milliners bazaar, described by one of the traders as the Dome of Hats and Cap Sellers.

By the end of the day I was satisfied with my efforts, which numbered: the Karakul Gate, one of the few gateways still standing in the city wall; the Mausoleum of the Samanids; the Minaret-Kalyan 145 foot high and impossible to miss; and the Mausoleum of Chashina-Ayub, also known as Job's Spring as it was built, so legend has it, on the site of healing water emerging from the desert when Job struck the ground with his staff. Other *medrasas* and mosques brought my whirlwind tour to an end.

The evening remained warm; one final wander and I came across a long, noisy, colourful procession with seemingly hundreds of flaming torches, two horns between ten and fifteen feet in length, and an instrument that sounded to my western ears like a badly played bagpipe. The procession, which took over half an hour to pass, was a wedding march leading the bridegroom to his bride. I'm ashamed to say I couldn't spot the groom and was unable to decide whether it was a Jewish, Islamic or Persian ceremony - maybe a mix of all three, or perhaps simply a local custom.

Tashkent, like Samarkand and Bukhara, is an oasis town which in 1930 became the capital of the Republic of Uzbekistan, taking over from Samarkand. My knowledge of Tashkent was limited to the severe earthquake in 1966 in which many thousands were killed and enormous damage done, Tashkent being at its centre. At the time the Russians remained silent and it was some days before the disaster was admitted – but its severity was denied.

At my first meeting at the Paediatric Research Institute my heart sank, but in fact it proved to be more down-to-earth and useful than the Institute in Moscow. Both Professor Kodyrova working at the Ministry of Health, and Professor Muhamedov a local paediatrician, were relaxed and well-informed regarding my questions, and three hours soon passed. My programme for the rest of my stay was then divulged: visits to the Medical Training School for Nurses; the General and Paediatric Hospital No. 2 which had finally been repaired and rebuilt following the earthquake; and Paediatric Polyclinic No. 14.

The Paediatric Polyclinic 14 had been recently rebuilt on the outskirts of new Tashkent, which was an extension of the more affluent Russian part of the city, as opposed to the old town composed mainly of Uzbeks.

A general feeling of cheerfulness pervaded the place, added to by the colourful decor and paintings done by the children. The polyclinic lay within the grounds of Paediatric Hospital 5 and I was interested to note that other polyclinics within the area were also supervised by the same hospital. Polyclinic 14 covered a *rayon* (local area) divided into eighteen *uchastoks* (districts) and was responsible for about 16,000 children. Operationally the doctors and nurses from the eighteen *uchastoks* provided the service; home visits were considered essential and carried out by both doctors and nurses. ECG and simple x-ray equipment were in situ but all pathological/laboratory work was carried out in the hospital. The physiotherapy department was a surprise – every possible bit of equipment both essential and unnecessary had been installed.

The General and Paediatric Hospital 2 took referrals from all over the country and was clearly a prestigious place. I trailed around all the departments trying to look impressed but all the time resenting what I felt was really a waste of time. However, during the discussions at the end of the visit I learned something of importance and great interest; the senior paediatrician let slip the fact that the *uchastok* paediatricians working in polyclinics were not sufficiently trained to take on much clinical responsibility, most of their time being spent on routine developmental examinations, health education for the mothers and the dispenserisation scheme. Treatment was only provided for minor illnesses, the rest being referred directly to hospital. A child under two years with a fever that had not responded to treatment within twenty-four hours ended up in hospital, although in reality it was sooner than that. Any clinical problem not immediately diagnosed was also immediately referred. Inevitably this led to a very high admission rate and the need for more beds; the bed ratio to population was higher than in any western country.

The senior paediatrician was by now becoming irritated with my questions and her answers became increasingly obscurantist and aggressively defensive. I wondered if perhaps this was the first time she had been really challenged or made to think about how she and her colleagues worked and how their services were run.

The Medical School for Nurses also included the education and training of physiotherapists, occupational therapists, radiographers, speech therapists and *feldschers*. The training of general and paediatric nurses was separate, thus anticipating the UK by more than twenty years. The majority of personnel in training in the Medical School were female.

Rachel and I had decided I would send a telegram (which proved to be difficult) when I reached Tashkent, which would be as far east as I was going. Being slightly disconcerted by the pamphlet *Security Advice about Visits to Communist Countries,* we decided our telegram would be such that even the smartest KGB Intelligence officer would not be able to decode it in the unlikely event I was being watched and followed. We resorted to a common acronym seen every day on a patient's notes – BOR meaning bowels open regularly. To Rachel's amusement the cable BORWJS arrived safely in Wells on 27 September. Unfortunately it wasn't true.

In the centre of Tashkent I came across a wonderful camping/boy scouts type of shop where I bought a dozen steel *shashlik* (skewers) – six were 27 inches long and six were 23 – yet I was able to openly carry them around tied up in binder twine. Whether I was in a train, bus or on a plane, on the streets or at Moscow's Sheremetyevo International Airport and even at London's Heathrow, nobody ever questioned me. At the time international tensions were running high and the Cold War was very much alive; today in any part of the world arrest and probable imprisonment would certainly be the result. How times have changed.

'It's a small world' is a well-used cliché but that doesn't mean it's over-used or isn't true. As I entered the rather small, very crowded, very hot, unpleasantly smelly and uncomfortable departure lounge restricted to foreigners at Tashkent airport, I struggled to find somewhere to sit and ended up next to the Military Attaché and his wife with whom I had enjoyed dinner in Terry Garrett's flat in Moscow (the Attaché commented on the skewers!). They were in transit to Kabul and had already been waiting two hours – not a happy situation with two small children and they were having difficulty even finding drinking water. Less than an hour later I was on my way to board the plane to Armenia whilst they continued to wait, goodness knows for how long. They must have thought I had all the luck – not only allowed to travel around independently but not even having to wait for my plane.

The flight to Yerevan was quite extraordinary. It was routine on all internal flights for the Aeroflot personnel to sort out the foreigners and get them on the plane first – pretty aggravating I would have thought for domestic travellers. I was the only foreigner so I quickly boarded and sat down with a sigh of relief, putting my hands on the mahogany arm rests to ease myself into position. As a sort of reflex I raised my arms only to find both arm rests came away from the seat. Embarrassed, I quickly fitted them back as quickly as possible hoping the cabin staff hadn't noticed.

By this time the locals were striving to get on board, a stream of brightly-clad Uzbeks of all ages struggling with their luggage – hardly a case to be seen but every conceivable type of holdall, plastic bag and sacking all tied up with string or straps and impossible to fit into the overhead lockers. It was spread into the aisles, where there was standing room only for about a dozen without booked seats. The pièce de résistance were the animals – chickens and ducks and rabbits in metal containers along with three dogs and two goats. It was more crowded than any bus or train I'd ever been on. About halfway through the journey, the final surprise: two stoves looking like primus stoves were lit at the rear of the plane in a circular area of the central aisle, to the total unconcern of the flight attendants. My general impression was that the children didn't seem to whine or grumble. They just wandered up and down the aisles whilst the babies were happy at their mother's breast. Any noise came mostly from the animals. The smell from the cooking started to make me feel hungry.

We didn't seem to reach any great height and visibility was excellent as we flew west for about 800 miles. The ground below was mainly desert, first reddish then mainly black, the surface curiously pitted. On the left there were always mountains in the distance with an occasional river, small lakes and oases. This continuous range of mountains separated the Soviet Union from Afghanistan, Iran and Turkey. Flying over the Caspian Sea I glimpsed again oil rigs extending out from Baku and along the coastline as far the eye could see. As we continued west, the Caspian Sea was left behind and immediately the Caucasus mountains appeared to our right before we came in to land at Yerevan.

The Republic of Armenia is known in the West for a number of reasons. One is the series of massacres by the Turks, the first in 1890 and the second in 1915 when at least a million Armenians died. Gladstone is remembered in these parts just as he is in Bulgaria for his outspoken opposition to the Ottoman Empire at the time of the 1890 massacre. Debate continues to this day as to whether the description 'genocide' is appropriate or not.

The next reason is that Armenia along with Georgia was the first of two nations to embrace Christianity; Armenia in 301 AD, ahead of Emperor Constantine's *Declaration of Christianity* in York in 306 AD, so the monument in York tells us, and Georgia's conversion in 330 AD.

I was met at the airport not by an Intourist official but by Dr Stefan Dilamion, a gynaecologist temporarily attached to the Ministry of Health. He spoke and understood English and was involved in the International Relations Department. Interestingly he had no say in his transfer from clinical to administrative work and was angry that he couldn't continue his clinical work. A fat jolly fellow, he was married with two children. He explained that he intended to give me an introduction into the rural health service if I agreed, which of course I did. We dropped off my luggage at the Intourist Hotel Ani, picked up two colleagues and off we went, no waiting around.

His plan was to combine work with showing me as much as possible of his beautiful country. As we drove east out of Yerevan the landscape was wild with bare rugged hills, flocks of sheep and herds of cows. The valley we were travelling along was fertile, and en route he pointed out a number of collective farms. Soon we reached Garni, about twenty-five miles from Yerevan, where the local collective farms had an attached medical centre and a small hospital. I was briefly introduced to Dr Kina Vardanian and we departed almost immediately, the doctor looking almost as confused as I was. I realised eventually we would be coming back later.

As we returned to the main road dramatic mountains came into view and suddenly we turned off onto a narrow road that took us up to a remote valley to see what was clearly one of the jewels in the crown of the tourist trade – Gheghard Monastery standing at the top of this wild valley surrounded by jagged cliffs: a desolate and dramatic spot. This remarkable and unique building had been carved into the mountain. The interior was lit only by candles and it was difficult to see much, but it was still a working church so we went across to talk to two priests in long black robes sporting splendid black beards.

Back then to Dr Vardanian and the medical centre and hospital. In reality the centre was just a room and whenever possible patients went directly to the hospital. Vardanian was single-handed and looked after the entire workforce of the collectives and their families, about 3,500. She took us over to the hospital, which had an out-patient area, thirty-five beds in three wards and a delivery room. The beds were for medical and midwifery work. All surgery, both emergency and routine, was taken to Yerevan. Around 130 to 140 babies were born there each year. Six nursing auxiliaries and six *feldschers* made up the nursing staff.

Although most patients were encouraged to get to the hospital, Vardanian stressed that home visits were done too, initially by the *feldschers*. Thus there were two stages to the provision of care in rural areas, the first being the responsibility of the *feldschers* or midwives and the second that of the doctors. Two ambulance cars were available for transporting patients or for the doctors' use.

All my questions and the subsequent discussions with Vardanian and several *feldschers* were relaxed, very different from Moscow and even Tashkent where the need to stick to the rules and regulations was paramount. Stefan Dilamion and his two colleagues also joined us and Moscow seemed a long way away.

The collective farm was on the edge of Garni, a large area surrounded by old buildings to keep the cattle in during the winter and to store whatever cereals had been grown. I could see small tractors and other farm machinery rusting away in various corners.

The workers lived in the neighbouring villages but Vardanian's home was on the road close to the hospital. It was a two-storey house, larger than the rest, and had a decent-sized garden with flowers, vegetables and fruit bushes. She was a keen gardener and we compared notes.

We left the hospital, crossed the road towards her house and climbed the concrete steps up to her front door – I hadn't realised she had invited us for a meal. This invitation and the wonderful welcome from all, including her family, was the only occasion I was asked into anyone's home during my travels in the Soviet Union. Frank Ošanéc told me that in over thirty years and many visits to the Soviet Union he had never had an invitation. I wondered at the time if Vardanian and the other health workers as well as Stefan and his colleagues might be questioned; in the '70s speaking to a foreigner, particularly from the West, could still give rise to difficulties.

Inside, two of Vardanian's three children had just come home from school and were eating in the kitchen. The main room was dark with heavy wooden furniture, dark curtains, rugs on the wood floor and a large table laden with food – traditional Armenian bread, meatballs wrapped in cabbage leaves, salad of all descriptions, tomatoes, peppers and goat and sheep cheese. The elderly grandmother in peasant clothes was in and out of the kitchen and very much part of the scene. Soon she was encouraging her grandchildren to tuck into the food and making sure the *feldschers* and nurses, whom she seemed to know well, were also enjoying themselves. Everyone was happy and soon the homemade brandy and vodka flowed. As we were leaving I noticed two religious icons and a carved wooden figure of Christ on the wall.

How much we don't know or understand.

Stefan had apologised to Vardanian about being late in returning to see the collective farm and the hospital; he explained we had been too long at Gheghard although actually it had been barely an hour and a half. In truth a whole day there wouldn't have been too long. Stefan wanted me to see another Armenian treasure, the restored remains of a Roman temple, later to become a fortress and finally one of the residences of the Armenian royal family which had suffered earthquake and endless fighting for over a thousand years. But the rush of twentieth century life was stamped on all of us and time was our enemy. Gheghard and Vardanian's wonderful hospitality had filled a perfect day for me, so a brief glance from the car was all I was able to see of the completed restoration high up on a spectacular promontory of rock. In fact I much preferred the food, drink and hospitality to any further sightseeing although I kept these thoughts to myself as we turned back along the Azat valley in the fast-fading autumn light.

Yerevan had five paediatric hospitals each with over two hundred beds and each with its own specialty – No. 2 cardiology, No. 5 allergy, respiratory diseases and ENT, which I was visiting. Having already been around paediatric hospitals in Tashkent I was hoping to concentrate on women's health or the Industrial Health Service, or at least get a more comprehensive understanding of how the polyclinics functioned. I needed to tackle Stefan about my future plans: certainly no more paediatrics.

In the discussion at the end of my visit to No. 5 where I had been shown around by Professor Astratsaturian, the Director, I began to see more clearly the strengths and weaknesses of the Soviet system, so the visit was proving to be more useful than anticipated even if women's health remained a mystery.

Astratsaturian strongly reinforced the views of Tashkent, that the work of *uchastok* paediatricians involved routine examinations, immunisations and health education whilst clinical work was restricted to first-aid and transferring sick children to hospital. My analysis concerning the limited care carried out by *uchastok* paediatricians was accepted, but Astratsaturian and his colleagues were less willing to agree that their education and training fell well short of what should be expected from general practitioners or paediatricians working at the coalface. Repeatedly I had to keep reminding myself that I was in the USSR to find out as much as I could and not to let discussions end up in fruitless argument. I had not been invited to give advice or to criticise.

Seventeen paediatric polyclinics, five directly attached to the five hospitals, all referred patients to whichever hospital they preferred, usually the nearest. In Yerevan 1500 paediatric beds for a population of 700,000, in Bristol 210 paediatric beds for a population of 430,000. This provides 1 bed for 466 patients in Yerevan and 1 bed for 1654 patients in Bristol. The facts speak for themselves. The cost implications were never mentioned and I believe were not even considered.

Another glorious day, cloudless sky, hot but not too hot. Stefan had agreed to concentrate on medical services for women. I thought he would be really enthusiastic as he was a gynaecologist and I was keyed up waiting for him. He never arrived. Instead an official from the Ministry of Health turned up who explained that Stefan had been told on arriving for work that he was to give up his arrangements for the day and go to a meeting fifty miles from Yerevan. I asked her to return to the Ministry and see if something connected with medical services for women could be arranged. She returned within the hour, the answer being '*Nyet*' (No). I was furious, particularly when I heard that the Ministry had made no attempt to organise anything connected with primary care; instead they would provide a car, and the official from the Ministry would act as my guide and take me to Etchmiadzin, the place where Christianity took root in Armenia. I thought it strange that in a communist country the first idea that came into the Ministry's head was a visit to the most religious place in the land. As we drove away from the hotel it occurred to me that the car and guide were being provided gratis so I might as well say *spahsseebah* (thank you) and enjoy myself.

The monastery of Etchmiadzin, commonly known as Holy Etchmiadzin, is only twenty miles south of Yerevan. Within its huge walls is the cathedral, the seat of the Katholikos (archbishop), leader of the Armenian Church worldwide. Historically the Church was independent of both Rome and the eastern Roman Empire of Byzantium and has remained so ever since. Three other church buildings complete the ecclesiastical complex, which is a perfect example of Armenian church architecture – a simple cross and a central dome, solid and unadorned, giving a sense of permanence and indestructibility, a sort of forerunner of European Romanesque. My guide, whom I'm certain had Christian beliefs, insisted I fully understood that this was the first time a circular dome had been constructed on a square base.

Even on such a short visit, or perhaps I only saw the best, Yerevan seemed wonderfully attractive. In the evenings there was plenty of noise coming from the restaurants and bars, but during the day the streets were quiet yet full of people, young and old, simply promenading – thoroughly civilised. It was known as 'rosy Yerevan' because many of its buildings were constructed from pink, sometimes reddish-yellow tufa, a type of porous rock. Wide avenues and streets, often tree-lined, large public squares and parks with fountains and small lakes, added to its charm. An hour or so before I had to get to the railway station I sat in the enormous Lenin Square, walked up through the parks and gardens and finally reached the hill at the top of the town. From here I had a magnificent clear view of the twin peaks of Mount Ararat directly south and close to the Armenian/Turkish border. Yerevan is about 3,500 feet above sea level and looks across to the highest peak of 16,900 feet. I could almost believe this was the traditional site of the final resting place of Noah's ark.

The train for Tbilisi left punctually at 7.20pm. As I stood on the platform, Mount Ararat seemed close in the warm evening light as did the mountain ranges to the north that separated Armenia and Georgia. I found the third-class sleeping compartment which I was sharing with two elderly peasant women and a young dental student and her boyfriend. I offered my bottom bunk to one of the old women and we were immediately friends for the journey, she even making up my bed for me. Stefan had alerted me to the custom of sharing food – everyone offers a bit of what they have and all is laid out. My contribution was bread, garlic sausage, cucumber and some ghastly white wine. It was all most enjoyable and certainly more companionable than any other train I've travelled on.

Another custom involved the women making up their beds first and changing into their night clothes whilst the boyfriend and I stood in the corridor; then the roles were reversed – except not quite as the women didn't stand in the corridor but lay on their beds. I slept in my trousers and took my shoes off.

The boyfriend turned out to be a medical student. He and his girlfriend both studied in Yerevan but lived in Tbilisi. I couldn't decide if they were Armenian or Georgian. The evening soon passed and just before bed the young man asked if I knew anything about Radio Armenia. I replied 'not much', but 'nothing' would have been the honest answer. He explained it was an imaginary mythical radio station that people in the Soviet Union as well as Armenia contributed to in the form of political jokes against the regime, trendy jokes and really crude *double entendres.* This explained why a number of allusions and comments made by Stefan had made no sense to me.

The train arrived in Tbilisi exactly on time at 8.20am. What differences would I notice between the Republics of Armenia and Georgia, lying next to each other in the dramatic mountainous beauty of the Caucasus? Both countries, at least superficially, had experienced similar histories with seemingly endless invasions and occupations by the Greeks, Romans, Mongols, Turks and Russians. Both countries were proud of their separate language and culture and that they were the first in the world to embrace Christianity.

As I was saying goodbye to my fellow travellers, all of us standing rather awkwardly in a little group, a striking-looking woman came up the platform and spoke to the students. To my great surprise she turned to me and introduced herself:

> "I am Tamara. I am to be your guide while you are here. I am at your disposal."

Instead of being grateful and pleased I was immediately on my guard. Perhaps she was a temptation sent by the authorities – I had been explicitly instructed by the Ministry of Health that on my arrival I must contact them and not the reverse. It is with some shame that I write this now because nothing could have been further from the truth. She was charming, vivacious and intelligent. I believe she was also a good interpreter although I have no way of proving this. She could and did become emotional but her behaviour was never provocative or suggestive. I wonder now if she wanted to defect and regarded me as a possible contact for her. Subsequently on 6 January 1974, the Feast of Epiphany in the West and Christmas Day in the Eastern Orthodox tradition, I received a Christmas card from her telling me she had left Tbilisi a year before, giving me her address in Moscow and asking me to write to her. This I did immediately, but sadly I never heard another word.

The Georgians were a noticeably good-looking race – dark olive skins and black hair. Pretty and lithesome young girls, middle-aged women with the hauteur of Parisians, and smartly-dressed elderly women competing with their hats could be seen promenading along the fashionable leafy Rust'avi Prospect between Lenin and Rust'avi Squares. The men were mostly handsome, of athletic build with prominent hawk-like noses. One thing was absolutely certain, fashion and style were the prerogative of the local Georgians and not the ethnic Russians.

Tamara took me to the Hotel Tbilisi, one of two Intourist hotels build by the Russians at the turn of the 20th century. It displayed an utterly delightful pre-revolutionary style and the interior didn't disappoint either, being a haven of old-world charm. As instructed I contacted the Ministry of Health. Tamara spoke to Professor Givi Jbaltvadze and arranged an immediate meeting. He was a charming man and showed no embarrassment or guilt that nothing had been arranged for that day. In fact he gave the impression that this sort of thing was routine in that part of the world. I had been told the Georgians were the Irish of the Caucasus, full of blarney and charm. I told Jbaltvadze it was most important for me to study the medical services for women – it was my priority, but could I be certain it was going to happen? As I was leaving, almost as an afterthought he told me that Tamara was to be available to me for the day and would collect me from the hotel later in the morning.

She was a little late, clearly flustered and had obviously been crying. It transpired that she had been visiting friends on account of a frightening dream she had had the night before; she was dying and surrounded by three icons and much else she couldn't or wouldn't describe. Her friends insisted she visit a church as soon as possible and light three candles.

> "I am not religious but I think my friends are right. Who knows, perhaps one day in the future I will start to believe in God again . . . I think."

By this time we were in the car and she asked if I objected to her going to the church first before anything else. To my surprise the church was Catholic, although as I understood it the Georgian Church was in communion with the Armenian and the Eastern Orthodox Churches but not the Catholic Church, and in Tbilisi itself they were a small minority. We arrived just as service had finished and quite a crowd were mingling and chatting outside including more young people than I would have expected. Inside I sat at the back while

Tamara lit three candles and placed them in different parts of the church, each time going through the same routine of kissing the wall and floor and repeatedly crossing herself: all in all about half an hour. Returning to the car in silence, once inside she immediately told me she was pleased she had come. She then asked me what I would like to do; on being told I'd like to see the sights of Tbilisi she asked the driver to take us to the cable car railway, after which we wouldn't need the car any more.

Tbilisi, lying along both sides of the fast-flowing Kura, is dominated by a number of hills, the most prominent being Mtatsmunda or Sacred Mountain, also known as David's Mountain standing about 2,500 feet above the town. We agreed this would be a good place to start. The views going up and down on the funicular showed the town to be surrounded by hills and vast areas of forest. On two occasions the cable cars passed almost within touching distance of two church towers and other buildings. Halfway up, St David's Monastery was easy to see nestling into the wooded hillside. At the summit a large park had been laid out and we had lunch just taking in the stunning views, Tamara identifying what she could.

What next? I explained that I didn't need her for the rest of the day – one half of me regretted this but I really wanted to wander around by myself, particularly through the old town of which I had had tantalising glimpses from the cable car.

The atmosphere of the old town was enchanting. Most churches were open and in use. The church of Meteki Virgin was the first one to catch my eye as it stands on the very edge of high rocky cliffs which form part of the bank of the Kura. Looking from the church across the river was a ruined Persian fortress at the top of Sololaki Hill. Just as the old town clings to the Sacred Mountain, so it is with Sololaki Hill, a labyrinth of steep cobbled streets and alleyways winding up to the forests and a jumble of small houses miraculously built into the steep slopes. I was able to watch two old men fishing in the Kura using very long rods, as in France, with live bait, mostly worms. I inspected their catch of only seven small fish, which wasn't surprising given the rapid rate at which the Kura was flowing. Like fishermen the world over they tried to explain why they had not been more successful. Needless to say I didn't understand a word but nodded and smiled sympathetically.

In the lower parts of the town the streets were wide enough for the sun to shine on the cobbles. The houses were mainly of sun-baked mud bricks, two storeys high with wooden balconies, and verandas with intricate metal railings and often a metal spiral stairway leading to the first floor. Washing hung everywhere, from every available hook or nail or post. Children were playing, the girls giggling and shouting, the boys with footballs. Climbing shrubs were everywhere – clematis, jasmine, bougainvillea, roses and honeysuckle, with willow herb and ragwort growing out of every dusty crack and crevice.

At the end of the day I returned on my own to Tamara's church and to my delight the baptism of a small boy was taking place. A large family group incorporating every generation was present and the service was being taken by the Bishop. The little boy's trousers had been rolled down so the sign of the Cross could be made on his forehead, chest and bottom in rapid succession. After the service I managed to buttonhole the Bishop and we had a stilted conversation in French and German. He was very pleased indeed to have his photo taken and asked me to send him a copy, which I did.

Early on the Sunday morning the sound of tolling bells woke me. I was intrigued. By ear rather than by eye I found the church quite near the hotel in a confusing maze of alleyways, which made me a little anxious in case I couldn't remember how to get back to the hotel where Tamara was picking me up later that morning. It was a Georgian church and the service had already begun with a congregation of about thirty, mostly old, peasant faces although a dozen teenagers arrived about the same time as I did. Three of the girls were determined to light candles and then got involved in the Mass; the boys remained nervously at the back in a side aisle. The service continued for another half an hour so by the time I had followed the teenagers to a nearby café for some sweet tea I was late back at the hotel. Tamara was waiting for me with two doctors from the Ministry.

My request – almost a demand – to concentrate on medical services for women had been agreed, only to be told by the two doctors that the plans had been changed. First we were to visit Hospital No. 2 and then go on to Mtskheta, the ancient capital of

Georgia about twenty miles north of Tbilisi, then on again to a rural hospital where I could talk with health workers from a rural setting. I was speechless.

No. 2 was a teaching hospital with roughly 300 students per year. Two polyclinics were attached to the hospital, one almost literally in the same grounds and the other in the same *uchastok*. I persuaded both Professor Chachava, Director of Surgery, and Professor Aladashvili, Director of Internal Medicine that I didn't want to look round the hospital but would much prefer to discuss with them and other of their colleagues about the relationship between primary and secondary care, concentrating on the two polyclinics and No. 2, and to hear their views on the success or otherwise of the emergency-call service and, if time, discuss health education.

Both Chachava and Aladashvili were senior men who spoke from experience and were totally at ease in talking about the cons as well as the pros of the Soviet system. As I had found in Armenia, openness prevailed with no concern that they might be reported to the Ministry for being so frank with a foreigner.

Interestingly Chachava had visited the Brompton and Hammersmith hospitals in London in the early 1960s and had retained contacts with the Royal College of Surgeons. It was difficult to believe he had also met Michael Wilson, one of the surgeons who regularly did out-patients and operated at the Wells Cottage Hospital where I worked; a very very small world indeed. Contrary to what I expected the hospital visit was a complete success, absolutely invaluable.

Before departing we all went back to Chachava's room for champagne and grapes. It was barely midday but they wanted to forget medicine and find out how much I knew about their beloved Georgia, its literature and poetry. Obviously disappointed and surprised by my ignorance, Chachava browsed along the bookshelves and found what he wanted – Shata Rust'avi's *The Knight in the Panther's Skin,* an epic poem from the $12^{th}/13^{th}$ centuries considered by Georgians to be the greatest romantic poem ever written and which in 1968 was translated into English in perfect poetic style. It was quite impossible to hide the depth of my ignorance so I asked them to join me in toasting Rust'avi and Byron – not that I was knowledgeable about Byron either but Chachava and his friends seemed to think he was one of the most famous of English poets. To my further embarrassment Chachava then presented me with the book in the earnest hope I would read this epic work. The book is still on my bookshelf and alas is still unread. Inside the cover is Chachava's message and the date, 3 October 1971, along with his home address.

To reach Mtskheta we drove along the Georgian Military Highway following the Kura river until it joins the Aragvi river at Mtskheta. I realised then that the visit had a number of purposes: one was to try and satisfy my request to study primary medical care, conveniently forgetting they had ignored my main request; second was that Mtskheta was a place they wanted foreigners to visit; third was to demonstrate that politics in Georgia was different to Moscow, in particular Stalin's association with Mtskheta and his continuing popularity; and finally such an event was a good opportunity to demonstrate Georgian hospitality, especially as it was all paid for by the Ministry of Health, which of course accounted for the number of colleagues who had joined us by the time we were ready to eat.

The meeting was held at the local hospital: 120 beds for internal medicine, paediatrics and surgery, and 40 beds for obstetrics and gynaecology. This covered the town's population of 10,000 and a further 20,000 in the surrounding villages and countryside. There were also two rural hospitals with 40 and 50 beds, so with 250 beds for a population of 30,000 there was certainly no shortage, in fact quite the reverse.

Primary care was provided by one polyclinic within the town while the rural population was served by twelve medical centres each with one doctor and dentist, six *feldschers* and six auxiliary nurses. Unbelievably, then, twelve doctors, twelve dentists, seventy-two *feldschers* and seventy-two auxiliary nurses were caring for a population of roughly 20,000. How these health workers found enough work to keep them busy remained a mystery; during discussions this 'mystery' was ignored or side-stepped, as was the cost, which concerned nobody. As I was finding out in my travels through the Soviet Union, it was considered to be the duty of the state to find the money.

Dr Giorgotiani Zugal, the Director of the hospital, was in charge of the whole set-up. He exuded energy, enthusiasm and optimism, while Dr Olag the chief surgeon was phlegmatic, happy with the status quo and not happy to answer my questions. Both men clearly got on well together, enjoyed their present life and were united in refusing to see any need for change.

The confluence of the Kura and Aragvi had been the perfect spot to build and develop the future capital of this region. The kings of Georgia had been crowned in the cathedral of Sveti Tzkhoveli – the Twelve Apostles or the Tree of Life – and buried there for hundreds of years, the last in 1801. Mtskheta was steeped in history and even in the atheistic Soviet Union the cathedral, still a working church, was held to be a place of great significance. As we arrived, the small congregation all dressed in black were just coming out, outnumbered by grazing sheep and playing children and equalled in number by tramps, often called Holy Beggars. We only had time to peer briefly into the dark, incense-filled interior, barely able to see anything with eyes accustomed to the brilliant sun and blue sky.

A little distance from the cathedral was the church and convent of Samtavro. Again both were in use and the convent was allowed to function as a community for the teaching of Christianity. Certainly since reaching these two Caucasian Republics I had been astonished by the freedom enjoyed by Christians – so many churches open and used for worship. In the West only the trials and tribulations of the Church in the Soviet Union and Eastern Europe were mentioned and curiously it was as though Armenia and Georgia didn't exist.

Tamara and I were on our own, which was excellent as she was as interested in these churches as I was. The rest of the group shambled along seemingly bored and uninterested. Suddenly Zugal decided he had had enough and called us over; it seemed we couldn't waste any more time looking at these old buildings, we needed to get to where we were to have a meal.

We drove over to the edge of town to a picturesque stone-built country house with a pretty covered veranda, surrounded by trees and shrubs and grasses being cut back with a scythe. It was the house of landed gentry before the Revolution and sixty years later was now a restaurant with a storage cellar for some of Georgia's famous red wines. The entrance to the restaurant was almost blocked by hovering waiters. Inside were strong wooden tables surrounding an area for dancing and a small stage for the band. The place was full but we were expected and there was much back-slapping between Zugal, Goguadze and many of the locals they knew. Ten of us plus Tamara sat down to eat; conversation almost ceased as we sat down and Zugal seemed not quite in control any more. Tamara whispered to me:

"Ask something about Stalin and see what happens."

It was as if I had thrown a firework into the room. Everyone wanted to tell me he had been born in Gori only twenty miles away, that the small house in which he had been born was now a museum and that the massive bronze statue of the great man still stood in the square opposite the town hall. Tamara was kept busy as only two spoke English and all wanted to have their say – how Stalin trained to be a priest, what he had accomplished for the Soviet Union, how the Great Patriotic War between the Soviet Union and Nazi Germany had been won almost single-handed by the local hero, and finally how wrong Khrushchev had been at the 20th Party Congress in 1956 to denounce Stalin as a criminal and paint his years in power as the most dreadful time of terror and starvation. As far as everyone at that table was concerned, he remained a hero in Georgia and would never be forgotten. I couldn't believe what I was hearing.

The table groaned with food and was continually replenished, a feast for a king, or certainly Stalin. I had been warned about toasting by Terry Garrett and in particular the problem of being the only guest as you have to respond to every toast, unlike your hosts. The toasting remains as much in my memory as the political support for Stalin; as soon as I had asked my question about Stalin, Zugal raised his glass for the first toast to Britain and the Soviet Union. I responded by taking a sip of my drink, which provoked shouts of *'do dna'* (to the bottom) from everyone, including everyone else in the restaurant.

The toasts continued for nearly three hours – to peace, to our wives, our mothers and fathers, the Queen, Brezhnev, Gagarin and all cosmonauts, doctors, nurses, Shakespeare, Tchaikovsky, Tolstoy, Rust'havi – anyone or anything. I was getting desperate and after about three-quarters of an hour Tamara managed to persuade Zugal and his friends to break with tradition; *'do dna'* was no longer possible for me thus confirming what they always knew – no foreigner could compete with a Russian. Vodka continued to be dispensed liberally by waiters who made sure your glass was always full. When we got up to depart I counted sixteen empty bottles of wine and a large basket full of empty vodka bottles.

As Tamara thanked everybody on my behalf I was sure the toasts were over, but I was wrong and the day was brought to a fitting conclusion with a final toast to Stalin from everyone in the restaurant accompanied by much clapping and shouting and more calls of *'do dna'*. I obliged by ostentatiously asking a waiter to fill up my glass which I downed in one gulp. A great cheer went up. An astonishing day!

The Experimental Polyclinic for Adults had been a recent innovation and the time spent with Professor Kipshidze proved really valuable as he was able to fill in some gaps and point out where I had misunderstood things. He understood and spoke English quite well and had a number of contacts in the UK.

Patients from all over Georgia were referred to the polyclinic. The main research concentrated on three areas of medicine: coronary artery disease, its aetiology, prophylaxis, emergency care, subsequent treatment, rehabilitation, and the time taken to get people back to work; respiratory diseases – asthma, bronchitis, emphysema and cancer of the lung – concentrating mainly on treatment; and diseases of the liver and gall bladder. Here again the main focus was on treatment, and the effects of alcohol and diet were being studied rather belatedly – and ineffectively judging by the number of drunks to be seen staggering about or lying in the streets even early in the morning.

It was a good end to my stay in Tbilisi.

Tamara took me to the small airport for the flight to Odessa; she mentioned keeping in touch but made no specific arrangements.

My original idea had been to continue travelling by train along the Black Sea coast to Odessa, but a look at the map showed that this was impossible, so the 'romance' of the railway was exchanged for splendid views of the snow-capped Caucasian mountains ending on the shores of the Black Sea with a glimpse of the Sea of Azov before landing at Simferopol in the Crimea for a short stop before continuing on to Odessa. The weather had changed and was now cloudy with a strong, cold northerly wind and spotting with rain.

What would the return to European Russia feel like? Would it mirror the change in the weather? Armenia and Georgia had left me with the feeling that both Republics were less hidebound by the Party, and less fearful of informers who might turn out to be a colleague, friend or even a family member. The availability of food and the standard of living was also a surprise. I should have been prepared for the diversity of culture but I think forgiven for not anticipating the comparative independence enjoyed by the Church.

The diversity to be found in Uzbekistan, Georgia and Armenia was not a feature of the health service – quite the reverse, with a uniformity of organisation which was possibly the only way of providing health care in a country of this size, particularly starting from the chaos and destruction of the First World War, the Revolution, and the subsequent Civil War to be followed by the Great Patriotic War of World War Two.

The visit to the Republic of Ukraine involved the capital city Kiev, but first the famous port of Odessa in the north-west corner of the Black Sea. It had been agreed that the rural service would be excluded. The only hotel for foreigners was in a perfect location on the wide, tree-lined Primorsky Boulevard overlooking the Black Sea. It was a traditional mid-19th century neo-classical building, its interior retaining the feel of another age. Turning left out of the hotel, crossing the boulevard to a wide promenade then walking for a few minutes, Odessa's most famous tourist site comes into view – the impressive flight of 192 steps from the promenade to the dock area, the Potemkin Steps (originally the Richelieu Steps named after the Duke of Richelieu, the first Governor) made famous by the film *The Battleship Potemkin.*

Whatever thoughts I might have had about this unique architectural wonder, twice as wide at the bottom as at the top and yet both sides seeming parallel, was quickly destroyed by the arrival of two coach loads of East Germans being supervised and herded around by their minders and blocking the view of the steps. 'Lumpen proletariat' was the perfect description of this group of workers and their wives who had been allowed to come and experience the delights of the Black Sea and Odessa, its wonderful Mediterranean climate, the tree-lined streets and many parks, the attractively-painted buildings and the cosmopolitan atmosphere of a busy port.

What a disappointment it must have been, this promise of golden beaches – instead a rocky coastline, and as the tide went out only smaller rocks and pebbles revealed. The walk along the shore, a mile or so, displayed trashy attractions – stands full of kitschy plastic souvenirs, shooting galleries blaring pop music, and the odour of cheap fatty sausages and bags of barely warm floppy chips. Inevitably there was rubbish everywhere being collected by the ubiquitous band of hard-working, middle-aged women sweeping slowly and methodically with their old-fashioned besom brooms. Such street cleaners were one of the commonest sights in the Soviet Union.

On subsequent visits to Odessa, one of the saddest sights, at least to me, was to watch the holiday makers proudly carrying their buckets and spades, full of expectation and laughter but with no chance of building a sandcastle. I suppose I was just comparing our own beautiful coastline and thinking how lucky my kids and their friends have been.

Apart from the East Germans only four other foreigners were staying in the hotel – two oil workers from Romania and a most interesting middle-aged British couple who were travelling by car. They had been regular visitors to the Soviet Union since the early '60s and had a complete grasp of all the difficulties and some of the delights that might be encountered.

It took a little time but eventually the meeting at the Department of Public Health with its Chairperson Dr Nestova took place. We discussed health education and preventive medicine and in particular how this might affect patients' attitudes towards polyclinics. Following on from this and questions about the Industrial Health Service about which I understood little, Nestova agreed to devote the whole of the next day to the Women's Health Service.

A Women's Consultative Clinic provided clinical and preventive care although in reality such a clinic was just another name for a specialised polyclinic. The normal catchment area was for populations up to 200,000, but the clinic I visited was unusual in two ways; first the catchment area was only 52,000, and second it was directly connected with Maternity Hospital No. 7. Future policy was to build clinics attached to maternity hospitals wherever possible, which it was hoped would be built as one unit. There were two intentions. The first was to encourage a greater exchange of staff with a view to improving morale and the quality of care. Obstetricians working in the clinic would attend a Women's Hospital twice a month to attend confinements, whilst a *uchastok* paediatrician would also visit the hospital before the mother and baby were discharged. In this way some continuity of care would be established, combined with the compulsory home visits after delivery. As well as ante-natal care that prepared mothers solely for a hospital confinement, and the usual post-natal care, all investigations and treatment of gynaecological problems would be linked between the Consultative Clinic and the Women's Hospital. The second intention was that patients should be helped by everything being carried out in one place.

One area of women's care was a big surprise to me and in this perhaps the Soviets were years ahead of the UK; routine screening for cervical cancer was performed twice a year from the age of twenty up to sixty. The procedure was carried out either in the consultative clinic or, for working women, in the industrial polyclinics. Routine breast examination – not mammography which had not then been invented – was taught to patients but was also carried out every year by doctors. Were such numbers of cervical smears and breast examinations necessary? Almost certainly not, and unfortunately in the USSR where so many examinations were carried out, no evaluation of the collected statistics was ever made: an enormous opportunity lost.

Requests for abortion formed a large part of the service. Abortions were not free and were not actively encouraged, but they were available 'on demand' – a patient could not be refused. A number of gynaecologists had spoken out about their worries concerning the medical complications and emotional problems that arose, and the three gynaecologists I spoke to were in total accord in their disquiet.

Unfortunately, for most women abortion was the main form of contraception. I met one woman who had had ten abortions, which she didn't seem to regret, and apparently such numbers were quite common. Wide variations existed in other Republics – in Uzbekistan, Armenia and Georgia, for example, in order to raise the birth rate women were discouraged from seeking abortions, whilst many, particularly in rural areas, either for religious or cultural reasons, preferred to accept 'the will of God'. I imagined that Azerbaijan and Kazakhstan and their neighbouring Asiatic Republics would be in this category too.

Contraceptive advice was available in theory but it didn't seem to be requested or dispensed. Condoms, caps and spermicides were available and the intra-uterine device had recently become popular. The oral contraceptive pill was regarded with suspicion by both doctors and patients, and the doctors' doubts about its long-term safety were passed on to their patients. I felt pretty certain that once lower dose pills became available, pressure would be exerted by those patients who could afford to pay (the OC pill was not free).

The Women's Maternity Hospital No. 7 had 100 obstetric and 60 gynaecological beds and about 3,000 births a year. Both forceps rates at 2 percent and caesarean section at 0.5 percent were extremely low compared with the UK, whilst the usual stay after delivery was on average seven days. The shortest time for a multipara was six days even though the majority of women wanted to get home much sooner. Neonates were examined every day by a neonatologist until the day of discharge; again no research was carried out as to whether this was necessary – another opportunity lost.

About 1,800 abortions were performed each year, and all the medical staff I spoke to agreed it was strange that in a country which placed such a high premium on prevention, abortion remained the commonest form of contraception.

The final visit of the day was to the maternity department of a rural hospital which, along with what I had already observed in Hospital No. 7, provided an unfavourable memory of the rigid rules imposed on mothers and babies: every four hours with no flexibility whatsoever babies were fed, then separated from their mothers and taken to the nursery where they were all tightly wrapped and placed in their cots, all lying on their same side. My enquiry about relaxing the routine was dismissed: 'there is no need'. And in fact an unexpected and surprising observation was how little I heard the babies crying – with such stringent regulation I would have expected the opposite. It was mystifying – did wrapping a baby up like a parcel provide a feeling of security?

The weather had been exceptionally unseasonable for Odessa, flurries of snow at the beginning of October almost unheard of. By the time I boarded Train 56 I was hoping for warmer weather in Kiev. But of more immediate interest was who would be my travelling companions. Unusually the train was not packed and the six-bedded compartment was only half full – myself and two massively fat middle-aged women, not from the countryside but pale-skinned townies, whether from Odessa or Kiev I never discovered. As soon as I entered the compartment I knew I wasn't welcome, whether because I was a foreigner or because I was male I didn't know. Luckily I had eaten at a buffet at the station so I remained in the corridor for as long as possible before re-entering the compartment, but found myself just as unwelcome. Naturally I slept in my clothes. I woke early and immediately escaped to the corridor to stand gazing at the flat agricultural land that lay close to the railway. It was dominated by endless cabbages and a landscape that undulated gently and disappeared into the mist; everything was covered with a powdering of fresh snow.

Kiev has been described in many ways – the Soul of Mother Russia, the Jerusalem of Russia, the Holy City of Kiev, the Cradle of Russian culture – and I wondered if this historic city would live up to expectations. Initially my hopes were dented. Hotel Dneiper was a good example of Stalin's early 1950's architecture, not the 'wedding cake' variety of the City Hall in Warsaw or the Hotel Ukraina in Moscow, but just drab and uninspiring with large ill-proportioned Corinthian columns hiding half of the ten-storey building. The interior was dark and utterly functional with a curious smell of disinfectant and cheap perfume. The girl at the reception desk, on the other hand, turned out to be bright and cheerful and happily carried out my instructions to contact the Ministry of Health.

"Yes, they're expecting you and have organised a programme to visit hospitals and research institutes."

She was crestfallen when I said I wasn't pleased and to contact the Ministry again to remind them they knew my interests. A meeting was eventually arranged for later in the morning and after some haggling I agreed to an emergency care centre and an adult polyclinic. That only took me up to midday so I asked about the rest of the day; nothing had been arranged and I was free to do what I wanted.

Vladimirskaya Hill is close to the hotel and an easy climb to its summit through parkland and small open spaces where children were playing and the elderly sat and chatted, some playing dominoes or chess. From the top there was a view across the Dneiper with a pedestrian bridge to Trukhanov Island, a sandy area in the middle of the river used by locals and tourists alike. On the far side I could see vast housing estates and factories reminding me of Buda and Pest and Elizabeth Island in the middle of the Danube. Turning slightly to the right I looked down on the huge bronze statue of Prince Vladimir, known as the Baptiser of Russia; one side of the substantial pedestal was decorated with a story in bas-relief of the baptismal scene as ordered by the Prince in 988 AD.

Whether you were christian or not, communist or not, atheist or not, it seemed that all Russians recognised the conversion to Christianity in 988 AD to be one of the defining moments in Russian history, when Orthodox Christianity and the chronicles of the country became inextricably bound. Somehow Lenin, Trotsky, Stalin, Khrushchev and subsequent leaders were unwilling or unable, even afraid, to break this connection. One only needs to recall how Stalin asked for the support of the Patriarch of All Russia and the Orthodox Church during the siege of Moscow in the winter of 1941/42.

The Orthodox Church representing the Greek-speaking Church of the Byzantine Empire had split off from the Catholic Church in Rome representing the Pope. Prince Vladimir decided against Rome. It has been recorded (whether true or just apocryphal I don't know) that within a week of this decision the entire population of Kiev was ordered to be baptised in the waters of the Dneiper.

Beyond the statue and on the same bank of the Dneiper a collection of golden cupolas could be seen. It turned out to be the celebrated religious complex of Lavra Pechersk, or Cave Monastery, on the steep edge of the river. It is a huge area dominated by two hills separated by a valley, and contains the site of the famous caves originally inhabited by monks and hermits. As I approached the entrance to this amazing complex I was spell-bound by the beauty and variety of the architecture, the beauty being magnified by the natural woodlands surrounding it. It is difficult to comprehend the sheer vandalism of the Nazis as they blew up much of Lavra Pechersk in 1941.

Nobody has doubted that at least sixty percent of Kiev was destroyed between September 1941 and November 1943, partly due to hand to hand fighting but mainly due to the dynamiting of the old city as the Nazis were preparing to leave – priceless churches, concert halls, museums and most of the University. Two hundred thousand citizens were killed and over one hundred thousand deported to Germany.

The Emergency Medical Service was completely separate from hospitals and polyclinics and functioned in urban areas only; the separation referred to the staff, a distinct group of doctors who were specially trained for this work.

Emergency Care Centre No. 1 was the main centre for Kiev through which all emergency calls were filtered to eight satellite centres in different parts of the city. With a population of 1,250,000 Kiev had nine such centres, Moscow with a population of 6,500,000 had thirty-three. Emergency calls were received from the general public, from the police and fire service and from doctors, the commonest emergencies being accidents, resuscitation, myocardial infarcts, pneumonia, labour and other obstetric problems, acute psychosis and poisoning.

Physicians were not accepted for training until they had worked for at least three years at a postgraduate level, not including the initial year after graduation. Once accepted into the service, for two months every year they would return to hospital for continuing education and training. The two exceptions were cardiologists and anaesthetists working in the coronary care ambulance as they were already working full-time in hospital.

Whilst we were in the control room four messages were received: someone found unconscious in the street had been reported by a member of the public; a myocardial infarct was reported by a *uchastok* physician; a stroke was reported by a member of the family; and a woman in premature labour was reported by her mother. I was disappointed that my visit to the control room had come to an end before I knew the outcome of the messages.

I returned to the Director's office for coffee, cakes, fruit and cigarettes. I could only state the obvious and comment on the excellent organisation and some first-class equipment and incubators for neonates. I was genuinely impressed but had no way of knowing if Care Centre No. 1 was unique or how well the Emergency Medical Service covered the rest of the USSR.

Polyclinic No. 22 was attached to a district hospital with 200 beds and supported a population of 50,000 living in 18 *uchastoks.* Dr Vasiljevna, the Director, proved to be not only a fund of information but was happy to answer my questions and eager that I should meet as many of her staff as possible.

Uchastok therapists divided their time between three and a half hours' consulting time and two and a half hours carrying out home visits – the patients were the elderly and the chronically ill, no workers and no women. Trained nurses, called doctors' assistants, worked with the therapists. Domiciliary care was different. The Red Cross provided nurses with only a limited one-year training. They were used to help the elderly with general care, washing, housework, cooking, collecting medicines and routine 'popping in' – in many ways similar to a Home Help in the UK. Acute domiciliary care was provided by *feldschers.*

Dr Vasiljevna had introduced a new psychology department in No. 22. The work concentrated mainly on young people, giving guidance about finding work amongst other things. She and her colleagues were adamant that such an approach was necessary; this seemed bizarre to me as nobody was allowed to be unemployed within the Soviet Union or Eastern Europe and officially unemployment did not exist.

With regard to traditional psychological problems such as anxiety, depression, neurotic illness and the like, Vasiljevna was unable to convince me that such conditions were not as common in the USSR as in the UK; certainly she could not supply any compelling evidence.

*

I had been successful in buying a Russian guidebook and map of Kiev, but anyone with the slightest knowledge of how things work in the Soviet Union will be familiar with their obsession for changing the names of cities and streets: St Petersburg to Petrograd to Leningrad to St Petersburg; Stalingrad to Volgograd; Nizhny Novgorod to Gorki to Nizhny Novgorod; Ekaterinburg to Sverdlovsk to Ekaterinburg; and so it goes on in almost every city, town and street. Both the map and the guidebook proved to be of little help and frequently it was virtually impossible to work out where you were. Sometimes a changed name was not altered on the map or guidebook or had been changed on one and not the other. From my personal point of view the refusal sometimes to call a church a church or a cathedral a religious building was absolutely maddening.

Before leaving Kiev I wanted to see three churches. St Sophia's Cathedral can be seen from almost anywhere in the city with its spectacular golden cupolas, although the notice board outside it stated: The State Architectural Historical Sofisky Monument Museum. Opening times were plain to see (it closed one day a week). The building is immense with a magnificent central dome and fourteen smaller cupolas where the gold had only recently been restored. The separate Bell Tower added to the splendour.

Inside an explosion of colour greeted me and as always the iconostasis caught my eye as well as the frescoes, murals, paintings, icons, manuscripts, and the painted ceiling, which beautifully completed the picture. Without doubt this was a museum and not a church.

St Vladimir's Cathedral was built in the middle of the nineteenth century to commemorate the 900th anniversary of the conversion to Christianity. No notice to indicate if this was an active church or not, but there were notice boards indicating it was an art museum. Outside, a collection of old women dressed in black and wearing black head scarves were sitting or leaning against the walls of the church alongside a dozen or so beggars and drunks. I assumed there must be a service due to begin and after about half an hour the west door was opened. The old women moved quickly to get inside to kiss the walls, the floor, pictures and icons whilst repeatedly crossing themselves and mumbling prayers as they wandered around lighting candles. Young girls holding hands and a few young men and young couples as well as middle-aged folk rushing in from work, completed the congregation. The clergy appeared briefly through the iconostasis, swinging censers and seemingly remote from the people, almost indifferent to them. Throughout the service two elderly priests sat on either side of the west door receiving apples and plums and *kopeks* from the old women. They wanted to be blessed or just spoken to by the priests, but the priests ignored them, barely even acknowledging their presence. It was a sad, shameful spectacle of which the Church could not be proud, never mind that it was to some extent redeemed by the beautiful orthodox liturgy.

Little time remained for St Andrew's Church, a jewel of Baroque architecture, painted blue and white with golden domes surrounded by five smaller golden cupolas. It was an enchanting building reached by a long straight stairway. The notices were clear, showing opening and closing times as a museum and information about concerts of Russian music being performed on Saturdays and Sundays. Again there was no indication whether it was a working church and I had no time left to go inside.

All three had been declared ancient monuments during Soviet rule – whether before or after the Great Patriotic War I never found out.

Hospitality had been spontaneous. One evening I went to the Ukrainian Folk Dance Theatre with colleagues from the Ministry with whom I had initially had an argument. A convivial evening ensued in a small café – much vodka but happily no toasts. The Director of the Emergency Centre and a couple of her colleagues pressed me to go again to the folk dancing on the following night, but I sadly declined as I would be waiting for a call from Vasiljevna. They seemed genuinely disappointed as I was when her call never came.

Later that same evening I met an interesting young nuclear physicist from Tbilisi and we were joined by a Sudanese who was in Kiev to be instructed about aircraft engineering and construction. Both were quite relaxed about talking to a westerner.

On another occasion, whilst having an early supper in the virtually empty restaurant before catching the train to Moscow, I was joined by a Dutchman. We were enjoying a pleasant chat when suddenly a four-man band arrived on the stage followed by a huge wedding party, the bride in the whitest of white gowns and the relations and guests in traditional Ukrainian costume. The success of a Russian band appears to depend on creating a lot of noise and this group were clearly a success! Almost as quickly as the wedding party had arrived so it started to depart, but not before playing and then singing 'Auld Lang Syne', Robbie Burns being, and I think still remains, the most popular foreign poet in Russia; at least half the wedding party knew the words and everyone got to their feet singing and shouting and clapping and dancing. I couldn't believe it – it was like the end of a traditional Burns Night supper except that vodka replaced whisky.

Train No. 16 left for Moscow on time and as I settled down I wondered if I had been in the heart and soul of Russia – looking in my diary later I had written 'I feel much at home', so perhaps I had.

I woke in the morning to miles and miles of silver birch woods, occasional small villages of typical wooden blue- or ochre-painted houses with smoke already curling out of their chimneys, farmland, a few cattle and sheep, and horse- or bullock-drawn carts with motionless farm workers holding the reins. It seemed a long journey, but 537 miles in twelve and a half hours averaged almost forty-five miles per hour. I had forgotten Train 16 was a 'fast train' – meaning simply that it stopped at fewer stations.

On the flight home I realised that important gaps remained in my grasp of primary care. Furthermore, Tashkent was still only a third of the way across the vast limitless expanse which had always saved the country from invaders. Gradually I came to accept that a second visit would be necessary and by the time I reached Heathrow my mind was made up. The only problem was how? . . . and when?

Everything proved to be easier and more straightforward than I had thought possible; in November 1971 I had been awarded a Nuffield Foundation Travelling Scholarship to study the Health Service in Japan with particular reference to primary care, and crucially my fare there and back was included.

My plan would be to return overland via the Soviet Union. On the advice of the Japanese, autumn was the best time to visit there, thus limiting when I could revisit the USSR; it would have to be either late summer/early autumn or in the winter. I remember hearing a well-known writer, whose name I have forgotten, insisting you couldn't say you had really and truly visited a country unless you had experienced its hottest or coldest time of year. This tied in exactly with my own thoughts, so winter would be my choice to experience the Soviet Far East and Siberia. Each of us has our own image of this land of snow and freezing temperatures, the vast desolate landscape, the taiga, the huge rivers and the tales of exile, political prisoners and labour camps both in Tsarist and Soviet times.

I couldn't do anything until my report on the USSR had been completed and it was not until early 1972 that the report was sent to Dr Eristavis at the Ministry of Health and Terry Garrett at the British Embassy with accompanying letters setting out what I wanted to do. Within about three weeks Terry Garrett replied, saying Eristavis had decided to distribute the report to Uzbekistan, Armenia, Georgia, Odessa and Kiev and 'he would be glad to grant me a visa and arrange suitable visits in the Soviet Far East and Siberia'.

This was more than I could possibly have expected; it was unbelievable, too good to be true, no hassle, no endless waiting at the Soviet Embassy in London, no prevarication or mindless bureaucracy – all so straightforward. Obviously this opportunity had to be seized before anything unforeseen could happen – after all, no one knew when the next bunch of Soviet diplomats might be thrown out.

My departure from Tokyo was unusual and frankly rather embarrassing. The flight to Khabarovsk had been in operation for less than six months with only two flights a week. My flight was called and I found myself the only passenger on the Boeing 707. I could see the air hostesses twittering away like little birds at the front of the plane and to my consternation four had been allocated to my block of seats. One of the most ludicrous moments involved one of them standing in front of me and going through all the emergency procedures as though the remaining 189 seats were all occupied. Food and refreshments were served with the exquisite politeness of the Japanese – mercifully the air hostess was not on her knees as she served me! As I stood up to go to the toilet one of them rushed down to make sure I was alright and after I had explained my purpose she backed up the gangway bowing all the way. As I returned to my seat the size of the plane and the sight of 189 empty seats was simply mind-boggling; it was no surprise that less than a year later Japan Airlines ceased flying to Khabarovsk.

As soon as the plane came to a halt I knew I was in a different world; there was thick snow on the ground and immediately the door opened it let in a perishing wind, an armed soldier and an Intourist official – quite a reception for a single passenger. The walk along the icy pathway been piles of snow was difficult – no question of being taken in a bus. Once inside the terminal, passport and customs went without a hitch. Mind you, even the Soviets couldn't have organised any problems under the circumstances.

It was forbidden to bring in any currency and I was whisked through so quickly that I forgot to ask if there was a currency exchange bank, so as soon as I sat down in the taxi I knew there would be trouble. True to form the bureau de change in the hotel was closed but opened quickly when the taxi driver started shouting and thumping his fist on the reception desk.

After the absolute cleanliness and simple tasteful decor of Japan, Hotel Khabarovsk seemed to be in urgent need of redecoration, whilst the dreadful landscape pictures and plastic flowers to be found in every room confirmed its uniform monotony. At least it seemed functional. But I was wrong – there was no bulb in the bedroom and both hot and cold taps produced barely a trickle, but I didn't grumble as at least the radiator was more or less hot which it needed to be with sub-zero temperatures outside.

My stop-over in Khabarovsk was not connected with primary care. I had been asked to visit the Department of Pharmacology at the Medical Institute to gather as much information and as many documents as I could regarding herbal and folk medicine and its use within the Soviet health service. John Massey Stewart, a fluent Russian-speaker, writer, freelance journalist and photographer, had recently published *Across the Russias*, but when in Khabarovsk he had been unable to meet Professor Fruentov. Subsequently they had been in correspondence and Fruentov had agreed to meet me.

On waking early on the first morning I knew something was different from yesterday: no traffic noise, and silence except for the crunching of footsteps on hard snow. Breakfast in the buffet reminded me of the dreary wartime British restaurants which continued until the early 1950s – little choice of food and what there was being poorly cooked.

The Intourist guide turned up about 9.30. She was pleasant and spoke English well. She said she had a great disappointment for me and was full of apologies; permission had not been granted for a visit to the Pharmaceutical Factory but I could go to the Pharmaceutical Institute instead. This was all rather confusing as I had never asked to visit the factory, so I was able to respond by saying how pleased and grateful I was.

Professor Fruentov spoke little English so my guide came into her own and the meeting went well. Fruentov proved to be the Soviet authority on ginseng, which was one of Massey Stewart's particular interests, almost an obsession. Was it really the elixir of life? Could it solve the many personal problems that are part and parcel of life? How well had it been tested by modern pharmacological techniques? One thing was absolutely certain – it was sold and used extensively by the general public throughout Siberia and the Far East (and perhaps the rest of the Soviet Union) and had a tremendous reputation as a 'good tonic and pick-me-up', particularly after a long winter. It was also reputed to be an excellent sexual rejuvenator for both men and women. Interestingly, about this time ginseng was becoming trendy and fashionable in the western world.

We parted after tea, chocolates, cigarettes and vodka plus two small bottles of ginseng as a gift for Massey Stewart and myself as well as a pile of literature and a book he had written. How I was going to carry all this plus my Japanese stuff I had no idea.

Khabarovsk was founded in the middle of the nineteenth century at the confluence of the Amur and Ussuri. For 800 miles until it reaches Khabarovsk the Amur forms the border between China and Russia. It then flows north-east for another 900 miles until it reaches the Sea of Okhotsk. The Ussuri flows north from its source near Vladivostok and is also the border between these two countries. The locals were keen I should appreciate the greatness of the Amur and were equally determined I should understand I was not in Siberia but in the capital city of the Soviet Far East. The Amur was over a mile across and completely frozen (usually for about five months). The great majority of rivers in Siberia and the Far East flow slowly and freeze easily. What caught my eye were the clusters of fishermen each fishing through a hole in the ice and hunched around an open fire. I didn't see a single fish caught. Looking back at the river as I walked back to the hotel, the round red ball of the sun was dramatic and caused intense reflections off the ice.

The numbers of soldiers around had been instantly noticeable, giving the impression of a garrison town, and looking across the Amur to China I could see why. The majority looked smart with good quality uniforms, heavy greatcoats, quality boots and warm fur hats in a variety of colours, perhaps denoting different regiments or corps. Their behaviour and discipline were professional, very different from other parts of the country. I asked my guide and others how much they feared living so close to China; it didn't seem to worry them and the general feeling was that Moscow worried more than those living on the spot, although they agreed in the end that the number of first-rate troops in the town gave them a sense of security.

A few pre-revolutionary buildings remained along with the ever-expanding, always-present blocks of grim modern flats. Nonetheless a provincial atmosphere prevailed, due in part to the town having been built on three small hills along which the main roads ran, and in part to areas of picturesque wooden houses each with windows and front doors framed by delicate carving, almost like lacework. Most too had their own gardens, now filled with snow, surrounded by a wooden fence. These traditional *izbas* (traditional Russian countryside dwellings) were what I had been hoping to see, but they were what the authorities did not want foreigners to see and alas the bulldozers were at work. I suppose the communist party believed they demonstrated backwardness and poverty and did not belong in a modern State. When I asked the locals and my guide about the bulldozers they just shrugged their shoulders in an expression of 'what can we do?'. Later, on the train to Irkutsk, I was relieved to see the *izbas* everywhere in the small towns and villages.

In spite of all the red tape and officialdom and sometimes the bad service or just bloody-mindedness, I couldn't help liking the Russians.

In a department store what a contrast with Japan, one full of everything one could possibly want (or not) and the other half empty. Was I happier with the consumer madness of Japan or the drab austerity of the Soviet Union? I really didn't know, although I was certainly happy to be back in contact with the history of Europe. Even the sight of a non-functioning Orthodox church with its golden domes rather than the mysterious beauty surrounding a Japanese Shinto shrine, made me feel I was not in a foreign country. Curious, really.

A couple of events made me realise there are decent people everywhere and the third showed that we're really all the same. The first was after I had exchanged some travellers cheques and had stopped at one of the many kiosks selling toothpaste, hair grips, nail varnish, picture postcards, combs and of course cigarettes, and bought some cards. I had wandered back to the hotel only to find I didn't have the envelope containing the roubles. It was late and everything was closed. Early next morning more in hope than expectation I returned to the kiosk and the elderly lady running it saw me coming and waved the envelope. She explained in sign language I had dropped it on the pavement and her next customer had picked it up and given it to her.

The second event occurred while in the post office where I left my small instamatic camera on the counter. It was not of any value to anyone seriously interested in photography, nonetheless it was valuable to me. I returned a few hours later and again it had been handed in to the cashier.

Finally, on a different tack, I was wandering around in a sort of supermarket just trying to judge how well or how poorly it was stocked. I came across the half-empty alcohol section where one shelf was advertising in Roman script, 'Vin Superieur de Haute Taiga'. I couldn't believe it, such delightful snobbery being universal.

Like so many things in Russia, the Trans-Siberian Railway was not just a simple matter of travelling from Yaroslav station in Moscow to the great naval base of Vladivostok on the Sea of Japan, an immense distance of 5,810 miles passing through nine time zones and arriving in Moscow or Vladivostok, a journey of eight days. That is to say, it was simple for Russians but certainly not for foreigners.

Train No. 2 travels west to east and Train No. 1 from east to west – no problem travelling in either direction if you are Russian, but if you are a foreigner Vladivostok is out of bounds, *zahkrittah*, closed. Who knows, you might see a warship or take a photograph or even be a spy. Between Moscow and Vladivostok there are nearly a hundred stations, the railway is truly the lifeline for people and goods, but only three stations are open to foreigners – Novosibirsk, Irkutsk and Khabarovsk. You can of course get off at the other ninety-seven stations provided you don't move from the platform. Foreigners coming from the west are obliged to get off Train No. 2 at Khabarovsk if they want to see the Sea of Japan, and get as close as possible to Vladivostok. The journey must then be continued on the local night train, the *Vostok*, to Nakhodka, a small port about thirty miles from Vladivostok. This was a port for foreigners but of no practical use because there were no boats. In spite of being so close to Vladivostok, which could easily be reached by car or taxi, you are not allowed even briefly into this great naval base. And so the only possible way to start the journey from Nakhoda is to wait four to six hours wandering up and down the platform, for the return of the *Vostok*. Clearly, unless you are the most determined and patient of travellers, there is no point in catching the *Vostok*. In retrospect I was relieved that I had no idea of the problems I was to encounter in Khabarovsk.

In 1972 Trains No. 1 and 2 ran a First Class only service known as the *Rossiya* – the Russians and Chinese had organised this weekly service so that the Chinese didn't have to change to get to Peking. Both these services were far superior in comfort and restaurant facilities than the normal 'hard' and 'soft' class trains. Mistakenly, in much of the talk about the Trans-Siberian, the *Rossiya* is thought to be the everyday train.

My guide, who accompanied me to the station, couldn't have been more helpful and considerate and was well aware of the problems that arose. I felt genuinely sorry for her because I couldn't help wondering how much of the stock-in-trade Soviet propaganda and the Soviet version of history a young person like her really believed. How much did she know about Stalin, about the Gulags, about the political trials of the late 1930s? I didn't have the courage to ask.

The train was already half an hour late and I was repeatedly looking at the station clock; it showed Moscow time whereas my wristwatch was local time. All timetables and clocks at airports, railway and bus stations use Moscow time but this did not apply if your journey was local. Yet what counted as local time in a country so vast? It was all rather a pain in the neck and something I could have done without – after all, how far out of Khabarovsk did 'local' apply, ten miles or a hundred?

My guide began to worry that my booked compartment might not have been booked on the correct train – this really worried me too.

"Perhaps the train we're waiting for may be only for Russians."

Of course at the time I had no idea this could be a possibility.

The platform was crowded with young soldiers going home for New Year's leave and there was an air of expectancy with much shouting and laughter filling the station. At last the long dark-green train arrived, sixteen coaches pulled by two large diesels which were immediately replaced by steam. Within seconds of Train No. 1 stopping and before the waiting soldiers could climb aboard, hundreds of sailors jumped off to create utter bedlam.

With great relief and a broad smile my guide found my two-berth compartment, soft-class. I asked her about food and she assured me that it wouldn't be a problem as there was bound to be a good restaurant car on the Trans-Siberian. We said our goodbyes and I looked around my compartment. I was pleased to find I had no companion and spread my stuff around. My passport and ticket were scrutinised and one of the conductresses (there were two to each coach) showed me the boiling samovars at each end of the corridors, plus sugar and tea. All the windows and exit doors were locked and the conductresses had the keys. The train started without warning and soon we were crossing the Amur, slowly progressing onto the longest girder bridge imaginable, and along the Chinese border.

Time to stretch and find the restaurant car. The corridors were perishingly cold with a frightful wind blowing through the ill-fitting connecting doors. Snow blowing through the rickety connection between coaches turned to ice and lay on the floor of the corridors. My heart sank on reaching the restaurant car – it was small and packed with soldiers and a few remaining sailors. The radio blared, everyone was drinking and smoking and shouting and chaos reigned. All I could do was return to my compartment, stumbling over the piles of coke and wood that half blocked each end of the coach. By this time a couple of coaches were full of fumes as the conductresses stoked the boilers. What a contrast to the Bullet Express between Osaka and Tokyo.

By early evening I was really hungry so, bundled up in my overcoat and scarf and gloves, I returned to the restaurant. What a pleasant surprise – it was less than half full and I could actually see half a dozen tables and two waiters. A young fellow asked if he could join me. He was a civilian travelling to Ulan-Ude, the town where the Trans-Siberian and the Moscow-Peking Chinese service part company. He explained that the restaurant had already run out of beer but vodka, tea and coffee were still available and – yes, there was a little wine too. I thumbed through the seven-page grandly set-out menu with the aid of my dictionary and my fellow traveller who was smiling and trying to explain something. The waiter turned up and as I leafed through the pages and pointed to some mouth-watering item the answer was always '*nyet*'. My companion ordered borscht, a scraggy chicken leg, potatoes, cabbage and some dessert; I followed suit. Eventually he managed to explain that in spite of nothing being crossed off the menu, only one thing was available. At this time it was common practice throughout the country, an absurd game between customers and waiters/waitresses creating the illusion that all was well.

On the first night a terrific noise woke me. The train had stopped and it transpired that empty buckets were being thrown from each coach onto the platform whilst a tractor and trailer progressed slowly along the platform with full buckets of coke. These were taken on board by the conductresses and emptied into the storage areas; the dust in the morning was unimaginable.

On returning to the restaurant car in the morning I found it semi-closed, the only food it supplied being black bread, hard stale cheese and the inimitable Russian garlic sausage, quite revoltingly fatty. However, all was not lost as twice a day a large, friendly peasant woman brought round steaming hot borscht served into army billy-cans, plus bread, stale cheese and sausages. I couldn't decide if this was an arrangement with the restaurant or an example of free market enterprise. Whatever it was I was really grateful, as I was too for the inexhaustible supply of hot sweet tea from the friendly samovars. I jumped out at most stations during daylight hours hoping to find food to buy, but with no luck; perhaps in the spring and summer small market stalls would have been on the platforms.

I felt fairly well prepared for two and a half days and three nights on the train – a pack of cards, a travelling chess and draughts set, and *War and Peace*, having only read about a third whilst in Japan.

To the south and west a range of mountains separated us from Manchuria and Mongolia and initially the countryside close to the train was flat and treeless. It was often difficult to distinguish roads and rivers as a thin layer of snow covered everything. There was hardly a village and certainly no town at which the train didn't stop – forty-five between Khabarovsk and Irkutsk, a distance of 1,500 miles. The little villages contrasted well against the drabness of the towns. They were mostly the traditional *izbas*, each with a wooden fence enclosing a garden, painted in the usual ochre or bright blue or green, the domestic scene completed by a bulb or paraffin lamp showing behind the neat lace curtains. I felt I could almost smell the reassuring smoke issuing from every chimney.

On this particular cloudless, windless Monday morning, each home had washing hanging on the line, this being the traditional day to do the washing the world over before the obsession for using a washing machine every day, or even more often, had affected the United States and the well-off in the rest of the world. It was somehow heartening to see this and I could imagine every piece of washing being brought in freeze-dried by the winter sun. Country folk were much the same the world over at that time and lived a simple life close to the natural world, something denied to urban dwellers.

Sometimes a tract of half-tarmacked road would cross the rail-track, disappearing on both sides into nothingness. Sledges pulled by horses, Alsatians, husky-type dogs or human beings, were the only transport except for the very occasional tractor. The only cars were in towns such as Chita or Ulan-Ude where new high-rise blocks of flats created the usual monotonous scene. Most people when we stopped at stations long enough for me to observe them looked well, and were well-clothed. This was a surprise as their lives were very hard.

Throughout the second day we seemed to be slowly climbing – endless vistas of fir and pine-clad hills and many small woods of birch and silver birch. The sun, shining from a cloudless blue sky through snow-covered branches created an enchanting scene. Contrary to what I had anticipated – absurdly I had imagined the railway line would be almost straight – the train twisted and curled its way as the terrain became more hilly and the valleys deeper, and wide rivers had to be crossed. Throughout this infinite snow-covered landscape I saw very little wildlife, just rooks and crows, ravens and magpies, and of course lots of *lbjs* (little brown jobs): unexpectedly no birds of prey.

To be able to watch from the comfort of my compartment this massive, powerful steam locomotive hauling the train with its sixteen coaches to the top of the next gradient was like a boyhood dream for me: smoke billowing, steam hissing, sparks flying around and dying in the snow as they landed, and in the opposite direction goods trains with over sixty wagons as well as the Trans-Siberian and other passenger trains adding to the wonder of it all.

On the third night we followed the southern shore of the famous Lake Baikal before descending slowly in the darkness of early morning along a pleasant wooded valley into the outskirts of Irkutsk, the capital of Eastern Siberia. On one side a dense mist was rising from the near-frozen river Angara.

Snow on the platform and the streets outside and a biting wind, yes, this was Siberia. A soldier in the next compartment kindly helped me with my heavy luggage – two large suitcases and two substantial holdalls with much of the space taken up by precious (to me at least) notes and information about the Japanese health service.

Even at this early hour the station was teeming with people. The central foyer was dimly lit and packed with families lying on the floor or on benches wrapped in coats, wearing every type of hat, mostly with ear muffs, and covered with blankets and rugs or anything else they could find to help keep warm. Their luggage was just bundles wrapped in brown paper and tied up with string, black plastic bags, and the better off with well-used carrier bags and the occasional suitcase. It was almost silent, just a few low murmurs and every now and then a baby crying or a small toddler shouting. The dirty, poorly-lit bulbs hanging from the ceiling made me wonder how they could put up with this dreadful squalor – after all, they weren't in the middle of a revolution or at war. Those who were not lying around hoping to sleep were stamping their feet and swinging their arms or struggling to get somewhere – I joined them.

I never saw a single trolley at any train or bus station, only at Sheremetyevo International Airport in Moscow, but at least my luggage didn't cry or shout or argue. What it must have been like struggling with a baby or a small child or argumentative teenager I couldn't imagine: a total nightmare I suspect.

Whilst looking in vain for an Intourist office I eventually found a queue for taxis and a woman in the queue told me the name of the Intourist hotel – not bad considering she spoke no English. About seven or eight people were waiting ahead of me in the queue. After a few minutes I realised that the few taxis there were had gathered about fifty yards further up the street. It was perishingly cold and I was regretting my clothing which was more suited to a Japanese autumn than a Siberian winter. Interestingly quite a few of the locals thought the same for as they walked past they remonstrated and pointed at my shoes and coat and in particular my uncovered ears.

I have usually found ordinary folk in most countries to be friendly. They try to be helpful, and Russians were no exception, particularly on this freezing morning. After about twenty minutes, to my astonishment a truly enormous woman with the almost statutory steel front tooth, whom I had seen serving hot tea from a kiosk, strode towards me and waited for the next taxi. She shouted at the driver much to his confusion and then pulled me across to the taxi and started banging on his window. She pointed at my coat, ears and shoes, opened the door, got me inside, picked up my two heavy cases and pushed them onto the floor. The whole thing was just bizarre and I wanted to hug her but my arms wouldn't have stretched even halfway round. All I could do was shout out of the window *'spahsseebah, spahsseebah, spahsseebah!'*

The Hotel Angara was a modern building looking rather second-class. A stony-faced receptionist, a lift which threatened not to reach the required floor, and the ever-present *dezharnaya,* who never smiled, confirmed my impression. The receptionist eventually gave the key to the hall porter and we went along to my room. He was clearly dissatisfied with my tip in spite of the fact he had been carrying the two lightest pieces of luggage.

Not a good beginning but I thankfully shut the door. After the smoke and dirt of the train all I wanted was a bath. But it was not to be, only a shower. This was a bent metal pipe with a garden watering can-type nozzle that never produced more than a trickle, even if I was using both hot and cold handles together. A single rusty tap above a small basin without a plug was no better and a cracked lavatory with a few *Izvestia* and *Pravda* (Russian political newspapers) for wiping completed the amenities. It was well over an hour before I managed to wash and shave without a mirror.

The restaurant was like a canteen; six waitresses were sitting at a table. Their heads didn't turn and neither did their eyes flicker as I sat down – they simply carried on talking and listening to a gramophone in the corner of the room. It repeatedly became stuck in the groove, much to their irritation, forcing one of them to get off her backside to adjust it. Finally another came across with a menu and showed me what was available – at least there was none of the nonsense I had experienced on the Trans-Siberian.

The Department of Public Health contacted me and apologised for not meeting me. They explained that the Intourist guide had been at the station in plenty of time but had been told the train was late et al – enough of the excuses, what had been arranged for the afternoon, I enquired – apparently a visit to a *feldscher* training school. I explained that I had already discussed *feldscher* training and wanted to see them at their place of work. More delays ensued, but at least the Regional Health Authority was contacted and later:

> "Yes, arrangements will be made. You will be picked up early in the morning."

All I could do was hope and meanwhile have a wander around Irkutsk.

The hotel stood on the edge of Kirov Square, the centre of the city. The main building, the House of Soviets or Headquarters of the Party, had been built in the 1930s on the site of Kazan Cathedral which had been demolished. There were three churches close by. The red brick Polish cathedral built in the nineteenth century by exiled aristocrats and intellectuals was now closed and starting to be used as a film studio. The Spasskaya church, about two hundred years old, was also closed and being converted into a museum. The third was falling down and hardly recognisable as a church, being a bakery.

It was early afternoon, the wind had miraculously dropped and it didn't feel so cold. The lowest temperature I experienced was -36°C and I was surprised it was that cold. A doctor who had worked on the building of the Bratsk hydro-electric scheme on the Angara said temperatures reached -60°C but caused few problems for the workers because there was no wind or damp. Much more trouble was experienced in the summer with mosquitoes and midges. He had been brought up in Leningrad where the temperature rarely fell below -10°C but it was always windy and damp and much more unpleasant than his time at Bratsk. Another surprise was how little snow there was around Irkutsk, but Eastern Siberia is one of the driest areas of the USSR both in summer and winter.

The Angara was awe-inspiring and the flow staggering. Lake Baikal is 390 miles long and in places 50 miles wide with more than 300 rivers flowing into it, but only the Angara flowing out. No wonder the Angara is the only river that never completely freezes over. In Irkutsk about a hundred yards into the middle of the river was a raging torrent with a thick cloud of mist rising from it. It was impossible to judge the thickness of the ice on either side of this explosion of water. The noise was frightening and the ground vibrated under my feet. Dramatic and breathtaking is a quite inadequate description.

The bright sunshine added to the pleasant atmosphere of the city with its wide tree-lined streets, its parks and gardens and buildings from the late-nineteenth and early-twentieth century still standing. Of course the usual post-Second World War blocks of flats extended to the outskirts of the city. I was able to stand in the middle of Karl Marx street as there was so little traffic about; all I could hear was the crunch crunch crunch of pedestrians.

Two-storey wooden houses with their carved windows, door frames and balconies were a reminder of times past – the merchant houses of Turgenev and Chekhov. Traditional *izbas* could be seen in the side streets and everything seemed very different from

Khabarovsk where destroying the past seemed to be the policy of the authorities. Traditionally known throughout the nineteenth century as a place of political exiles, the historic feel of the city was powerful. In addition it had been one of the main trading posts between China and Western Russia and the present day commercial area was still active.

Seven or eight orthodox churches were still standing although I only found one open for religious services, and interestingly it was not just the elderly wandering in and out; neither were the beggars and drunks pestering people. Krestovskaya church with its golden domes looked perfect against the cold blue sky.

Medically speaking the three days spent in Irkutsk proved to be the most useful of all the time I spent in the USSR. Dr Boris Problinkov, Deputy Director of the Regional Health Service and Dr Valentina Litvinova, Director of the District Rural Health Service, along with my Intourist interpreter, were a great trio. Problinkov and Litvinova had read my requests carefully and converted them into action.

A rural hospital and a *feldscher*/midwife post were on the agenda for the day. Urik village, about thirty miles from Irkutsk, was not an easy drive on a steeply cambered road at -30°C. The fifty-bed hospital was large for the size of the community it had to serve, a population of about 6,000. About half the beds were occupied and I was assured that normally it would have been filled, although such a claim was manifestly absurd. In addition to medical, gynaecological, obstetric and paediatric wards, a polyclinic/outpatients faculty was attached. An interesting statistic for 1971 was twenty-four births and thirty abortions, confirming what I had been told so many times.

Whilst we were talking in the patient waiting area of the polyclinic I had noticed a young woman and child sitting quietly and patiently. Suddenly she crossed over to us and asked if I was an English delegation. I replied that I wasn't a delegation but yes I was British. She explained she taught English and French in the local village school and wanted to practise her English. She was quiet and impressive and I just couldn't imagine any rural primary school teacher in Britain teaching French and Russian. She asked how foreign languages were taught in Britain. I managed to sidetrack this as I was too embarrassed to tell her the truth; I continued talking so that at least she was practising her English.

After the doctor had seen and examined the teacher's daughter she informed us it was time to eat. She was a happy homely middle-aged lady with two grown-up sons who worked in Irkutsk, and a daughter aged ten; there was no mention of a husband. She had worked in the rural service for twenty-five years and in this hospital for fifteen years. I asked her if she missed city life. Her response was 'Good gracious no'. The thought of going into Irkutsk filled her with horror because it was so busy.

Lunch was in the Director's room – Siberian soup, meatballs and black bread, with champagne for the ladies and vodka for the men. Wonderfully, no toasts. As we all sat down, including a couple of nurses, I could see through a window our driver sitting in the car with the engine running. I have always enjoyed making societies that consider themselves strongly egalitarian feel guilty so casually I asked where our driver was going to eat. There was general consternation and after attempting to explain why he was sitting outside at -30°C he came in and joined us. Utterly confused to be eating with the medical staff he looked rather uncomfortable, but it didn't stop him from eating as much as he could as well as enjoying the unrestricted vodka.

The alcohol loosened everyone's tongue. We chatted about politics, in particular Northern Ireland. All of them were very pro-IRA and greatly influenced by what they saw and heard on their televisions. They wanted to know my hopes and fears, my likes and dislikes – it was very hard for my interpreter but the atmosphere remained relaxed and friendly. As we prepared to leave a little conversation took place:

"Have you heard of the Decembrists?
"Yes"
"Would you like to see their graves?"
"Yes I would."

With considerable difficulty we walked towards a stone-built orthodox church, passing on the way beautifully carved and decorated peasant *izbas* – I couldn't believe my good fortune. A few villagers were out and about, bent old men struggling with their sledges, and two horse-drawn wooden wagons with their wheels replaced by wooden skis. Unfortunately it was too cold to linger but long enough to find the stone memorial to some young cavalry officers from St Petersburg, and to aristocrats and intellectuals thought to be from Moscow. The burials took place in the late 1820s but I forgot to ask when the memorial was built and by whom.

The *feldscher*/midwife post was in the village of Smolenskina about seven miles from Irkutsk, but unfortunately in the opposite direction to Urik; the journey was more than nerve-racking with a driver full of vodka, and Problinkov repeatedly had to ask him to slow down.

The post was run by two splendid women who had worked in Smolenskina for sixteen years, knew everyone in the village and much more besides. They had an excellent rapport with the patients, but above all, according to the patients I spoke to, the continuity of care they provided was particularly valued. On average twenty patients a day would be seen as well as two or three home visits carried out – on the previous day they had done six. As all deliveries took place in Irkutsk they were only involved in ante-natal care and the obligatory post-natal visits to the mother's home; much of the work concerned prophylaxis and health education.

It had been a great day. I had been able to gain an understanding of the value – and sometimes the limitations – of the medical care being provided by personnel not qualified as doctors. It was clear that the success of the *feldschers* in rural areas depended on the support and supervision provided by the local rural hospital, although if Urik and Smolenskina hospitals were anything to go by the numbers of beds and staff could have been reduced by half and the money saved used in a different way. As usual no one mentioned, thought or worried about costs.

It is the intention of the Soviet Health Service to eliminate the *feldschers*, apart from in very remote areas, as quickly as possible as it is felt they represent everything that is backward and out of date. Even though they are considered by many patients to be one of the most valued and successful health workers, the bureaucrats refuse to listen. A few health workers agree with the patients and think that with better training the *feldscher* could flourish, and I would certainly agree with this opinion.

On returning to the Regional Health offices, the Flying Doctor Service of Siberia and the Soviet Far East was outlined; fifteen main centres associated with the main urban areas provide the service and each main centre is responsible for smaller facilities – all straightforward and uncomplicated. All personnel have further accident and emergency training with additional study on the effects of long polar nights and the intense cold. It was a great surprise to find how little they knew about the Australian Flying Doctor Service, which emphasises how cut off they were from the outside world.

A fascinating day concluded with Problinkov presenting me with a handsome piece of Siberian agate/quartz 'as a memory of wonderful Siberia'. It was rather embarrassing; I felt the roles should have been reversed and wished I had something to give to the trio with my sincere thanks.

The next day two industrial polyclinics gave me some idea of how privileged groups got special care – not surprising even in an egalitarian society. Polyclinic No. 3 was restricted to scientists and the staffs of institutes of research and colleges of higher education, a small population of roughly 7,500 who were covered by six *uchastok* therapists, and twenty specialists alongside the usual diagnostic departments. An average of twenty home visits per day were carried out by the therapists and nearly thirty by qualified nurses.

Polyclinic No. 1 supported a population of 40,000 working in heavy industry, light engineering and plastics. Fourteen *uchastok* therapists looked after about five times the number of patients; in other words, one group of *uchastok* therapists cared for roughly 1,250 patients while the others were responsible for 2,860. Interestingly, home visits were rarely carried out. Both No. 3 and No. 1 polyclinics provided better care compared with a normal polyclinic..

By the end of the day it had been admitted that other groups such as coal miners, railway workers and sportsmen had even better arrangements. It was then agreed that the most privileged of all were the high-ranking military and their families, politburo and the senior politicians throughout the country. No one disputed that the general public were angry about this disparity and thought it was simply unfair.

In the hotel a leaflet with an English translation caught my eye; it concerned the Irkutsk Symphony Orchestra and a coming concert.

On enquiry it transpired that during the winter months conductors from the main orchestras in Moscow and Leningrad toured the country to provide tuition to local orchestras, after which they conducted a concert. It seemed an interesting idea but I couldn't get a ticket, so I was told to simply turn up. On arrival a solid mass of people were standing outside the concert hall with snow falling and impatience rising. The holdup was caused by everyone having to divest themselves of their hats, scarves, gloves and overcoats in a totally inadequate vestibule – the chaos involved in collecting your stuff afterwards can only be imagined. No one was allowed into the hall unless partially undressed. I managed to get a ticket although I forget how, perhaps from a vestibule attendant. Mercifully the concert started nearly half an hour late.

An excited audience, young and old, poorly dressed or still in working clothes, filled the auditorium, even sitting on the steps of the aisles. A Mozart overture, a violin concerto with a young Czech violinist, and a Rachmaninov symphony were conducted by the conductor of the Leningrad Symphony Orchestra, a fierce-looking man with closely-cropped black hair (unfashionable in those days) and an upright stance. The audience were most attentive and wildly enthusiastic.

Walking back to the hotel through the barely lit streets with snow falling more heavily and only the occasional bus or taxi, a provincial atmosphere prevailed, reinforced by barking dogs and smoke rising slowly and almost vertically into the windless black sky. The newest of new moons illuminated nothing and the curtains, often just blankets or rugs, hid the occupants of these humble homes. The silent darkness allowed me to ponder on this remarkable evening; I couldn't imagine the conductors of the London Symphony, the BBC Symphony, the Hallé or the Scottish National orchestras providing a similar 'winter tour' to Plymouth, Carlisle or Inverness.

At my final meeting in the Regional Health office with Problinkov I was able to clear up a couple of queries. But most of all I wanted to thank him and all his colleagues for the excellent three days they had given me. As we parted he suggested there might be a problem at the airport due to the weather overnight and the heavy snow now falling and freezing hard. Certainly the drive to the airport was slow and somewhat nerve-racking.

At the airport I was told the flight to Novosibirsk had been delayed by eight hours, then delayed indefinitely, then it had taken off from Khabarovsk, then finally the airport at Novosibirsk was closed but I might be able to fly the following day when Irkutsk re-opened.

"Could I please go back to the hotel?
"Nyet"
"Could I change flights and go to Moscow?"
"Nyet"

The information was supplied by an impenetrable Aeroflot official; as yet I had still not understood the futility not to say stupidity of asking questions; it didn't dawn on me until I noticed that the locals rarely asked questions and nobody seemed to get impatient or angry unless they were drunk. There were two Russians on my flight who spoke a little English so I asked them:

"What do you think about the delay and when do you think we'll depart?"

Not even a reply, just a shrug of the shoulders. Really it was so much less hassle not to ask because the locals know that nobody knows anything including the officials so the only response to questions is a shrug or upturned hands – best just to keep quiet.

I had been put in a small room kept separate for foreigners and again I was the only one. After half an hour or so I decided to wander around. The room was on the first floor and looking over the balcony I could see my luggage, which was easy to spot as one of my cases was of green metal with a leather strap tied tightly round it. There was no other luggage, which I found strange – and worrying.

By mistake and by chance I walked into the Aeroflot staff area where cabin crews and pilots were sitting around half a dozen small tables drinking beer and vodka. Included in this group were three older men all showing four gold rings on their sleeves – senior pilots I presumed. None was visibly drunk but most were the worse for wear so I really hoped my flight would be delayed for another six hours by which time, hopefully, they would be sober.

The Aeroflot official was waiting for my return.

"Where have you been? Why did you leave the room without

permission? Your flight is to leave in fifteen minutes."

As we passed the balcony I stopped to point out my luggage which was still on the floor. By this time an Intourist interpreter had arrived and I told her I wouldn't get on the plane unless Aeroflot guaranteed my luggage would be on my flight. The Aeroflot official promised it would be moved, and although I continued to ask repeatedly about it as I walked across the tarmac I eventually accepted it was futile to argue any more. Many soldiers were standing around in the freezing weather and I was told to hurry up as they had been waiting for the bl — dy foreigner who couldn't be found. As I was climbing into the plane I found I was on a different flight which was already half full of the Red Army which had been allowed on board ahead of the bl — dy foreigner. From my point of view it had not only been a total shambles but I also realised I was now in real trouble. By take-off the Ilyushin 18 was packed, not as bad as Tashkent to Yerevan, but standing room only and every available space filled with army rucksacks and equipment – no concern about weight or anything else. At least there were no animals or primuses for cooking.

My luggage was not on the plane. It was now early on Wednesday morning and I was due to leave Moscow for London on Saturday. The heavy snow and the strong wind which was causing much drifting added to my anxiety as to whether Novosibirsk airport would be closed.

The hotel was in the centre of the city just off Lenin Square. My room had a bath and the restaurant had food, which was all a great improvement as was the help I received from the receptionist. I explained my problem with the luggage and she immediately contacted Intourist; within an hour a representative had arrived. Olga contacted Aeroflot and was given the run-around.

"It has been sent to Khabarovsk – "
"It has been sent to Sverdlovsk – "
"It has been sent to Krasnoysvsk – "

I asked to speak:

"Why the hell hasn't it been sent to Novosibirsk or Moscow?"

The response:

"Don't you realise how difficult it is at this time of year?"

Olga decided to take me to the Intourist main office to meet two of her colleagues. By this time I could think of nothing else but my luggage and the certainty that once I had left Russian soil my luggage would be lost forever and it would be impossible to write the report on Japan for the Nuffield Foundation.

The three Intourist girls continued to try and help. They telegraphed Aeroflot in Irkutsk and Sverdlovsk but had no response. I wondered why they couldn't phone, but it seems it was not permitted even though I offered to pay – such were the rules and regulations. Olga in particular remained sympathetic, but their oft-repeated 'everything will be alright' merely increased my doubts.

Suddenly they decided to take me to Akademgorodok as a sort of occupational therapy for me and a break for themselves as they were at their wits' end knowing what to do with me. Novosibirsk had been built in the late nineteenth century and was now the largest city in Siberia. It couldn't boast any building of much interest and had been taken over by Akademgorodok, or Academy City, created following the 20th Party Congress in 1956. It was to be the centre of scientific research as well as being the focus of planning for the future development of Siberia. Situated about twenty miles outside Novosibirsk it had been literally hacked out of the Siberian forest.

Largely hidden amongst the trees, the buildings and the residential areas were better constructed and more attractively laid out than anything I'd seen before. The homes of the chief academicians, technocrats and such-like were substantial and well-hidden, rather like the Party hierarchy. Neither the Intourist girls or anyone else I met thought this was unfair, nor the considerable difference in wages for those in Academy City – 800 roubles or more per month compared with 70 - 80 for the average worker.

Back in Novosibirsk it was suggested I might like to go shopping whilst they continued their efforts on my behalf. They stipulated I must try to return within the hour. This instruction intrigued me and I subsequently found out I was the first Englishman they had met and they wanted to listen to me speaking as I was easy to understand! The occasional Australian, New Zealander and American passed through but they spoke so differently – 'not like English on our gramophone records'. I was surprised and slightly flattered, but forty years later

I can't imagine the next generation of Intourist guides would care a damn or notice any difference.

The snow continued falling as I meandered rather aimlessly thinking of little else other than my luggage. Then two things interrupted my obsessive thoughts. A small bookshop caught my eye; it was simple inside, small and warmed by a paraffin stove. The owner was friendly and spoke and understood English. It was like a good second-hand bookshop in Britain. There were a number of British authors on a couple of shelves – Greene, Dickens, Galsworthy, Burns, Scott and others, but no Shakespeare as far as I remember, and a number of books by Russian authors had been translated into English. I didn't have much time, but as I was leaving I spotted a book of poetry by Ho Chi Minh entitled *Prison Diary*. It was the translated poems of the late President of North Vietnam describing his capture and imprisonment by Chiang Kai-Shek's forces in August 1942. It seemed a little off-beat, particularly in the middle of Siberia, but I bought it.

As I left the shop a wonderful aroma of *shashlik* wafted down the street. Following the glorious smell I rounded a corner to find a bit of open wasteland where two Uzbeks from Tashkent wearing full Uzbek dress were standing in the snow gently turning skewers of sizzling meat. A crowd of locals had gathered to enjoy the warmth and bargain over the *shashliks*. I just paid and enjoyed this almost unbelievable occasion.

Back at the Intourist office there was still no news of my luggage although I received confirmation my flight to Moscow was due to arrive on time. A few hours remained and the girls decided they would take me to the pictures to keep me calm. The four of us set off. The film was a light-hearted, apolitical, rather garish musical with the hero an obvious heart-throb. Olga and one of her colleagues must have irritated the people sitting close to us as they tried, quite unsuccessfully, to explain the jokes.

As we trudged back to their office they talked and asked questions non-stop and I felt rather pleased that I might be helping them. Still no news however, so Olga and I walked back to the hotel to collect my bag and pay the bill. Just as we arrived her colleague rang to say the flight was leaving in forty minutes. If this was true I couldn't possibly catch it as the airport was ten miles out of town and the roads were icy and badly rutted following a dramatic drop in temperature. We arrived an hour late and were calmly told the flight was not now leaving until 8pm (Moscow time) or midnight (Novosibirsk time) arriving in Moscow at 2am (6am Novosibirsk time).

Olga was a little emotional as we parted company; she gave me her address and asked me to write and let her know how things had gone and to keep in contact. I had understood that Intourist personnel, unless ordered to behave differently, were expected to remain distant from their customers and if it was discovered I was writing to Olga I wondered if she would get into trouble. But presumably she knew what she was doing.

I was determined not to go back to the Hotel Ukraina or get booked into the rather grim Hotel Metropole in the centre of Moscow, and happily the Intourist office in Novosibirsk had booked me into the National. Built at the end of the 19th century on the corner of Prospekt Marksa and Gorky Street on the edge of the huge Manezhnaya Square overlooked by the walls of the Kremlin, it had a wonderful fin de siècle feel about it. The interior had retained a bygone elegance and grandeur. My room was large, had a bath with a plug and both hot and cold water and, as I was quickly to find out, a really helpful Intourist bureau.

I explained the problem of my missing luggage and following a number of phone calls by these attentive women they were able to tell me that it had reached Novosibirsk – they had no idea where it had come from but it should be in Moscow by the evening. Too good to be true and so it proved to be.

In the early evening I was watching the television foreign news which was largely focused on Northern Ireland. The UK was portrayed as an imperialist power indifferent to the sufferings of its own citizens. The footage was routine with a series of photographs: two fully-armed British soldiers aggressively patrolling a deserted, rain-drenched, wind-swept street - cut; a group of Catholic residents – men, women and children, chatting on a poor run-down housing estate – cut; two bodies, a mother and child lying dead in a pool of blood – cut; two fully-armed soldiers walking away from the camera – cut; only one conclusion was possible for the average Soviet viewer.

Just as the tv news came to an end the phone rang: bad news, my luggage had been sent to Krasnoyarsk in the Urals. The good lady could give no reason, no explanation, and was extremely embarrassed. The bureau was closing but to my amazement she promised to phone me around midnight from her flat as soon as the flight from Krasnoyarsk had arrived.

"I'm sorry your luggage hasn't arrived."

She did her best to reassure me it would arrive on the next flight in the morning.

"Anyway I promise to phone you."

Around 8am the phone rang:

"Your luggage has arrived and I'll make sure it gets to the hotel before you leave."

There was about three hours before I had to set off for the airport and if it were to arrive I felt I could again believe in miracles. It was a close-run thing.

Whilst waiting on the tarmac at Sheremetyevo airport two unconnected thoughts crossed my mind: how odd it was that after these two visits I hadn't seen Leningrad, the 'Venice of the North' which according to Baedeker and many others was 'one of Europe's most beautiful cities' and to most westerners the most sought after tourist attraction in the Soviet Union. Even stranger had I but known, it would be another nineteen years before my wife and I would arrive in Leningrad on 9 September 1991, the day the city was again renamed St Petersburg.

Airborne at last, I thumbed through my passport and realised it hadn't been stamped; there was no evidence I had visited the USSR. I recalled now that it was the visa which got stamped, the USSR being the only country to issue the visa as a separate document, which they then retained. Presumably it must be in a file marked W J STEPHEN on Dr Eristavis's desk at the International Relations Department at the Ministry of Health in Moscow. What a mysterious country.

*

In February 1973 I received a letter from Olga. I had written as requested and sent *A Concise Oxford Dictionary* which incredibly had arrived without the parcel being opened. She wrote:

> "I am very glad everything finished happily. Now I can tell you frankly I was almost sure that you wouldn't get your luggage in Moscow because the day before you were leaving the USSR it was somewhere far from Moscow and as you remember the weather was bad to fly. Your trip in our country was like a tale with a happy ending. Usually such a tale finish 'All is well that ends well' . . . This (dictionary) is just what I dreamt of. I never expected to get such a wonderful dictionary! Beside it was delivered as a letter and I paid nothing for it!!!'

Olga asked me to write again and I did so a number of times over eighteen months but heard nothing further.

11

ASIA

The fall of the Berlin Wall in November 1989 followed by the Declaration of Independence by the countries of Central and Eastern Europe, the Baltic States, Armenia and Georgia, finally led to the collapse of the Soviet Union on the last day of December 1991 and the formation of the Commonwealth of Independent States (CIS) – the ten former Republics of Azerbaijan, Belarus, Kazakhstan, Kyrgyzstan, Moldova, Russia, Tajikistan, Turkmenistan, Ukraine and Uzbekistan becoming independent countries.

Almost overnight the unknown names of the former republics of the USSR along its southern border forced many of us to search for our atlas. Kazakhstan, the largest of these countries, bar Russia, stretches nearly 1,900 miles from the Caspian Sea in the west to China and Mongolia in the east. Its borders are protected in the south by Turkmenistan, Afghanistan, Uzbekistan, Tajikistan and finally Kyrgyzstan in the Tien Shan range of mountains adjacent to the north-west corner of China and Mongolia. To the north just one country, the Russian Federal Republic, extends along the entire frontier. All these countries have their separate and distinct languages, culture and customs as well as a variety of religious beliefs.

It had been my intention to coordinate visits to Kazakhstan and Mongolia, but this proved to be impossible. With regard to Kazakhstan I was interested to find out what changes, if any, had taken place since my previous visits to the former Soviet Union some twenty years earlier.

Mongolia had remained a largely unknown land which for many years had been sandwiched between China and the USSR, but in the late 1980s and early '90s I was intrigued by positive whispers in the UK about its health service and I wanted to find out if they were true.

12

REPUBLIC of KAZAKHSTAN

I was staying in Moscow with our friends Ali and Valentina. It was exactly a year since Rachel and I had been staying with them just before the breakup of the Soviet Union. At that time they and their friends had been moderately confident and optimistic about the future. Now, however, it was all gloom and doom with uncertainty about the economy, the political situation and, surprisingly, about the influence of a number of religious groups from the United States who were running three of the five television stations; everything was in a mess, they felt, and nothing worked. The recent hero Gorbachev was now blamed for everything.

Alma Ata, the capital of Kazakhstan, was difficult to reach by air and the most direct route was via Moscow. However, I had promised Rachel not to fly – since the collapse of the Soviet Union, Aeroflot's record had taken a knocking, particularly in relation to internal flights. The International Air Transport Association (IATA) was responsible for their international but not their internal domestic flights where maintenance and inspection was poor and sometimes non-existent. As a consequence the number of domestic crashes had significantly increased, the figures only representing the accidents that were officially reported. Hence the reason for being in Moscow.

The alternative was to go by train, but buying a ticket in the UK proved impossible as I was not able to book a seat and without a booked seat you were not allowed on the train. I had expected Gorbachev's glasnost and perestroika to have taken care of such bureaucracy ; how wrong I was. It took two days for Ali and Valentina and Samir, an Iraqi friend and refugee from Sadam Hussein, and others to beaver away on my behalf before the ticket problem was at least half-solved. The Moscow to Alma Ata ticket was fine, but they couldn't purchase the return ticket because my address in Alma Ata wasn't known. Regulations stipulated a ticket could be bought no sooner than ten days before departure and furthermore an address was needed so the ticket could be delivered to me by an Intourist agent from Tashkent (Uzbekistan) as there was no office in Alma Ata! To add to the difficulties, the Intourist Ticket Centre no longer sold train tickets and Samir was sent to another office which he couldn't find. There were no telephone directories in Moscow so he couldn't phone either. Eventually a friend of a friend of Valentina's found us the address, by which time Ali had joined Samir. This was how the first day of this bureaucratic nightmare unfolded. You couldn't have made it up.

I had a further plan for after my return from Kazakhstan, which was to visit a friend, Vladimir and his family, in Minsk on my way back to the UK via Prague. Vladimir had been in charge of a group of children on a visit to Wells following the Chernobyl disaster. The next day Ali and I discovered I couldn't buy a ticket direct from Moscow to Prague via Minsk (virtually a straight line) but would have to travel via Warsaw which would require a Polish transit visa taking at least two weeks to be issued. Air flights were very expensive in this part of the world and in the end Ali had to get me a return Moscow-Minsk-Moscow and Moscow-Prague direct, which he did while I was in Kazakhstan. Again, bureaucracy truly beyond belief.

Throughout my brief stay in Moscow, Ali and Valentina, Samir and their friends, did their best to dissuade me from taking the train – it would be difficult, it would be unreliable, it was dangerous particularly for foreigners as the trains were full of criminals, there would be little food and the toilets would be disgusting: by this time I was beginning to have doubts myself!

Ali and his son Omar helped me with my luggage on the Metro to Kazan station. The train was waiting – twenty-two coaches, half of which were sleepers. This was my first long-distance train journey since the Trans-Siberian. We left exactly on time at 6.30pm. It was Sunday and we were due to arrive in Alma Ata around 7am on Thursday, a total of three days and four nights. My companion in the first-class compartment (two berths) was a computer programmer in an engineering company in Saratov, a large industrial city on the Volga. He spoke little English and we simply enjoyed sharing food before settling down for the night.

The sheets and towel were clean, but Valentina's prediction of disgusting toilets was spot on. The lavatory and washbasin at the end of the corridor were dirty even before leaving Moscow. The basin of course had no plug and precious little water – no hot and only a trickle of cold, and the handle to turn the water on and off did not operate from side to side but by applying upward pressure. I was sure it had been designed by a dyslexic engineer. It certainly made shaving impossible and trying to wash was hardly worth the effort. By the time we reached Alma Ata the state of the lavatory can be imagined, with only a trickle of water even to flush. It was just filthy. Valentina was right, this aspect of the journey was grim. However, the ubiquitous samovars with a ready supply of sugar and tea and a constant supply of hot water made one feel almost civilised. The coal/coke bunkers were already full but as yet the stoves were not in use even though it was pretty cold at night.

Contrary to another of Valentina's predictions there was a restaurant car with basic food which, like the beer and vodka, was easily replenished at the next station. Twice a day, as on the Trans-Siberian, a peasant woman passed slowly up and down selling sweet pastries and biscuits, but no borsch or anything savoury. She was definitely not connected with the restaurant as I saw her purchasing her supplies from the many stations en route – a straightforward capitalist entrepreneur.

The railway was an integral part of every town and village and most stations looked like a local market, piled with salad and fruit as we passed through on a pleasant sunny autumn afternoon. Tables of bread, cheese and salami were laid out the length of the platform and the wonderful smell of cooking *shaslick*, meat and chicken filled the air. The platform seemed in fact to be one of the main streets in town, and sheep and goats, geese, ducks and hens wandered freely around. One of the most noticeable changes since 1971/72 was that smoking was now only permitted in the corridor at the end of each coach and this, plus the lure of the cooking, quickly emptied the train. Groups of old men, mostly smoking pipes, chatted and played draughts while everyone waiting for the next train to arrive. The whole scene mimicked descriptions by Turgenev, Chekhov and Tolstoy.

At the small village stations or stops where nobody seemed to get on or off I felt we were travelling through the world of Edward

Thomas and *Adlestrop*: the poem was written during the First World War and not published until after he had been killed in action at Arras in April 1917. Surely 'No one left and no one came' can only be a reference to those who did not return, and both the Russians and the British have a deep understanding of what he was writing about.

Yes. I remember Adlestrop -
The name, because one afternoon
Of heat the express-train drew up there
Unwontedly. It was late June.

The steam hissed. Someone cleared his throat.
No one left and no one came
On the bare platform. What I saw
Was Adlestrop - only the name

And willows, willow-herb, and grass,
And meadowsweet, and haycocks dry,
No whit less still and lonely fair
Than the high cloudlets in the sky.

And for that minute a blackbird sang
Close by, and round him, mistier,
Farther and farther, all the birds
Of Oxfordshire and Gloucestershire.

Three days gave me plenty of time to observe, but it wasn't until the second day I noticed the big difference between the railways of the former Soviet Union (FSU) and the UK. The great majority of workers were women, including drivers. Station masters were station mistresses, signalmen were signalwomen, the level crossings were manned by women and the majority of maintenance workers were women. Two or three times a day a platoon of women would slowly make their way along both sides of the train tapping the wheels with heavy hammers. They were formidable women resembling East German Olympic shot-putters, and likewise they would do the heavy lifting that was required on goods trains and at stations.

Size seemed to matter and it was impossible not to be aware of the length of the trains – passenger trains between 18 and 24 coaches, and goods trains between 50 and 60 trucks.

I often saw a great number of open wagons containing mostly

potatoes and cabbages standing in the sidings of many stations, just rotting in the rain or ruined by the blazing sun and never any sign they were going to be moved. There were also hundreds of rusting wagons and cattle trucks; presumably no one was in charge or willing to take responsibility. Seventy years of communism had certainly left its mark.

The people I met were the real interest of the journey. The computer expert got out at Saratov early on Monday morning whilst it was still dark. After the war the city had become part of the Soviet Military/Industrial complex and was a closed city. It was interesting that even in 1992 the train only stopped there when it was dark so that nothing could be seen on the hills on the far side of the Volga, which continued to be occupied by the military. I'm almost certain I would have needed a special visa had I wanted to get off the train there.

I was joined by a young man who had recently left the army and was really pleased to have finished his compulsory military service. Ethnically Russian, he and his family lived in Kazakhstan although he was now going to work in Ukraine. We were together for two nights – I enjoyed his beer and he enjoyed my cup-a-soup and Nescafé – and both evenings we drifted down to the restaurant car for stale bread and a lump of cheese.

Gradually as we approached Kazakhstan the steppe began, rocky barren scrubland and sandy stony desert. Every river or stream was barely flowing and was covered with an evil-looking grey sludge. If I had been on the train fifty years before, the track would have run along the edge of the Aral Sea, but today there was nothing but the dried-out seabed as far as the eye could see. Occasionally a few scattered houses and rusty boats would remind the traveller that the Aral Sea had once boasted both a thriving fishing industry employing thousands, and a small but successful agricultural sector. Some surviving reed beds were the only indication of where the shoreline had once been.

The diversion of the rivers Ama Darya and Syr Darya had reduced the size of the Aral Sea by more than eighty percent over the past thirty years, and the man-made ecological disaster had finally been admitted, and shamed the new generation of Russian scientists.

Beyond the Aral Sea as we travelled south the barren desert became even more bleak and grey, the monotony fortunately relieved by hundreds of camels wandering freely, unexpected flocks of magpies roosting like swallows on the telephone lines, and clusters of houses appearing in the middle of nowhere surrounded by gardens of colourful wild flowers and cultivated fields of cereals and vegetables. Water is very much the key to everything and I wondered if fifty to a hundred years ago travellers would have seen many more small villages with agriculture flourishing and colourful domestic gardens carefully tended.

As I stood in the corridor gazing out of the window or wandering up and down the train, the criminals my friends in Moscow had warned me about never appeared, and I never felt as though I was being watched or felt threatened in any way. However, if I'm honest I was pleased I was sharing the compartment with Russians. If my companion had been another westerner perhaps the story would have been different – foreigners were considered easy to attack and my friends in Moscow assured me they would! Thankfully I never found out.

The young man departed at Chimket, an industrial town in the south-west corner of Kazakhstan. By this time it was early Wednesday afternoon and another young man filled the vacant berth. He was a Kazakh, spoke no English and little Russian, but was friendly. We had settled down to slices of his large water melon and the cooked meat and bread I had just bought at the station, when a sound like a rifle shot rang out. The carriage window was shattered, covering both berths and the floor with glass. Amazingly neither of us was cut or even seriously scratched but it took a long while to pick out the slivers of glass from each other's hair and clothes. Within minutes the sun began to set and I realised how cold it was. The noise had been loud enough for the carriage attendants to appear and for a number of passengers to come and have a gawp. Being a foreigner was for once an advantage and within half an hour my luggage had been moved to another compartment. Its occupant was a young Russian woman in her late twenties who was obviously surprised and clearly annoyed to find I was to join her. Soon however the camaraderie of the long-distance train took over and we were sharing her food and my cup-a-soup and Nescafé; what a godsend they were proving to be.

To the casual observer Russian society appears – at least to the outsider – to be rather prim and proper, holding hands in public but little more, so mixed sleeping compartments on trains continued to be a surprise. I knew the bedtime routine so whilst I was waiting in the corridor I thought I might as well go and see how the young Kazakh was faring. Attempts had been made to block up the badly damaged window with cardboard, slats of wood and blankets, but it was totally ineffective. The young man, wearing all his clothes and wrapped in additional blankets was frozen and looked totally dejected. I felt genuinely sorry for him and was certain that had he been a foreigner another compartment would have been found. With difficulty I forced the reluctant sleeping car attendant to come and see how cold he was and a fellow passenger who understood a bit of English explained to the attendant I thought the young man should be moved. I soon realised it was a hopeless idea, but how I would like to have shaken that unhelpful and uninterested attendant who, needless to say, was warm as toast in her cubicle next to the samovar.

On getting back to my compartment the young lady was in her pyjamas and had made up my berth rather artistically with the sheet and blanket intertwined around the pillow. They really are an extraordinary people – they can be so rude and unpleasant in public but in private so different. The compartments on either side of us wanted to celebrate the last night so the six of us moved into one compartment to share the remaining food. I couldn't reciprocate, but the cup-a-soup and Nescafé again turned up trumps whilst the samovars provided as much hot water, tea and sugar as we wanted . . . and naturally no shortage of vodka.

It was early in the morning so few people were about and as I got off the train I was relieved to find two young ladies carrying a modest placard JOHN STEPHEN. Dr Sadykova, President of the Association of Physicians and Pharmacists of Kazakhstan, and an interpreter, took me to the Sanatorium Kazakhstan where I was to stay. Cardio-vascular disease was its main interest but employees of the Ministry of the Interior were also housed there – an extraordinary combination. As we were driving to the Sanatorium Dr Sadykova spoke rather sternly to me:

"You must behave. It will be full of secret police."

Quite what she thought I might be up to I don't know. I was

completely confused, although from a personal point of view I was delighted when Sadykova informed me that the cost of staying there would be less than half that charged by the cheapest hotels. In 1992 B & Bs were some years off.

Endeavouring to get my visa stamped confirmed I was still in the world of the Soviet Union. Sadykova and I visited three different police stations all of which refused to stamp it until at last Sadykova was told that the Association could do it themselves. Why life continued to be made so insanely nonsensical and complicated nobody was able to explain.

The first evening provided the final touch. After four nights on the train I needed a wash, preferably a bath; the shower unit was a shallow tiled area no more than six foot square with no curtain or glass to prevent the carpet getting wet. A watering can-type nozzle from which trickled a drizzle of barely warm water, plus of course no plug for the basin, and no lavatory paper, completed the picture. The light bulb was of such overwhelming dimness that reading was virtually impossible. I certainly didn't need reminding that the influence of the Soviet Union remained in Kazakhstan.

The Association of Physicians and Pharmacists had been founded in Moscow in 1990 and had spread in an inconsistent manner throughout the USSR. Following the break up in 1992, Kazakhstan decided to form its own association, quite separate and independent, under the Ministry of Health in Alma Ata.

The WHO Collaborating Centre had been set up in 1980 following the WHO/UNICEF International Conference on Primary Health Care held in Alma Ata in 1978. Primary health care was declared to be the key to achieving an acceptable level of health for the majority of the population, and it was from this conference that the famous slogan 'Health Care for All by the Year 2000' had rung around the world and been accepted by the vast majority of members of the WHO. Sadly the cynics and sceptics – some would say realists – have proved to be right – progress has been painfully slow.

By 1992 eight Collaborating Centres in Primary Health Care and fifteen Collaborating Centres on Nursing had been set up worldwide, but Alma Ata remained the only joint venture between the two disciplines. The purpose of the centre is to concentrate on research, training, the dissemination of information and the encouragement of collaboration within the health services of individual countries.

The Association of Physicians & Pharmacists organised my first week and the WHO Collaborating Centre the second. I couldn't quite decide how much collaboration there had been but the result was excellent.

There was no love lost between Dr Sadykova and Dr Karagulova the Deputy Director of the WHO Centre, a tension simmering below the surface. Again I couldn't decide whether this was simply a matter of nationality – Sadykova was Kazakh and Karagulova was Russian – or maybe it was just a female thing. Looking back I think it was mainly Kazakhs versus Russians as they equally made up eighty percent of the population, the remainder being Germans, Byelorussians, Ukrainians, Uzbeks, Turks and Azerbaijanis. Before Independence both Russian and Kazakh were spoken although less than ten percent of Russians spoke Kazakh, and it seemed as if the importance of the Kazakh language was now becoming a major issue; meanwhile the remaining twenty percent were making it clear they wished to speak their own languages and retain their own cultures.

In 1926 when Kazakhstan was incorporated into the USSR, the rural population had been virtually ignored and by the time of my visit virtually all Russians lived in towns and industrial centres whereas the majority of Kazakhs still worked in agriculture with its traditionally poor wages.

Since the fall of the Berlin Wall and the breakup of the FSU the history of the last seventy years was openly talked about and resentment about the Stalin era grew quickly. Pockets of industrialisation along its southern border combined with the exploitation of considerable mineral resources only profited the Russians. To the outside world Kazakhstan was the far-away country where Gulag camps had been built and to which hundreds of thousands, probably millions, from Eastern Europe, Byelorus, Ukraine and Caucasus had been deported and hidden away. It was as though Kazakhstan and not the USSR had been responsible for all the horror and financial rape of the country.

The organisation of primary care both in urban and rural areas was much the same as when I visited the USSR in 1971/72 and in my opinion it remained sound. This was an unfashionable view at the time and contrary to the views of many foreign advisers. Certainly the polyclinic had come in for some justifiable criticism over the years, not for its principles but for the way it was staffed, and especially for the poor training of doctors, but there was no reason to throw out the baby with the bathwater. En passant, it is worth mentioning that the polyclinic had a great deal in common with the *Dawson Report* (Lord Dawson of Penn) 1920, which is now acknowledged to have been one of the most visionary documents ever produced in the UK during the twentieth century relating to health care. In the ninety years since its publication a constant stream of articles, discussions and conferences have focused on the need to improve communication between primary and secondary care as well as highlighting the obvious advantage of providing both, as far as possible, within the same building. This is exactly what the polyclinics attempt to do.

Visits to polyclinics, women's consultative clinics, *feldscher*/midwife posts, an emergency call centre, regional, district and rural hospitals, a regional diagnostic centre as well as meetings at Medical and Nursing Schools (attached to Alma Ata university) had been arranged for me.

Alma Ata and the city of Dzhambul, a highly polluted centre of the chemical industry, were the urban settings for visits while the villages in the Ilinsky *rayon* of Alma Ata and the Sverdlov *rayon* of Dzhambul provided the rural scene. Both Sadykova and Karagulova had made a considerable effort on my behalf.

Feldscher/midwife posts remained one of the most valued health facilities for patients and had stayed unchanged since my visit in 1971/72. The Kazakh authorities, as in the FSU, viewed *feldschers* as being evidence of backwardness compared with advanced western societies, a thing of the past and something to be ashamed of. Their popularity with patients was obvious but ignored. *Feldschers,* midwives and nurses had usually been in post for many years and were well-known in the community. Not only did they live locally, but more importantly they provided continuity of care which was much appreciated and led to confidence between patient and health worker. Young doctors who by law had to work in the rural service or the poorer areas of towns and cities, resented spending two to three years in this activity; their ambition was to return to hospital and be trained in 'proper' medicine.

Simple research into patients' attitudes to the three essential features of primary care – continuity, availability and accessibility – would be immensely valuable and would have much to tell planners and academics, provided they were prepared to listen. An added bonus – such research would cost virtually nothing.

A new facility, the Diagnostic Centre, had been introduced in Kazakhstan in 1998, the first in the FSU (although this was not quite accurate as a similar facility had been up and running in Moscow since the '50s and '60s for members of the Politburo, the top echelon of the communist party, and the top military). By the time of my visit a further six had been opened and three more were planned in Kazakhstan. On first being told about this I was surprised and impressed.

In the Diagnostic Centre I visited, two new departments had been quickly introduced. As well as the usual diagnostic/investigative departments a separate department screened the majority of patients on their initial referral. The accuracy of the diagnoses from the referring doctors had been found to be so poor that the department had been expanded to reduce inappropriate and unnecessary investigations being carried out. The main complaint from patients, many of whom had been under treatment for years, was that they felt no better, but nobody would listen to them. They had not only lost faith in the polyclinic doctors but now experienced little difference in the Diagnostic Centre. The second new department had proved successful. This was the Psychological Department, its purpose being to deal with the anger and frustration of patients, as well as saving them from repeated pointless investigations or treatment, particularly the elderly.

All this tied in with what I had been told by my interpreters, their families and friends and a number of staff at the Sanatorium. Two further criticisms which are in no way confined to Kazakhstan came top of the list. First, the education and training of doctors left a lot to be desired, so in desperation many had turned to private medicine in the hope the doctor would be more likely to listen and give them time.

Those without money just 'kept clear of the system' or 'hoped for the best'. Second, as in all countries doctors and nurses could be rude, dismissive and uncaring – in Kazakhstan being drunk on duty was an additional complaint. The best hope of finding a sympathetic listening ear was bribery, which appeared to be very common.

The Hospital for Nursing Care had only been opened since June 1992; it presented a new philosophy and emphasis on training. The Deputy Director was open about the problems he would face and straightforward about how much he would be allowed to accomplish. He was actually a doctor and it seemed odd he was in charge of a nursing project; he explained what I already knew, that nurses were held in poor repute – but it seemed to me that the same applied to doctors. Anyway, whether the attempt to change behaviour and be more polite, caring and sensitive would amount to anything more than window-dressing, I've no idea.

The elderly were considered to be most at risk, but from conversations with expectant and young mothers it was a different story – they were told what to do, their worries weren't listened to or were just ignored, and their opinions were never sought. Of course I could equally be describing patients' complaints about the NHS in 2015. It's easy enough to talk about high professional standards to improve quality of care while sitting in an office or on tv or the radio but virtually detached from the sharp end of clinical practice, and it's certainly easy to believe your own propaganda.

Just before I arrived, UNICEF and the WHO had found serious deficiencies in rural areas regarding the availability of clean water, and the extensive contamination of water in the countryside had caused great resentment in the population. Safe drinking water from deep wells and capped sources along the southern mountain ranges was being used exclusively for cities and towns. In rural areas more than thirty percent of the population had their drinking water delivered by tankers or horse-drawn trailers. The source of water came from the rivers originating in two small countries – Tajikistan and Kyrgyzstan, giving them power and influence in the region that also included Uzbekistan and Turkmenistan – thus a potential cause of instability.

In a cultural sense the difference between rural and urban areas was self-evident – no cinemas or libraries and suchlike – but in my very limited experience as we drove fifty or sixty miles or so into the countryside between Alma Ata and Dzhambul, I was surprised by the reasonable state of the roads and to find much of the land was being harvested – celeriac, maize, sugar beet , cabbage – and collective farms were still in operation.

I certainly saw water being delivered by tanker and bullock-drawn trailers, but in the rural hospitals and polyclinics water didn't seem to be a problem. Sanitation on the other hand was another matter with pit latrines being the only method except for dirty flush lavatories usually using a bucket in hospitals. Most of the buildings were old and poorly maintained. In 1990 a polyclinic had been opened in the small town of Byrynda in the *oblast* of Alma Ata, but architecturally and in design it could have been thirty years before.

Whether it was a small hospital or a village shop, food didn't seem to be a problem and bartering was the accepted way of acquiring what was needed. On two occasions I was given a traditional welcome, one of which was at a large collective farm. The ostensible reason for the visit was to show me the medical centre attached to the collective. The manager was married to the doctor, who was responsible for around 2,000 employees and their families. I pleaded with the doctor to show me the medical setup and to talk about the difficulties she experienced, but to no avail – everyone was on the starting blocks for food and drink. A large tented area, which appeared to be permanent, was as close as I was going to get to the medical centre. Inside were many tables laden with food, groups of musicians were ready to play, and the many groups of workers standing around were becoming increasingly impatient.

A feast is the only word to describe the scene, which unfortunately included endless toasts; on this occasion the honoured guest was not required to respond to every toast but was involved in a different unwelcome experience – I was honoured with the special delicacy, the boiled head of a sheep, the *pièce de résistance* being the eyes and brain. It took all my ingenuity to avoid giving offence as I restricted myself to a bit of burnt skin off the snout meanwhile surreptitiously depositing the eyes and brains on the ground under the table.

Amongst the professional people I met the majority were interested in the West (and the non-communist world), most just wanting to make contact – perhaps to find an opportunity or get an invitation regarding a joint research project; get advice about organising training courses; help in organising meetings and even perhaps exchange of staff. It would provide a lifetime of hope. Time and again both doctors and nurses reassured me that the mistakes of the past, the faults of the present and the difficulties in the future were acknowledged. Cooperation with the West and not being told what to do by the Russians was what they wanted.

Both the WHO Collaborating Centre and the Association of Physicians and Pharmacists knew what they wanted; all the West needed to do was listen. I tried to set out the main worries in the West which related not only to the government but to all levels of society. One of the main concerns was corruption; how could we be certain that the selection of doctors and nurses wouldn't be due to political influence and that departments that had been selected for research undertakings weren't involved in bribery?

On my return to the UK I was disappointed, frustrated and angered by the lack of interest and the excuses made by the Department of Health, medical schools, various institutes and some individuals about the state of medicine in Kazakhstan. After all, this was a part of the world where we were trying to expand our almost non-existent influence. It was immediately obvious that hospital medicine and little else was of interest to the Department of Health and medical schools; primary care was at the bottom of the heap. As far as I remember, three Departments of General Practice were interested but all advocated in one way or another the establishment of general practice à la UK in Kazakhstan – in my opinion an absurd suggestion.

The British Council did not wish to be involved in anything medical and the Know-How Fund was lukewarm. NHS Overseas Enterprise was a government setup to improve health in poorer parts of the world; in fact it turned out to be almost exclusively interested in the hospital sector and if possible high-tech medicine. Some interest was shown in public health. It took me some time to realise that finance was the main reason for the involvement of Overseas Enterprises. British companies along with architects and engineers were involved in the construction of a number of unnecessary and inappropriate hospitals in the developing world, and of course *pari passu* other companies were ready with as much equipment as they could sell, especially high-tech stuff.

I have no idea how it was possible for Overseas Enterprises to mislead the media and the general public and hide their activities from them; only the Department of Health and its consultant advisers know the answer to that.

> 'Hardly a plane touches down in Moscow or St Petersburg these days without at least one passenger claiming a special interest in the Russian health system. Ask an academic why he is on his fifteenth trip to Eastern Europe this year (and he is planning to annex Russia) and he will tell you it's for money (from lucrative prospects for aid agencies), foreign students and opportunities for research in what for Westerners is virgin territory. Whoever is to blame, there is general agreement that too many people have been going to Russia to catch up on what's happening. The question that these visitors rarely ask themselves is: what do Russians want from this invasion?'

So wrote the deputy Editor of the *British Medical Journal* in 1992. Similarly, from a report on Eastern Europe written by a Polish doctor who graduated in the UK, again published in the *BMJ* in 1992.

> '. . . your foreign advisers are all too often a great disappointment to us. They come over here and start out as if in deepest Africa, spending a great deal of time and money arriving at conclusions we ourselves reached long ago. Indeed the consensus of opinion in Poland is that too much loan and grant money from the European Community, the World Health Organisation and the World Bank, and other smaller agencies such as the British Know-How fund, is being misused or wasted, often squandered on unnecessary elaborate studies carried out by Western consultants.'

Information from Czechoslovakia as it then was confirmed a situation similar to that described in Poland and spoke of disillusionment and cynicism about much foreign advice and advisers.

What had happened in the FSU, Poland and Czechoslovakia could easily be repeated in Kazakhstan. Although I had hoped to help my colleagues in Kazakhstan and was dreadfully disappointed in the British response and felt I had accomplished nothing, it all turned out for the best – at least Overseas Enterprises didn't get involved and only one Department of General Practice made a brief visit, which was taken no further.

My thoughts regarding Kazakhstan were not primarily about medicine or politics or travel, rather they concerned the personal stories of interesting people.

I met Professor Alimkhanov in a meeting at the Institute of Postgraduate Training; psychiatry was his speciality and his expertise was postgraduate teaching/education in polyclinics. As the meeting broke up he asked if I would like to be shown some interesting things around the city. He was as good as his word and the following Sunday morning he turned up at the Sanatorium. He was steeped in the history of the place and our wander was utterly absorbing, but to me of even greater interest was what he recalled of his childhood.

He and his family had lived in a small village in the Albai district of the Region Semipalatinsk, the area in the FSU where all atmospheric nuclear testing took place between 1953 and '63. The village was about ninety miles from the testing area and on the day of each test his primary school would be closed but all the children would turn up so they could watch under the supervision of their teachers. Naturally the children were delighted to get off school and he remembered it always seemed to be a clear cloudless sunny day, at any rate on the three to four occasions he watched. They were all lined up, very excited about what they were going to see. The first thing to come into view were two distant vapour trails followed by the sight and sound of a massive explosion:

> "The sun looked like a dark almost black coin in the sky; none of us wore sunglasses or took any protective precautions and we were all so happy and excited. I'm rather ashamed that I can't remember what our teachers told us and it was just what small boys and girls thought was very exciting. We all felt the same."

He was about eight or nine at the time. Subsequently he became a member of the International Group of Physicists studying nuclear explosions. Whether it was a truly international group I don't know, but certainly some Japanese were included. As a psychiatrist he had concentrated on the effects on the brain, leaving the horrible physical deformities to the neurologists. Schizophrenia, epilepsy and suicide had been steadily increasing, according to Alimkhanov, but he had no information about the extreme west of China and Mongolia, which was on the border with Semipalatinsk. He maintained that in the Soviet era medical reports were vague but not actually disingenuous, and over the past few years, particularly since independence, there had been marked improvements in diagnosis, which he genuinely thought would continue.

Dr Alexei Ovsiannikov was the Director and Chief Surgeon at the District Hospital in Dzhambul. He was a charming middle-aged man of the old school with an obviously good relationship with his staff and patients. I had managed to restrict my visit to the obstetric, gynaecological, paediatric and emergency departments of the hospital and in spite of my showing no interest in the Department of Surgery he responded to all the questions I threw at him. My interpreter and I then joined Ovsiannikov, half a dozen colleagues and several nurses in his official office where a large table was laden with food; later a special bottle of champagne was opened, followed by vodka. Almost everyone smoked heavily. In any official building or office there would be a portrait of Lenin in a prominent position and Ovsiannikov's room was no exception. In all private houses Lenin was not to be seen but one or two Orthodox icons might be displayed. In this proudly atheist land the power of religion or spirituality or whatever you like to call it had not been destroyed. Interestingly it was the crucifixes and icons of Christianity that were visible; both publicly and privately Islam and Judaism seemed to have no place in contemporary society.

Vodka relaxed Alexei Ovsiannikov and he started talking about his training in the FSU and how, after qualifying, he had spent the statutory two to three years as a village doctor. I was keen to keep him talking and without really expecting anything I asked if he had ever heard of Solzhenitsyn whilst he had been in the Gulag. Alexei seemed a genuinely modest fellow so I'm pretty certain he wouldn't have mentioned Solzhenitsyn if I hadn't asked. No, he'd had no knowledge of him whilst he was a prisoner at Ekbastaz in the Karaganda region, one of the many labour camps in this remote area of Kazakhstan. However, their paths crossed later. In 1953 Solzhenitsyn was released from his Gulag imprisonment and after many stops and starts including a brief stay in Dzhambul with four or five other ex-prisoners he ended up in Berlik, a village in the harsh grey grassland of the bleak steppe cum desert in the south-west of the country.

It was here that the young Dr Ovsiannikov had been sent after finishing his year's training in the District Hospital in Dzhambul where he was now the senior surgeon. He had no idea who Solzhenitsyn was, how could he? He was just an ex-prisoner who had written nothing that had been published.

> "How I wish I'd known at the time how famous my patient was to become. I remember him as a quiet unassuming schoolmaster teaching mathematics in the local school. He seemed a bit of a recluse, rarely mixing in the village."

But Solzhenitsyn's medical history he remembered really clearly. Yes, it was true he had been operated on whilst still a prisoner in the Gulag; the operation was performed under local anaesthetic and was for a seminoma of the testicle. No, it wasn't cancer of the stomach as had been reported in the West, possibly on account of his novel *Cancer Ward.* After he had been in the village a little while he presented himself with a swelling in his groin and a slight swelling in his back. Alexei diagnosed a recurrence of the seminoma with probable metastases in the spine and retro-peritoneal tissues. Immediately he set about organising Solzhenitsyn's referral to the Oncology Department at the State Medical School in Tashkent. Although this was arranged expeditiously, the swelling in his back was much bigger by the time he had arrived. The reputation of the Soviet health service in the '50s was poor, but Solzhenitsyn's recovery definitely belies this, particularly as only basic x-ray therapy and drugs were available. It also says a great deal about the young doctor who organised the transfer from one Republic to another; one can readily imagine the bureaucratic obstacles that would have been put in the way of such a young physician.

Alexie repeated a number of times how he wished he had known that his patient would become one of the Soviet's most famous dissidents and would be awarded the Nobel Prize for Literature.

At the Sanatorium I had become friendly with a young Yugoslav. I had noticed him almost as soon as I had arrived, always on his own and eating his meals with a faraway look, unhappy it seemed. I joined him as he seemed anxious to make contact.

"I want you to understand how complicated everything is, nobody realises."

His story just poured out. He was married with two children and had left Yugoslavia and travelled to Kazakhstan ten months earlier. His wife and children still lived in Split in Dalmatia.

"Where's Dalmatia?"
"Oh, in Croatia on the coast."

His wife and family were Croatian and he was Serbian. Before he married he had lived with his parents in Sarajevo, gone to school there and found work there. When he was born, his personal identity card had been stamped Bosnia-Herzegovina although his parents were Serb; after his marriage he lived in Split and his passport was Croatian. If he joined the Serbian army, which his parents wanted him to do, he would be fighting against his wife and children and her family. If he joined the Croats he would be fighting against the Serbs and his parents. If he joined the armed forces in Bosnia-Herzegovina he would be part of a Muslim army utterly opposed to the Catholics of Croatia and the Orthodox Church of Serbia.

"What could I do? I see no hope. Do you understand?"
"Yes, and what do you think is going to happen?"
"I don't know. I just hope I see my family again."

He was utterly distraught the first time he told me but as he retold his story he became angry and sad.

What did I learn? Over the next few years, in fact until the present time, whenever I hear simplistic or confident authoritative discussion between politicians, diplomats, the military and journalists about the situation in the Balkans and in particular Bosnia-Herzegovina my thoughts always return to my Yugoslav friend, the complexity of his life and what happened to him and his family.

Svetlana was a Senior Interpreter/Translator at the Ministry of Economic Affairs. I never understood why she was staying at the Sanatorium which looked after patients with cardiovascular disease and provided accommodation for members of the Ministry of the

Interior as well as odds and ends like the young Yugoslav and myself. Anyway, it was of no consequence.

'For many years I have had much trouble with my back' was indicative of her interest in talking to me. An official government delegation from the Ministry of Economic Affairs was shortly visiting London and Svetlana was to accompany them – could I give her the name and address of a specialist in London whom she could contact?

The Yugoslav, Svetlana and I quickly became a most unlikely trio, always having meals together and on a number of evenings retiring either to Svetlana's or the Yugoslav's room (I have lost his name), but for some reason never to mine; always cognac and tea with Svetlana and vodka with the Yugoslav. Conversation was usually in English and this gave Svetlana the opportunity to complain that she had little chance to practise her English because so few British people came to Kazakhstan. She was a really tough cookie and demanded aggressively to know why this was; none of my answers satisfied her.

The medical service was discussed and she told us there was only one doctor she trusted, someone she'd known for twenty years. Again and again we heard about rudeness, the lack of respect for patients and low professional standards.

> "If you want to get a higher degree in medicine you must bribe – two sheep is the going rate at the moment."

Even if this wasn't true, people were prepared to believe it.

One evening, when we were having our meal, the conversation was all about the mess that used to be Yugoslavia and the mess that was now Kazakhstan; naturally Svetlana had strong views:

> "Nobody wants to work. Everybody wants to sell – they buy from state shops and then try to sell at a higher price and they think that's capitalism. Pensioners and people with poorly paid work don't like it, they want a return to the 'old ways'. The present situation is a mafia of old communists and free marketers and this makes a jungle."

The young Yugoslav and I simply paid attention and listened– once in full flow Svetlana was unstoppable – but he eventually managed to interrupt and tell us about the difficulty he had had in getting from Split to Alma Ata. He had barely begun before Svetlana interrupted and told him he could have flown there from Ankara. He just sighed, raised his eyebrows and explained that with a Croatian passport he couldn't even get a Turkish transit visa. She'd had no idea of the hurdles he had to face and for once was silent. He then proceeded to tell us about the extraordinary happening at Alma Ata airport.

According to the International Aviation Authority (IAA) international flights were forbidden (except to the Russian Federation) as the airport was not up to standard regarding its runways, air traffic control, safety arrangements and facilities for passengers. However, for one afternoon each week the airport was closed to domestic flights too, and the Kazakh authorities announced it was then opened as an international airport – but only for Turkish airlines. How this was permitted was a mystery and we all agreed that bribery must have been involved – undoubtedly more than two sheep.

One evening Svetlana divulged a family secret – a sort of confession, or the need to tell someone. It seemed she had been secretly christened as a baby; her maternal grandmother had taken her to an Orthodox priest. She hadn't been told until it was felt she was old enough to understand. Then at about age fourteen she was also instructed never to speak about it for fear her mother might lose her job.

> "I'm not really interested in religion but for some reason I've started going to church again."

She so reminded me of my guide in Georgia.

Svetlana was a caricature of someone who had lost patience with her country, could clearly see its many faults and was angry that so few people thought as she did. In fact she was not alone and I met many like her, a surprising number having an additional anxiety regarding the number of foreigners flooding into the country – such people were greedy and often ignorant. Svetlana was able to verify this:

> "What hope is there if an official in a high-level Iranian delegation thought Kazakhstan was an Islamic republic?"

When I was endeavouring to find the WHO Collaborating Centre when I first arrived, the address was Pasteur Street 15, and while I was struggling with a map a young fellow came up to help:

> "Oh no, Pasteur Street is no longer, it was changed a month ago."

It's a well-known and irritating obsession that the Russians have for changing the names of cities, towns and streets for political reasons, but what possible reason could there be for changing Louis Pasteur, the famous father of modern bacteriology, for the name of some unknown Kazakh or Russian politician? That evening I asked Svetlana why this sort of thing happened.

"The reason is simple – ignorant, stupid, political bureaucrats remain in charge."

And whether you are in a shop, bank, railway station – in fact any state-run organisation – idleness, indifference, rudeness, the shrug of the shoulder or the raised eyebrow were accepted as normal behaviour. For instance, at a smart hotel:

"Is your shop open?"
"No"
"Where is your shop?"
"Down the stairs"

– where I found the shop open; once in the shop the usual routine with the assistants reading or varnishing their nails, talking to each other, refusing to look at the customers, always reluctant to get off their backsides and finally, with much sighing, opening a cabinet or drawer to bring what you had asked to see, meanwhile continuing to talk to her colleagues. Banks were for me the worst with a perpetual expression of 'what on earth are you going to ask next?'.

Needless to say Kazakhstan had another side and one which I often experienced. The hospitality, kindness and embarrassing generosity of the families with whom I had become involved, and the consideration of the people I met – all were such a contrast to the official world. In the streets and parks unknown folk were ready to help, whether I was struggling with a map, having difficulty with my baggage getting on or off a bus or train, or whatever, and offering a simple smile as I walked around. Old men would give me a gruff but friendly nod and young mothers loved it when I peered into their old-fashioned prams and smiled at their baby or toddler. This was the other aspect of Kazakhstan.

13

THE PEOPLE'S REPUBLIC of MONGOLIA

'Do you remember where you were when . . . ?' is a frequently asked question: when Neville Chamberlain spoke to the nation on that Sunday morning and we knew we were at war with Germany; when President John Kennedy was shot; when within months of each other Martin Luther King was assassinated, followed by JFK's brother Robert; when Neil Armstrong set foot on the moon – and so it goes on.

I remember clearly where I was when Margaret Thatcher resigned – I was being driven down the Mall in a taxi on that Thursday morning 22 November 1990. The taxi driver suddenly turned round – he could hardly contain himself:

"D'ya hear that, guv? She's bloody gone."

He had to stop briefly and we had a chat while he recovered his composure. He was taking me to the Mongolian Embassy.

An appointment had been arranged with the Cultural Attaché who to my surprise was a lady, Mrs Balchiglin Bazarkhand; she proved to be a great help and full of useful advice. In order to get a visa I would need at the very least the agreement and support of the Minister of Public Health in Ulaanbaatar. She knew him and was able to tell me that recently he had been studying at one of the Medical Research Council Laboratories in London – as far as I can remember he had been awarded a British Council award. During his stay he had told the Cultural Attaché how well he had been treated in the laboratory – far better than he had expected, and as a result had a soft spot for Britain and great interest in the NHS, particularly the way primary care/general practice was organised and delivered.

Mrs Bazarkhand took me to the Ambassador, Mr Otehivbal, who was equally courteous and friendly and interested in my project. He promised he would write a letter of support to the Minister, which he duly did. I was somewhat mystified by the support of the Embassy and the apparently friendly attitude to the British.

On 10 December I wrote to the Minister Dr P Nymadawa and within a month or so I heard from the Embassy that my proposal had been accepted although no date had been suggested. So far so good, though my original idea of visiting Mongolia and Kazakhstan at the same time seemed most unlikely.

My knowledge of Mongolia was limited, but no worse than the majority of my compatriots. It consisted of: the Gobi Desert, Genghis Khan, the Golden Horde, and the reputation of the all-conquering Mongol tribesmen sweeping all before them and leaving many of the great cities of Asia, the Caucasus and the Middle East savagely destroyed until finally reaching the outskirts of Vienna close to what is now Poland.

Over a period of about 150 years the largest empire the world has ever known was built – four times the size of Alexander the Great's enormous conquests, twice the size of the Roman Empire, longer than the Ottoman Empire and covering a greater land mass than the British Empire – from central Europe to the Pacific coast of China, to many parts of the Middle East and the northern half of India including present day Pakistan and Bangladesh. Japan was never invaded. And then, when at the height of its power, in 1242 AD the Mongols suddenly returned home to attend a great gathering of tribal rulers to elect a new leader; this *quriltai* proved to be the most significant event in the country's history until the establishment of the communist party in 1921. The Empire was never defeated, it simply disappeared.

Mongolia was part of the Chinese Empire for hundreds of years and by the beginning of the twentieth century had suffered enough from the brutal treatment of their Chinese overlords. The failed Revolution of 1905 in Tsarist Russia, followed by the Revolution of 1917 and the subsequent civil war, coincided with the increasing anger of the peasants within both Mongolia and China. In 1921 Mao Tse-tung in China and the Revolutionary Party of Mongolia founded the communist party in their respective countries. In 1924 the People's Republic of Mongolia was declared and the country became the second communist country in the world (Russia being the first). It was not until twenty-five years later in 1949 that the Chinese People's Republic was declared and Mao became head of state.

From 1924 Mongolia became completely dependent on the USSR economically, politically and militarily, and was not infrequently referred to as the 16th Republic of the Soviet Union. Throughout all this time the country remained almost unnoticed by the Western powers. From the Soviet point of view this suited them well, providing a buffer zone first against the capitalist China of Chiang Kai-shek and then the political uncertainty of Mao's China. On its western frontiers the USSR had had to wait until the end of the Second World War for the countries of Eastern Europe to provide a buffer zone in the same way as Mongolia.

Mongolia is roughly three times the size of France, half the size of India and Pakistan; Russia forms its northern frontier (1,500 miles) and China lies to the west, south and east. The maximum distance between the northern and southern frontiers is about 890 miles. In 1994 the population, of which half were still nomads, was only 2.4 million making it one of the least populated countries in the world. Its society is basically homogeneous with the Kazakhs making up the only significant ethnic minority of about 5.5 percent; they live in the far west where the frontiers of Mongolia, China, Kazakhstan and Russia meet on a pinhead of land – interestingly this minute area had been the most northerly staging post of one of the historic Silk Roads between East and West.

An amusing way of looking at the statistics concerns the head of livestock – sheep, goats, horses, cattle, yaks and camels – which is roughly twenty-six million (this is generally reckoned to be a very conservative estimate) or more than ten times the human population. Only one percent of arable land was actively cultivated, mostly potatoes and wheat, both hugely affected by the short growing season. None of this appeared to worry anyone as the vast majority of people didn't like vegetables in any case. Some paediatricians and public health workers told me that trying to explain to women about the importance of vegetables was an essential element of health education.

Ulaanbaatar was divided into an inner central area and the surrounding environs that stretched out into the countryside. It was covered with thousands of *gers*, the traditional Mongolian felt tent; each *ger* was surrounded by a wooden fence or palisade creating a private area or yard known as a *tasha;* goats and sheep wandered everywhere with dogs endlessly barking. A settlement of up to two hundred *gers* was called an *ail.* No roads, only tracks criss-crossed these huge areas surrounding Ulaanbaatar. I quickly found out that urban families much preferred to live in *gers* than in the concrete flats provided by the Soviets at the end of the Second World War. Repeatedly I heard 'we're happier living like the nomads', which was a little surprising as although most had electricity there was no running water or decent sanitation.

Parts of the city centre could have been anywhere in the FSU – blocks of identical housing, grey and dirty with rotting balconies and hideously stained walls, foul-smelling entrances and chipped concrete stairways.

The main street was wide and spacious and lined with trees. The impressive central squares were surrounded by public/government buildings – the national parliament, palaces of culture, concert halls, and a quite outstanding museum of natural history containing the world's largest collection of dinosaurs. All were built in traditional Soviet style – I really felt I could have been in an outpost of the USSR with the ubiquitous large metal heating pipes (always above ground) with their serious rust problems and leaks zigzagging their way along and over the streets. How they could function in winter I had no idea; no wonder the women in the *gers* had told me how much warmer it was for them, and they had an additional back up as animal dung or *argul* was also used as fuel. And snow instead of water.

In a valley at the very edge of Ulaanbaatar, pollution from a coal-fired power station and two chemical factories climbed into the sky displaying all the colours of the rainbow. Curiously I found the city itself to be a blessed relief from the overcrowding and apparently unnoticed poverty of Hong Kong from where I had just come via Peking. The poverty in Hong Kong was hidden in the forest of high-rise buildings which concealed the tiny flats with no air-conditioning and not even a simple fan in summer, and blankets and rugs the only protection against the cold in winter.

Within forty-eight hours I had noticed a number of buses which had apparently been abandoned in the city. It seemed rather odd until my guide/interpreter explained, as we were following behind a bus which stopped suddenly on a gentle slope and all the passengers got out. The men proceeded to push the bus to the top of the slope, about a hundred yards, whereupon everyone climbed back in and the bus free-wheeled down the slope into the bus station in the centre of the town. No cursing, no threatening the driver, just an acceptance of the situation as something to which they were quite accustomed - it had run out of petrol. On numerous occasions a similar scenario played itself out except that the bus was only pushed if there was a slope, otherwise it was simply abandoned. Trolley-buses would suffer the same fate except that the cause was electricity cuts. In Ulaanbaatar and apparently in the rest of the country too, electricity and piped water were restricted to a couple of hours twice a day – but you never knew when that would be. The uncertainty was exasperating when in addition it could be cut off for short periods without any warning. In winter of course it was all a hundred times worse, making it impossible to warm your flat.

The shortage of petrol was obvious – long queues of lorries and a few cars waiting patiently at the few garages in the city. On a personal level, on a number of occasions the ministry car didn't turn up or was very late – either there had been difficulty in obtaining petrol or a problem getting the car repaired. It became rather embarrassing that we were being given special attention, and this became especially noticeable on our four-day visit to the Gobi to study the rural health service. On this occasion the Ministry of Health couldn't provide a car and it looked as though the visit would have to be cancelled. Finally they managed to borrow a clapped-out UNICEF Russian jeep and in fact the old banger did very well. At the facilities we visited – health centres and rural hospitals – one unvarying complaint concerned transport, the lack of fuel and the almost insurmountable difficulties in getting repairs done. Unemployment was a serious problem and I couldn't understand why vehicle repair garages were not being set up – certainly if you owned or worked in one you would never be unemployed again, at least for the foreseeable future.

On the second day an unexpected advertisement caught my eye. Peace Avenue, an impressive tree-lined boulevard with dualcarriageways and a central reservation of shrubs and bushes, was the main road running west. My hotel was on one side and on the other was an old, detached two-storey building set at right-angles to the road. The whole top floor was covered by a fading yellow advertisement for Lipton's tea written in English. Why such a traditional British company should have such a prominent site puzzled me. However, on reflection it was not as strange as I originally thought. Great Britain was one of the first countries to recognise Mongolia as an individual separate country and in 1924 was the first to exchange ambassadors. At this time the Empire was still an empire and its adventurers and entrepreneurs were still flying the flag and covering the globe. Sir Thomas Lipton, the Scottish businessman and philanthropist, had bought many tea plantations and rubber estates in India, so Mongolia would be an obvious outpost for his flourishing grocery business.

Until this visit to Mongolia I had always been on my own when involved in my study of PMC/PHC, but on this occasion it was different. I joined Dr John Birch, a non-medical NHS manager who had been asked by the Foreign & Commonwealth Office to go as a consultant adviser to access the progress being made following the recent introduction of the new Family Doctor Service.

John Birch's experience and expertise revolved around management within the hospital service; very late in the arrangements the FCO contacted me to say that Dr Nymadawa, through the Department of Health in London, had insisted I should accompany John Birch. I was extremely apprehensive about the whole venture and would have been far happier to be going on my own. I was certain John and I would have different interests – this was inevitable as he had no knowledge of primary care or family medicine, and I was concerned that time-wasting arguments and unavoidable compromises would result.

Three cities – Ulaanbaatar, Darhan and Erdenet – varying in population between 65,000 and 555,000 were Autonomous Municipalities which elected their own mayor and governed themselves. The rest of the country was divided into eighteen provinces or *aimags,* similar to counties in the UK, with populations of between 43,000 and 106,000. Each *aimag* was divided into between twelve and twenty-six *sums,* similar to district councils, and they were further sub-divided into an average of four *bags* with populations varying between 500 and 600, rather like a parish.

Aimags, sums and *bags* had corresponding health facilities to match the administration; in 1994 there were 21 *aimag* provincial hospitals, 328 *sum* hospitals and health centres and 1,249 *feldscher*/midwife posts.

In broad outline the health service was a mirror image of the USSR with city and university hospitals, separate women's and paediatric hospitals, emergency centres, polyclinics called district health centres, rural hospitals/centres/primary care units, and finally *feldscher*/midwife posts.

Following the demise of the Soviet Union all financial support to Mongolia had been withdrawn, just as in Cuba and South Yemen. Until then the Soviet Union had provided eighty-five percent of all development costs or, to put it another way, thirty-five percent of government spending. At the same time as Mongolia decided to break away from its former ally, in the field of health care even before 1990/91 a small group of Mongolian physicians led by Dr Nymadawa realised that the cost of the health service as a percentage of GNP was unsustainable. The most urgent problems were too many hospital beds, a low level of activity throughout the service along with the inefficient, inappropriate and ineffective use of both doctors and nurses, in particular the excessive number of so-called 'specialist doctors' working in district health centres (equivalent to polyclinics in the Soviet Union) and a similar state of affairs in rural areas. Dr Nymadawa and his colleagues realised it was going to be difficult to change the status quo and that great opposition would come from the medical profession.

As a consequence, but unwisely, the Ministry of Health rushed the introduction of the Family Doctor Service (FDS). It was set up initially in 1990 in Erdenet, the third largest city, followed in 1991 in selected areas of Ulaanbaatar, and finally on 1 January 1994, by ministerial decree, the rest of Mongolia was to follow.

I found it genuinely difficult to assess the real level of implementation of the FDS although the very poor standard of training of family doctors was painfully obvious. In the Han-nul district of Ulaanbaatar (one of the selected areas in 1991) nearly a hundred percent of doctors were unable to use simple medical instruments – auroscope, ophthalmoscope and vaginal speculum. However, there was ample evidence at least on paper of families having registered under the care of a named family doctor, and impressive risk factors colour-coded in their records plus the diagrammatic representation of blocks of flats along with the size and health status of each family clearly marked.

What proved impossible to discover was whether the family was seen by their named doctor or by any doctor who happened to be around, and how much home visiting actually took place considering the unreliability of transport and therefore the distance a doctor would have to walk – quite impossible in winter. I was told there was no need for me to be concerned . . .

In urban areas about eighty-five percent of family doctors were female. A stethoscope, a sphygmomanometer and a weighing machine were the only pieces of equipment I saw in a family doctor's room – no auroscope, opthalmoscope, vaginal speculum, simple reflex hammer or tuning fork to measure hearing or vibration sense. But while talking with these doctors, even had these tools been available none had been trained to use them. A direct consequence of this were the unnecessary but inevitable referrals to 'specialists' in a health centre who then just passed on the patient to a hospital. All ante-natal care (ANC) was referred to 'specialist obstetricians'. However, it is worth remembering that in 2015 all general practitioners in the UK (except a very small number in remote areas) take no part in ANC, which has been passed over to midwives.

As mentioned above, this rapid introduction of the Family Doctor Service was a mistake, and it was going to take many years to accomplish, while lack of re-education would continue to be a stumbling block. Admittedly since 1993, whenever possible, doctors with some training in internal medicine, paediatrics and obstetrics have been selected to become the first family doctors, but this couldn't be accomplished overnight.

The situation in 1994 was that the 'non-hospital' specialists were employed in large numbers in all types of facility and functioned at an extremely poor level of clinical competence. They were usually underemployed and had no experience of working in hospital or in the patient's home. In reality they were nothing more than an extra layer of an unnecessary and badly-trained workforce: a huge waste of time and money. The laboratory doctors I spoke to admitted they might carry out as few as one or two blood tests per day and often none. The presence of 'non-hospital' oncologists without any possibility of working in a hospital was just insanity. It was accepted that more than ninety percent of such doctors acted as nothing more than a signpost to the hospital. No thought had been given to the idea of hospital specialists working part-time in district health centres.

A small but increasing number of doctors were beginning to realise that a change to undergraduate education was an absolute necessity for an overhaul of the health service, quite apart from the new FDS. But there was an obstacle that hadn't crossed my mind – I was of course aware of the antipathy often existing between doctors working in primary and secondary care, but I hadn't expected or realised the great divide in Mongolia between medical schools and those working at the coalface.

Undergraduate teaching took place in district hospitals, but the doctors who were responsible for the diagnosis and treatment of patients had been excluded from teaching. This responsibility had been put in the hands of doctors at the medical schools who would be lecturing or researching on anatomy, physiology, pathology, epidemiology, public health and so on, but who had absolutely no direct contact with patients.

I attended one teaching session; patients were chosen by the medical school staff and brought into the lecture hall, usually on a stretcher. The students were given no opportunity to talk to the patients or take a history or carry out any physical examination: a total mad-house which I wouldn't have believed had I not witnessed it. This antipathy will take years to resolve and even when it has been overcome another hurdle of equal importance lies in wait. If the Family Doctor Service was to be the goal then postgraduate education and training would have to be shared between primary and secondary care, and family medicine or general practice would have to be accepted as a separate discipline, a new speciality. A formidable task.

At Maternity House No. 11, District Hospital No. 4 and Children's hospital No.4 there was general agreement that since the FDS had been introduced a deterioration in standards and care had been noticed with greatly increased numbers of unnecessary referrals and family doctors failing to visit their patients. This was particularly the case with those who had had operations, had serious respiratory and cardio-vascular problems, and mothers and babies immediately after confinement.

Ration cards for basic foods were introduced in 1992 because of shortages alongside rising prices. The ration card provided every family with the guarantee of basic food at an affordable price. A year later supplementary cards were issued to pregnant women and children under two – clearly the original card hadn't been sufficient. A further emergency measure was set up with extra milk being provided for children under five provided they had a note from the doctor. By the time of my arrival a black market with extortionate prices was flourishing. Here was a situation where nurses could get involved and take the lead in giving dietary advice and making sure the ration cards were being used correctly and the milk centres were treating the mothers fairly.

At the same time as Soviet influence started to decline, Buddhism started a resurgence with an increase in the numbers of priests and the building of new temples. Coinciding with this, alternative medicine and traditional healing began to flourish – for centuries it had been a central part of Mongolian culture. In the Sukhebaatar area a Buddhist-trained healer was working full-time in a health centre – he had been completely accepted by the medical and nursing staff and warmly and enthusiastically received by patients. I was very pleasantly surprised by what I found when I spent a couple of hours with him. His room was spotlessly clean as was the healer himself. On his desk were two telephones and on a nearby table a computer, printer and another telephone. A large glass-fronted cupboard held all the medicines, potions and ointments, and again was spotlessly clean. The whole ambience was of modernity and a great emphasis on hygiene. The healer himself was quiet and calm and created a feeling of security; all my questions he answered with consideration. As I was leaving he proudly showed me three folders containing beautiful coloured drawings of many of the plants he used in his work; sometimes he would show patients which plant he was prescribing. I could see why patients liked him.

Nurses had been established as a separate profession for many years so it was surprising to observe their lack of independence from the medical profession. As far as I could see there was no defining what work should be done by the doctor and what by the nurse, who was never allowed to stand apart as a practitioner in her own right; they lacked leadership and allowed themselves to be dominated by doctors. Admittedly I had only the briefest experience but it was clear that the Buddhist healer was more respected and given more independence than almost any nurse I met.

There were, however, some opportunities for nurses to work on their own. Primary care had for a number of years been concentrating on immunisation against TB, the triple vaccine for diphtheria, pertussis and tetanus, oral polio and, recently, measles. According to UNICEF coverage was satisfactory; this was just the sort of work that needed to be led by nurses so that the new family doctor could concentrate on diagnosis and treatment.

Maternity services in rural areas changed as a result of the introduction of a market economy. Until 1990/91 all agricultural cooperatives, similar to collective farms in the FSU, were basically owned by the government, which had accepted responsibility for supporting and maintaining maternity rest homes – their function being to provide care for pregnant women by admitting them one or two weeks before their expected date. The midwife would then be able to explain about the delivery, about breast-feeding and the general care of babies. By this it was hoped not only would mothers get to know the midwife in charge of her delivery, she would also meet the *feldscher*/midwife who would visit her and her baby when she returned to her *ger*, thus providing the all-important continuity. A statutory law stated that for the first year the baby should be visited every two weeks for the first three months and thereafter every four weeks up to one year old.

Unfortunately, after the cooperatives ceased to exist in 1990/91 no-one would accept responsibility for this excellent service and closure was inevitable. The doctors and midwives concerned with maternity work were united in blaming the closures for the recent increase in maternal and infant morbidity and mortality.

Sometimes however there was a beacon of hope and we found this during the visit to the Gobi; the Gov'Ugtaal hospital in Delgersts *sum* had set aside two beds to compensate for the closure of the nearby maternity rest home. This measure had proved to be perfectly adequate and had not added increased costs. It is to be hoped that more senior doctors will show similar common sense so that initiatives such as this could expand throughout the country.

These hopeful signs were in part due to the fact that the majority of recently selected doctors had originally lived in a rural setting and were enthusiastic to return and experience the increasing cooperation between the doctors and *feldschers*/midwives. I was given a good opportunity to talk with both patients and health personnel and all believed the situation was beginning to improve; patients felt the service was better and health professionals had greater job satisfaction.

A final comment on the maternity service and a tradition found in both urban and rural hospitals as well as in urban homes and *gers:* just as in Russia, babies were swaddled from head to foot for two to three months and thereafter for another few months from their waist to the tip of their toes. It was almost a full-time job for mothers to have to remove one, two, three or more layers of clothing in order to clean the baby. Eventually the baby was only swaddled whilst asleep. In winter swaddling was seen as the only way to keep the baby warm, with the addition of extra blankets to surround the little bundle. Obviously in the brief summer it was difficult to keep very small babies swaddled and cool. But in spite of these difficulties swaddling was accepted as normal and necessary.

Mongolia was not alone in being ashamed of the *feldscher*/midwife post – exactly the same attitude prevailed in the FSU and most countries behind the Iron Curtain. In any discussion about the future I was firmly told that the intention was to get rid of them. Officials would listen to me politely but weren't interested in anything I said, particularly in Mongolia when I suggested that in rural areas the new family doctor should be like a *feldscher*. In my report I strongly advised the Ministry of Health to re-evaluate and strengthen their training and continue to use this particular health worker. At the district health centre Sukhebaatar and the sub-district No. 15 the two senior doctors were most enthusiastic about the new family doctor service and also wholeheartedly supported my views on *feldschers* and how they could be used to their full potential. The problems connected with the new service had been accurately analysed by these men who surprisingly were thinking about the urban and not the rural service. What a refreshing change.

Four days were to be spent in the Gobi to give us as complete a picture of the rural service as possible. Our destination was *aimag* Dundgov, meaning Middle Gobi, and by the time we reached our hotel the vast emptiness and the huge overall distance as well as the distance between small *ails* and isolated *gers* (between twenty-five and forty miles) had truly sunk in.

On leaving the tarmac road, about half an hour from the outskirts of Ulaanbaatar, rutted tracks were visible as we passed through green pasture in a wide valley lined by gentle hills. The tracks soon petered out and an endless featureless landscape with occasional desert scrub and clumps of marram grass and one or two small rivers took over for the next six hours. Rickety bridges of unstable wooden planks lay over dried-up rivers; many unmarked cairns were passed or could be seen in the distance – one was draped with beautiful blue *khadags* (Buddhist prayer scarves). It was the custom at the larger cairns to stop and walk round them three times – I forget if it was clockwise or anti-clockwise, but I remember our driver telling us how important it was to go in the correct direction. Traditionally songs would be sung to the past travellers who had built the cairn and to bless our companions and to offer hope for a safe journey.

From the time we left the tarmac road and reached our destination only three lorries and one jeep passed us, travelling in the opposite direction, and we overtook one crowded and overloaded bus that looked as if it wouldn't make it to wherever it was going. Once or twice we stopped for the driver to take stock and get his bearings – how he decided which way to go he couldn't explain but never once did he make a mistake.

The wildlife was tremendous – hundreds of burrowing furry

marmots, which were eaten as a delicacy, foxes and other small mammals and groups of grunting yaks. The most spectacular sight was the herds of wild horses charging madly across the stony desert – on three occasions as many as fifty to sixty horses were under the control of two or three herdsmen or *arats* using long whips and lassoes; one group had young boys with them learning their trade – they couldn't have been more than twelve years old yet they were able to use the long whips and successfully lasso a specified horse – complete control. It was a really impressive sight as they galloped off with the herdsmen – they could take the Olympic Games by storm were they only able to get there! What a magnificent spectacle to see the Mongols, Arabs and Cossacks in a mile-long race charging round a stony circuit. Several times a very large number of horses along with their *arats* would be collected around a well with drinking troughs. Camels were lolloping around in their aimless way although they must have belonged to some nomads; sheep were always kept close to *ails* or a single *ger*.

The bird life was unexpected and to be without binoculars was frustrating; there were buzzards, black kites, eagles, vultures and other raptors, ducks and geese, storks, wheatears, larks and many 'little brown jobs'. The final delight was to unexpectedly come across clumps of wild flowers of many colours, the most common and the only one I could identify being the beautiful blue irises. If climate change were to bring regular showers of rain, what a wonderful sight this stony desert would be.

Studying the rural health service reminded me of the privilege of being a physician; very few jobs give you the opportunity to knock on the front door and find you are accepted and often even welcomed into the home, its occupants willingly talking to you about the difficulties in their lives, their anxieties about the future and in particular about the health of their children; someone asking if you would please listen to their heart or chest or feel their tummy or look at a rash or listen to them if they have a pain. I was given a glimpse into their lives and an opportunity to understand the hardships of such an existence.

We stopped and knocked on the front door of five isolated *gers;* barking dogs usually warned of our approach and then typically a man or a boy would appear. The *gers* would be surrounded by mainly sheep and goats but also horses and camels, never cattle as they were miles from any pasture. A motor bike was propped up close to one of the *gers* and at another a small, very old truck stood with its wheels nearly covered in sand. We asked if it was still driveable – in a flash the sand was cleared and the nomad proudly drove off without any problem.

Inside it was surprisingly spacious – all five were the same. The cooking and heating area was in the centre with an open chimney space in the roof. Outside, mounds of *argol* had been prepared for the winter and was being intermittently used for cooking even in the summer. Around the perimeter of the tent were rugs and cushions, mattresses and eiderdowns, children's cots, an occasional chair and low wooden benches for sleeping on. The floor was covered with felt matting and around the edge with bundles of sleeping bags. To begin with the children hid in the cooking area or behind the adults but quickly came out to stare. Always in every *ger*, almost before we had sat down, mugs of *tsai* (tea) were produced – Mongolians drank more tea than even the Russians but it wasn't so good. Tea was brought with either the leaves in the mug or what were called tea bricks which were lumps of what looked like mud or earth. These were extremely compact and needed a hammer to chip off what was required. *Suntei-tsai* or milk tea with added salt was the most popular and we would always be offered a second mug.

Sheep, and to a lesser extent horse, was the main food and appeared at breakfast, midday and in the evening. Every part of its anatomy including the head was used (the eyes being an especial delicacy) and only the stomach and upper intestine were thrown away, being full of undigested food. The mutton or horse-flesh and everything else – pancreas, liver, kidneys, lower intestine, bladder, ovaries, uterus, testicles and of course the brain – were always cooked in boiling or simmering water, never roasted, fried or grilled. To refuse to eat and drink this nauseating stew with fatty lumps floating about was tempting, but there was little else to eat. Other mainstays were very salty cheese and the very popular *airag* – fermented mare's milk or milk with added salt.

The smell of boiled mutton and horse was ever present and most unpleasant, but two customs helped to cover the odour. One of these was snuff taking, which was a traditional and frequent activity that usually left a powerful scent behind. Most middle-aged men carried the customary stone snuff bottle – I never saw a snuff box. The second custom was cigarette smoking – universal amongst Mongolian men, but in the *gers* long-stemmed pipes with smallish bowls were preferred. Without a doubt for me the smell of snuff or pipe tobacco was infinitely preferable to the alternative.

Home-made vodka or *shamiarikh* was made from milk – sheep, mare, camel or goat depending on personal preference and the availability of the milk. Commercial vodka or *arikh* could only be found in large towns and was exclusively imported from Russia.

The FCO was full of warnings about Mongolia – poor facilities, restricted travel and awful food, although they did add that people, especially the nomads, were hospitable and friendly. I couldn't disagree with the FCO and their warnings were not without reason as I found on this trip. We stayed in two hotels, both small single-storey buildings of concrete blocks clad in rubble and mud with corrugated iron roofs. The walls inside were cracked, full of holes and the plaster falling off, but at least there was a bed and a communal tap (for six rooms) in the corridor or attached to the outside wall. Ill-fitting door frames were a feature and in one room the rusting metal pipes circling the room ended with an open pipe hanging over my bed; nothing happened, maybe it had never carried any water, who knows. The communal lavatories were seriously ancient and chipped but surprisingly they half flushed in a trickling sort of way. No lavatory paper. The communal washing area at least had a cracked mirror and a basin. No plug. It was just impossible to imagine what it would be like in the winter – perhaps it would be closed. The food was grim.

Back in Ulaanbaatar the domestic scene was intriguing; it was the same as anywhere else in the world with families, the old and the young, wandering around. A large area of parkland was available for children to play and adults to amble and picnic *en famille*. In addition hundreds of folk gathered in a separate area of grassland to watch the two main sports – wrestling and archery. The wrestling was particularly exciting, bare chested, without shoes or sandals, just colourful shorts and depending it seemed to me on muscle and brute strength, so different from the obscenely-obese highly stylised sumo wrestling of Japan. The archery was impressive and as far as I recall was exclusively a male sport; in the adult section the distance was significant – as much as fifty to seventy yards.

The difference in clothing was instantly noticeable as most middle-aged and all the elderly of both sexes were wearing traditional clothes. These consisted of a *deel*, a calf-length embroidered tunic of yellow, deep maroon, red or green tied round by an orange or yellow silk sash. The men wore *gutals* – the typical boots with upturned toe pieces. The women covered their heads with colourful scarves and the men wore a variety of head gear –soft trilby hats with upturned brims, fur hats à la Russia, soft felt or woollen hats usually red, or the four-sided, pointed head gear which wasn't quite a hat or a cap. It isn't very often that the middle-aged and elderly add colour and atmosphere to the streets, but here they most certainly did.

The younger males wore jeans and T-shirts and the ubiquitous baseball cap that sadly had arrived with American culture. Teenage girls often wore jeans and a blouse, a few sported frocks. Small children were dressed like small children and pushchairs looked much the same as anywhere else in the world – the babies however looked different as they were swaddled from head to toe.

Did I have any regrets? Yes.

First I remember many occasions when doctors who had been showing us round their health centre or rural hospital or paediatric ward or delivery room would all say:

> "You won't forget us, will you? Experts come and we show them everything and they never come back."

They were almost pleading with us. I promised I would send information about my intended return but I never did because I didn't return. We promised to send our report to the British Embassy in Ulaanbaatar for photocopying and distribution. It was sent to the Ministry of Health by the Ambassador, but what happened then I've no idea.

Second, my reaction was anger and resentment more than regret. The British Embassy, the first foreign embassy to be opened in Mongolia, seemed to provide endless support to New Zealanders, Australians, Canadians and other Commonwealth nations who had no embassies of their own; most of these received plenty of cash and support for their projects and most of the individuals I spoke to were on their second or third visit to Mongolia. Our Embassy and its small staff had little money and not enough for even the smallest things. I asked the ambassador about providing weighing devices for checking a baby's weight, modern sphygmomanometers and midwives' maternity bags – nothing expensive and absolutely bog-standard; quite impossible, apparently. In no way did I blame the ambassador but I certainly felt that as a UK citizen I was the poor man of the Commonwealth and the ambassador was a poor man in his own Embassy.

Third, I wished I had explained more emphatically about the use of the title 'family doctor'. The Ministry in Ulaanbaatar had been led up the garden path or unwittingly didn't understand that the UK had given up the old family doctor service in the 1980s. Although we pretended we still had such a service the reality was different and now, in 2015, it is clear for everyone to see that our family doctors are now part-time GPs with no guarantee their surgeries will remain open for five days in the week, with no night work, no weekend work, and the patient generally registering with a practice and not an individual doctor. The Mongolians should have been advised to call their new project the General Practice Service – this would have had the advantage of being honest and would also have been easier to implement.

Our departure was somewhat unnerving. Time of takeoff was spot on entirely due to a large Chinese delegation; they arrived in a fleet of Soviet-style politburo limousines with blacked-out windows and the Chinese flag conspicuous on the bonnet. After much hand-shaking and bowing they quickly boarded the waiting plane.

The only runway had a significant slope with hills close by at the highest point. As the groaning Tupolev struggled up the runway it seemed we only cleared the hills with difficulty. After half an hour or so it was obvious we weren't gaining height and an announcement informed us there was a technical fault and we would be returning to Ulaanbaatar.

We watched the technical fault being repaired; an ordinary ladder was propped up against one of the wings and an 'engineer' climbed up to attack one of the engines with a hammer and screwdriver while his companion waited on the ground with a workman's bag and held the ladder. The ladder was moved around and different hammers and screwdrivers were tried, plus on one occasion wire cutters and pliers. Thus time passed, one and a half hours to be precise. It was all rather amusing, though it must be admitted also a trifle anxiety-making.

Mongolia Airways were known to have only three operational aircraft so the likely end to the predicament would be to wait until the next day for the second aircraft to arrive from Peking. But suddenly – great excitement as our aircraft was towed away and replaced by aircraft No. 3 which had been standing unnoticed behind a large shed. A silent three cheers for the Chinese delegation – everything had to appear to run smoothly for them and without them I am sure we would have had an overnight wait.

But to end on a sad note. In May 1995 I had written to Dr Nymadawa about my report, enquiring about any changes that might have taken place in the Family Doctor Service and saying I hoped to meet him when he came to London in 1996. A month or so later I heard from our Embassy in Ulaanbaatar that Dr Nymadawa had died unexpectedly and suddenly earlier in the year, apparently from food-poisoning.

14

THE THIRD WORLD

In the early 1950s the 'Third World' was first used to distinguish developing countries from the Capitalist and Communist blocs. Since then the 'Developing World' and the 'Third World' have been used synonymously, although other phrases have crept into the language – under-developed, less developed, even just poor and rich. At the same time a number of countries didn't wish to become associated with the labels of Third World or Developing country and set up the Non-Aligned group of nations.

By the middle of the 1970s the WHO, UNICEF, the World Bank, the International Monetary Fund, as well as individual governments and research groups such as Willy Brandt's *North-South: a Programme for Survival* had revealed the magnitude of the problem – 75% of the world's population received only 12% of its wealth. Since that time the gap between rich and poor has remained, and within the Third World itself the glaring contrast in living standards between the elite ruling class and the mass of the people is clear to see, even in the very poorest countries of sub-Saharan Africa and Asia. The corruption found in so many governments and societies coupled with the inequality of world trade leave most of us with a feeling of helplessness.

Poor health is a direct consequence of poverty so it is ridiculous to talk about the problems of health care in isolation; politics and health are inextricably interwoven. The basic problems of the Third World are well-known: lack of clean water; almost non-existent sanitation; poor housing and overcrowding; frequent famines from failing agriculture; war and the displacement of hundreds and thousands across frontiers into endless refugee camps completing the picture.

The most serious medical problems are equally obvious – high maternal, infant and early childhood mortality along with malnutrition and common diseases such as simple diarrhoea and chest infections. Throughout the twentieth century the introduction of vaccination and immunisation particularly of children has brought about encouraging improvements.

Since the end of the Second World War a serious mistake has been made by both politicians and health professionals – the focus on hospital building and the promise that the result of this building would benefit all patients. It is now accepted that the notion that a hospital would act as a referral centre for patients from every corner of a country is simply untrue. Examples are everywhere – in the Mulago hospital in Kampala, Uganda, 88% of all admissions come from the Mengo district of the capital in the immediate vicinity of the hospital; in the central hospital in Accra, Ghana, less than 10% of patients come from outside the capital. I could go on and on but there is no point as the principle is the same throughout the Third World.

President Nyere of Tanzania summed up the views of a few enlightened leaders in the Third World:

> "We must not again be tempted by offers of a big new hospital with all the running costs involved until at least every one of our citizens has basic medical services readily available to them."

The running costs now increasingly include high-tech medicine, which is entirely the responsibility of the medical profession. Sadly Nyere's advice has not been followed, but mercifully he died before he realised he had been ignored.

The study of primary care in two Third World countries was undertaken in 1974. Chile and Cuba had similarities: geographical location and similar-sized populations, and both had already developed some form of health service, Chile in 1952 and Cuba in 1959. But here the parallels ended and different political manifestos showed the consequences for patients.

15

REPUBLIC of CUBA

My first contact with the Cuban authorities was a surprise. I wrote to their embassy in London on 6 February 1973 and the Second Secretary replied immediately on 8 February suggesting we meet on the morning of 24 February – a Saturday. Never before or since have I ever heard of an embassy of any country being open on a Saturday, and certainly not for a routine appointment. I remember feeling vaguely optimistic, but it was premature.

Angel Dalmon passed on my request to visit Cuba to the Ministry of Health in Havana, but a year later I had still not received a reply. At this time Cuba's relations with many countries in the non-communist world were difficult and of course, with the USA, non-existent. Interestingly only citizens from Scandinavia, Canada, France and Italy didn't require visas. I had no contacts and neither had Frank Ošanéc in Prague. However, it turned out I had a contact on my doorstep.

Neville Butler was Professor of Child Health at the University of Bristol; over a number of years he had been in charge of a study looking into the causes of perinatal deaths in the UK and had become a WHO consultant adviser on the subject. In 1973 the Cubans had invited him to advise on neonatal and perinatal deaths.

It was purely by chance I heard of his Cuban connection during a lecture on perinatal deaths in the UK in which he briefly mentioned his work for the WHO, and his very recent involvement with Cuba. On 1 February 1974 he wrote:

> 'Just to let you know I had quite a successful time in Cuba and passed on your curriculum vitae and necessary details to Professor Jordan and also to the Chief Adviser in Obst and Gynae, Professor Lagonchere. I told them both how anxious you were to visit Cuba and I am sure they will do their best. Unfortunately I believe there has been a clamp-down on the number of visas given to British subjects and I heard from another source that unless one has a close relative in Cuba or is going on what they consider to be important national business, there seemed to be a long waiting

time. However, one can only hope that the mission you wish to accomplish there will have a priority!

My own work there as you know was concerned with analysing their one week national survey into births . . . and a three months' survey into perinatal deaths. I am going there again in the last week in September . . . I may have some further news for you when I come back if you have not heard before. Doubtless we shall be seeing each other long before that.'

A letter dated 22 March from the British Embassy in Havana showed Professor Butler's influence already having some effect and clearly, without his willingness to help, my visit would never have taken place. The Embassy wrote:

'You were of course very wise to have written about a year in advance (in fact it was nearly two years) of your proposed visit but I am sure you will understand that it was inevitably a little difficult to get anyone from here to focus on your proposal which when I last wrote seemed so far away. However, now that the time has shortened and I know that during his recent visit to Havana Professor Neville Butler spoke to Professor Jordan and a colleague about you, I think we should soon have something to tell you.'

It became a story of downs and ups. 17 April produced another letter from the British Embassy:

'. . . I am very sorry to have to report that to date there has been very little progress. We have repeatedly tried to get in contact with Dr Jordan but he appears to be out of Havana doing some short-term voluntary work in the countryside (as was the custom in Castro's Cuba) and repeated promises by his secretary that Dr Jordan would phone back as a matter of priority have come to nought. In fact it appears that the secretary herself is now out of Havana doing her stint in the countryside or whatever . . .'

Next some good news:

'. . . since writing on April 25th (a letter I never received) the International Relations Department of the Ministry of Health have replied to our enquiries to say they would be pleased to sponsor your visa application and give you every assistance when you arrive in Cuba.'

And on 20 June:

'. . . the Ministry of Health have said they will make the necessary reservations for you but we shall try to check tactfully that they have done this a few days before your arrival . . .'

Just over three months later on 22 October:

> 'You should by now have heard from the Latin American Department of the FCO that the Ministry of Health in Havana has informed us that unfortunately your proposed arrival date of November 13th would pose problems. The World Asthma Conference is taking place in Havana from the 3rd to the 9th . . . and its aftermath . . . puts them in a bit of a quandary . . . most welcome from November 20th onwards . . . they would be pleased if you would be willing to speak to groups of Cuban physicians . . .'

The change of date in fact gave me a lot of trouble as I needed to re-organise my NHS work in my practice and also had to contact Chile by cable in the hope I could change the date of my visit there. However, I awaited my visa without anxiety. Weeks went by and no visa although Angel Dalman at the Embassy assured me there were no problems. I was due to leave on 19 November and by 17 November there was still no visa although late in the evening a cable arrived from the British Embassy in Havana:

> 'Ministry assure us the Cuban Embassy in London have now been instructed to issue the visa.'

The next day I contacted Angel Dalman only to be told no instructions had been received – and then later in the afternoon he telephoned to say I could pick up the visa the next afternoon, 19 November.

Arriving at the embassy mid-afternoon, yes, the visa could be issued but, surprise, surprise, Angel Dalman had gone out and no one else could stamp it. Perhaps I could go to the Cuban Embassy in Madrid – at that time there were no direct flights to Cuba – travelling either by Aeroflot via Moscow or to Madrid and change to Iberian Airlines via the Canary Isles to Havana. I didn't know whether to scream or weep as I was due at Heathrow around 6pm. Dalman was finally contacted and soon after 5pm my visa was stamped and he agreed to take me in his car to the West London Bus Terminal. The flight left at 8.05pm with me on board.

I have gone into such detail about the difficulties of those days as few readers will have any idea or experience of the ramifications of the Cold War.

*

Arriving in Havana about 4.45am, to my astonishment I was met at passport control by someone from the Ministry of Health who whisked me through customs to someone else from the Ministry in the Arrivals waiting area. It was explained that all the hotels were full due to a Women's Congress (it was the United Nations Year for Women) as well as a ballet festival plus the aftermath of the World Asthma Conference. Whilst driving into town it was further explained that Yasser Arafat, the leader of the Palestine Liberation Organisation was also in the country. In the eyes of Castro and his government, Arafat was highly respected and his portrait hung from every dimly lit street lamp along with the ubiquitous portraits of Castro and Che.

I was taken to Protocol House, also called the Ministry Hostel for Health Workers, a large nineteenth century mansion in a pleasantly wooded area surrounded by a number of small houses. How lucky I was that all the hotels were full as the cost of the Ministry Hostel was a quarter the cost of the cheapest hotel and being a foreigner I would only have been permitted to stay in one of the two most expensive hotels in Havana.

My room was small and poky with peeling plaster and paint but it had a washbasin and a primitive shower area. I was ready for a good wash but the water was turned off. After a couple of trips down to the doorman he gave me a couple of buckets of water and an old enamel mug to use as a shower. Two barely functioning light bulbs lit the room and in trying to turn one off I had failed to notice it was attached to a bare wire sticking out of the wall – the electric shock was enough to throw me backwards onto the floor. I removed the bulb and didn't replace it. Eventually falling asleep I was suddenly awakened by a tremendous clanking noise as though someone with a sledge hammer was at work outside my door, but it was no more than the water system being turned on. This was a regular feature of the early morning as was the water being cut off in the early evening.

The women who served in the communal restaurant became extraordinarily friendly and helpful; they spoke no English and I spoke no Spanish yet they managed to understand the problems I was having with washing myself and my clothes. Using sign language they explained I must get a couple of buckets of water from the houses that surrounded Protocol Hotel when I returned in the evening. On one occasion I forgot to leave the buckets to be filled, so after the evening meal two of the women from the restaurant took me to the man in charge of the water pump and forced him to fill them – they were formidable and not to be argued with. The whole rigmarole seemed utterly pointless and was especially irritating as there was no shortage of water.

Food rationing had been a fact of life since the Revolution except for government officials or the use of bribery. Bread and milk daily, an egg twice weekly but no meat or chicken. Fruit was plentiful and cheap as was fish, but it seemed Cubans rarely ate fish. Considering the shortage of food this seemed very strange and I never found out the reason. It was suggested that the most plentiful species of fish was very bony. Each family had weekly ration cards for very basic needs and they were directed to specific shops. This enabled the official who was in charge to know the exact number of customers he would have each week. The system worked well and an almost-family relationship built up in the shops.

A couple of days after my arrival there was torrential rain in the night and I slipped as I was hurrying for the waiting ministry car. My trousers were smeared with mud so I quickly went back to my room to change. On returning that evening and wondering how on earth I was going to wash the trousers, I found they had gone. Early next day one of this band of wonderful women knocked at my door with the trousers washed and ironed; I was just bowled over by their kindness.

It seemed as if this Hostel for Health Workers had created a sense of equality and social cohesion amongst the workers, who were from every branch of medicine and nursing. Cuba was the seventh communist country I had visited and superficially at least it felt different – perhaps the climate and being part of the Caribbean was a factor but it wasn't the whole story. I had experienced help and kindness in other countries I had visited, but never communism where alcohol was actually enjoyed, with laughter and dancing and singing in a cafe or on the beach or in the streets. Always in the Soviet Union and in Eastern Europe alcohol was consumed seriously and in great quantities – mostly to shut out the grim reality of life and often just to survive the long winters. Cuba was communism with a smiling face – how long the smile would last I had no idea.

The Spanish Empire occupied Cuba for longer than any of the other countries in Central and South America, and it was not until 1899 that it experienced brief independence followed in the early twentieth century by protected status under the United States and was quickly proclaimed an independent republic. This proved to be a total fiction as the United States was able to intervene on almost any pretext and to put a stranglehold on Cuba both politically and economically.

The Cuban scene involved corruption, social injustice, nepotism, farmers, fishermen, tradesmen and a large number of unemployed; there was no middle class. Foreigners ran the economy and were mainly responsible for the poverty and for creating a haven for gambling, drugs and prostitution which satisfied the steady flow of businessmen from many parts of the world, though mainly the USA and South America – and tourists from the Americas and Spain.

Cuba was rotten to the core and was ready for revolution. 1959 was the year the country freed itself from the United States but became instead beholden to the Soviet Union.

Even the most fervent opponents of the Castro government could not disagree with the following assessment of health care at the end of the Batista regime. First of all a health service didn't exist and only about 25% of the population had private health insurance, so the rest had little hope of getting any medical assistance. Second, primary care was practised largely by specialists who were paid on an item-of-service basis. As a direct consequence the emphasis was on curative medicine and little thought was given to prevention. Third, the mal-distribution of doctors and nurses had left a large percentage of the population with nobody. Fourth, the hospital service was poorly organised leading inevitably to a duplication in some specialties and many gaps in others. Finally, medical education was divorced from the needs of the community.

By 1974 medical services had been organised à la Soviet Union. The post-revolution principles and objectives were clear. First, both curative and preventive care were to be provided free at the time of use; as in the UK, children, pregnant women and the elderly were exempt from prescription charges. It had been impossible to provide complete cover at a stroke so well-defined priorities and problems were the focus i.e. poor housing, sanitation, ante-natal care and the supervision of deliveries, neo- and peri-natal mortality and morbidity, childhood nutrition, and a concentration on the commonest causes of morbidity and mortality in adults.

Second, a redistribution of hospital resources took place; in 1959, 54.7% of beds were in Havana for 22% of the population and 15.5% of beds in Oriente Province for 35%. By 1972, 40% of beds were in Havana and 23% in Oriente with roughly similar populations.

Third, as most illnesses can be dealt with outside the hospital environment, the emphasis was placed on community facilities so that by 1971, 236 polyclinics had been built or adapted from old buildings and over 50% of these had been developed as rural hospitals. By the time of my visit further buildings had been completed although the exact numbers weren't available.

Fourth, the mass emigration of doctors at the time of the revolution had caused huge problems; in 1959, 6,300 physicians were working in Cuba and by 1962 more than 3,000 had departed, almost exclusively to the United States. Although a medical school had been founded in Havana in 1928, no further schools had been opened since, consequently it was hopelessly inadequate for coping with the post-revolution exodus. A second school was opened in Oriente Province in 1962 followed by a third in Villas Province three years later. By 1974 thirty percent of all university entrants were for medicine of which fifty percent were women. Nursing schools had increased from six to twenty-two with around three hundred nurses qualifying annually.

Finally, something unique to Cuba: the participation of the general public in the running of the health service. This appeared to have been more than a vague well-meaning promise and not an idle threat.

The revolutionaries believed that by actively involving the local population it would minimise the 'we' and 'they' philosophy and would diminish the constant carping from the sidelines which is common in any society. Complaints from the community would initially have to be considered by the community and would involve a variety of organisations – the Committee for the Defence of the Revolution, the

Federation of Cuban Women, various trade unions, and the Federation of Small Farmers. As I write now these organisations are still functioning.

Havana was a fascinating place, at least in parts. Spanish colonial architecture reigned in the old parts of the town with the main streets colonnaded in the neo-classical style, giving welcome protection from the summer heat or the wind and rain in the winter. Dilapidation was a feature of the old city – ancient courtyards with attractive iron balconies and intricately framed windows adding great charm, and despite these looking in imminent danger of falling down, children were playing and mothers and grandmothers sitting and talking and no one seemed to worry.

Walking through this rather sad scene of disrepair and faded elegance I found a number of churches open and I was able to visit freely; they appeared to attract quite large congregations. On the first occasion the church was close to Revolution Square and I had arrived about half an hour before early mass had finished; it was about half full of mainly peasant women of all ages.

I wanted to take a photo of a large portrait of Castro that almost filled one side of the square; I needed to take it early as my instamatic camera (equivalent to the old Box Brownie) was incapable of producing a reasonable photo unless the sun was shining directly on the subject – Castro. Several old women looked disapprovingly at me as I left before the service was over. There was no one about and I took my picture without difficulty, but as I walked away I sensed someone behind me and looking round saw an armed soldier hurrying to catch me up. He turned me round without speaking and pushed me back to his guard-post on the edge of the square. After a couple of phone calls an officer arrived. He understood and spoke English and I explained I was British and was studying their health service – that pleased him. I had forgotten my passport and couldn't recall Dr Roberto Sollet's name (he was in charge of my stay in Cuba); it was all rather embarrassing.

The officer made it very clear that taking photographs in Revolution Square was forbidden as was taking photos of Castro. He then reminded me never to go anywhere without my passport.

I realised I had been fortunate not to have had my camera taken, or worse.

Later that morning I returned to find matins had just finished; I was intrigued by a middle-aged woman sitting on her own by the west door holding a harmonica – she had been playing during early mass. She turned out to be an American and it transpired that at the time of the Revolution she had been living in Cuba, had been imprisoned for spying and sentenced to ten years. For the first few months she had been treated badly and then quite inexplicably everything changed and she was released after eighteen months – but forbidden to leave Cuba. Curiously she was allowed to train as a teacher and she was now teaching maths, English and Latin.

"Yes, I'm free."

But she was lonely and found life sad; few trusted her, even in the congregation.

"I hope one day they'll let me go back to the States."

After an early breakfast the following Sunday I returned to the church in the hope of finding the American. The congregation was much the same, but sadly there was no sign of the harmonica player.

I wandered along to another church I had noticed on the main road close to the Ministry of Health. As well as the church there was a convent and a large quadrangle surrounded by cloisters. The church was full – about a hundred – but only five men including myself. The women were well-dressed, wearing clothes and jewellery that looked pre-revolution. As I left the church I spoke to a number of people including two nuns. They were fascinated to have had a foreigner at the service and a small crowd surrounded me. Some in the group started to talk and the subject of communism and religion surfaced. I couldn't follow everything that was discussed so as I was departing I asked one of the crowd to tell me what they had been talking about; it seemed that the majority of them were convinced that religion, or rather religious people, were not made to be revolutionaries although it was agreed that Christ was the greatest revolutionary in history. They seemed happy to criticise themselves as they agreed that Christ's followers in Cuba didn't understand, or else chose not to understand, the need for continuous revolution in every generation. Christianity just provided comfort and reassurance for the well-heeled but nothing for the downtrodden. A quite unexpected and extraordinary chat.

In the late afternoon of the same day, by chance I came across multiple christenings taking place – eight babies and their families and friends, both men and women. I witnessed no harassment of the Roman Catholic Church, or perhaps it was just well hidden. But provided the Church didn't impinge on or interfere with the State, and didn't advocate revolution, I suppose all was well. At this point the reader may well be wondering whether it was primary medical care I was trying to study or the relationship between communism and religion!

Wherever you live in the world parents are always proud of their children. Early one evening by chance I met one of the Cuban health workers who was staying at the hostel and we came across a large rally outside a school. He was certain it was some sort of celebration connected with the Communist Pioneers (superficially similar to the Guide and Scout movement in the UK). The children looked enchanting, dressed in red and blue uniforms, both girls and boys wearing white skirts and white shorts with neat triangular scarves around their necks. The parents were barely able to contain themselves as their children marched up and down singing patriotic songs – it was a scene of unmitigated pleasure and happiness. As the parents and children drifted away a good crowd surrounded us clamouring to know who I was and to hear me talk. I asked my companion what nationality they thought I was – without exception they said Ruski. When I asked them if I could be French, German, Spanish or English – not possible; asked if I might be American – *impossible!* We were followed back to the hostel for a few blocks feeling for all the world like the Pied Piper. In ten days or so I was to have a similar experience in Chile.

Public transport was clapped out, unreliable and almost without timetables. It was often quicker to walk, even long distances. The majority of buses were British Leyland, reminding me of the huge controversy in 1964 with the renewed selling of buses, the first since the 1959 Revolution – before then they had been sold to the Batista regime since the early 1950s. Harold Wilson's government had given Leyland the ok, much to the anger of the Americans who were trying to impose a total trade embargo on the island. It had even been speculated at the time that the CIA had been responsible for the sinking of a large container ship full of Leyland buses in the Thames estuary. Private cars of which there were few were really old and equally clapped out – they were almost entirely American, reminding me of American films of the '40s and '50s with their conspicuous shark-fin tails. Petrol was both expensive and in very short supply so it was surprising these 'gas-guzzlers' were being driven at all, but then, there was really no alternative except for the occasional Fiat or Trabant.

Food shops were never more than half filled and there were always queues at the corner shops, even if they were nearly empty. Vegetable markets were rare and small and it was obvious why food rationing was still a fact of life.

In my ignorance I had somehow expected Cubans to be similar to the rest of the Caribbean and to the West Indians who came to Bristol in the '40s and '50s, or to the cricketers who subsequently ruled the world. Angel Dalman at the Cuban Embassy in London should have prepared me – he was the first Cuban I had ever met and he had ginger hair. The multi-ethnicity was immediately obvious and by the end of my visit it was clear no tensions existed, quite the opposite.

Cuba is barely seventy miles from the Florida Keys and the esplanade in Havana is directly opposite. Going there at high tide it was never crowded, just a few old men and boys fishing. I was interested to see if they caught anything, what they were using for bait, or whether they were just flinging out spinners onto the second or third line of breakers. By and large fishermen are friendly and so the Cubans proved to be. This was my second wander along the esplanade and I'd brought my camera – limited to sunny, cloudy and dull – which had caused so much trouble in Revolution Square. I was about to take my third photo of the three boys, who looked as though they knew what they were doing, when I heard a scream of tyres and a military jeep stopped close by. Out jumped two fully-armed soldiers shouting wildly and pointing out to sea and at my camera. An officer followed:

> "Don't you know it is forbidden to take photographs? Don't you know this is a military zone and America is over there?"

He asked to see my camera, which I had easily hidden in my trousers. I couldn't decide if he thought the camera was nothing to worry about or the latest in western spying technology. He certainly didn't believe I had been photographing the boys and removed the film from the camera. What useful information he thought I might be collecting I've no idea, but he left with a serious warning – next time I would be arrested.

The docks were full of Soviet oil tankers and Cuban cargo ships exporting sugar, tobacco, bananas and other foods back to the Soviet Union. Two cruise liners with tourists from East Germany and Czechoslovakia completed the scene. According to my Cuban colleagues the tourists would be middle-aged Party members or trade union officials, plus their wives: not a pretty sight.

Although it was on the outskirts of the city, the harbour was enclosed by some of the most attractive baroque and rococo buildings and colonnades – certainly comparable with the centre of the city. Narrow twisting alleys and small houses without windows onto the streets and corrugated iron roofs housed the poor.

Often when talking about health the conversation would drift onto education, which was so highly praised I found it difficult to believe. I asked to be taken to a secondary school. The one chosen was in the town of Artemis about sixty miles from Havana. An impressive new school with about 550 pupils, I was sure it had been handpicked as the school to show foreigners. On the way home I felt confident enough to explain my doubts and asked if we could stop at a village school. 'Of course, choose any village you want' was the answer. This I did and decided on an area that looked particularly run-down. Our interpreter got out to make enquiries and we quickly found the school about fifty yards off the main road.

It had been built since the Revolution but was looking in need of a coat of paint. Our interpreter came out with a young teacher and we were all introduced. She was clearly flustered and invited us in nervously. The school was bright and clean, the walls covered with children's drawings and pictures. There were two rooms, one the classroom and the other a rest room as well as somewhere to eat. There were also flush toilets and a kitchen. Around forty children of primary school age were sitting formally behind five rows of desks; all were in the uniform that was standard throughout the country. The teacher asked them to stand and welcome us to their school. This they did, first in Spanish and then in English, copying what the teacher said. Next I was invited to ask a few questions, to which they replied in English – I presumed the brightest children were asked. By this time the children were beginning to grin at each other and were relaxing; the teacher encouraged them to ask a few questions and this they did although very shyly at first. The teacher lived in the village, spoke Spanish, French and English but not Russian. By the time we departed she was quite relaxed and answered my questions readily. It was a really impressive time and this school had not been handpicked as it was in the middle of nowhere. My visit ended with them singing an English song that they had recently learned – I'm ashamed I can't remember what it was.

One of my lasting memories and something I had not expected was the ease with which I could be invited into people's homes, or with which we could talk openly in the street. Late one afternoon Roberto Sollet decided he would like me to experience how the locals enjoyed themselves. Our destination was Santa Maria beach about fifteen miles from Havana – miles and miles of white sand lined with coconut and date palms. It wasn't overcrowded, just families with picnics, boys kicking footballs, girls chatting and giggling and no sign of irritating teenagers making a nuisance of themselves. There were small bars selling beer and cocktails, stalls with ice creams and soft drinks, but nobody swimming – far too cold.

Just as I thought we were about to return home Roberto explained he had a good friend in a village farther down the coast and it would be good to see how ordinary people were living. This friend had been a guerrilla with Raol Castro at the time of the Revolution and was evidently held in high regard. So we all set off – Oscar Barros the driver, Horacio Fernandez my interpreter and a few others who had joined us on the way. His friend's house was a modest single-storey bungalow built of concrete blocks with a corrugated iron roof. Children of all ages filled the place and as it was quite obvious his wife had not been expecting us we all trooped off to the local bar/restaurant. Roberto explained that taking me out was in fact against the law, but he and his friends had decided I was sympathetic to their 'cause' and wouldn't be any danger to them. I didn't understand what he was saying or what the 'cause' was, but the alcohol flowed, some food appeared and the atmosphere was convivial, relaxed and embarrassingly complimentary – I felt I had almost become an honorary member of Raol Castro's original guerrilla unit as well as a signed up member of the 'cause'. A memorable evening.

Roberto and his wife were again involved in another visit to friends, this time in the centre of Havana – apparently no worry about breaking the law. The flat was in the old part of the town which in the '20s and '30s would have been a fashionable and desirable place to live; now it needed much repair and repainting. After we had negotiated the rather grand hall and the foul-smelling staircase up to the second floor the flat turned out to be clean though sparsely furnished, with two photos of Fidel and Che prominently displayed. Their friends tried their best to be friendly but they spoke little English and I spoke no Spanish, so communication was difficult. Homemade cocktails were quickly produced with Roberto and his wife debating what the mixture should be and the four of them sipping away until perfection was accomplished. In spite of the influence of the Soviet Union I was never offered vodka – I knew they considered themselves to be more sophisticated than the Russians.

On numerous occasions Oscar would drop off Horacio at his home before driving back to the Health Workers Hostel or to wherever I was to meet Roberto or other colleagues. Horacio had recently married and had small baby. Although they lived in a poor district of the city they just seemed pleased to have somewhere to call home. Neither Oscar nor Horacio were remotely embarrassed that I was seeing the really poor areas of Havana – a foreigner was merely seeing how the majority lived. They were quite open about it all and seemed to harbour no resentment.

In a similar open way it had been easy to listen to the American, harmonica-playing church-goer telling me her life story while sitting on the pavement for an hour or so; neither of us had looked round to see if we were being observed. Equally at the church with the convent many of the congregation, including two nuns, had smiled and spoken briefly to me as I wandered around. I was obviously a foreigner but nobody seemed concerned or worried about the military or secret police.

As promised I gave a number of talks to health professionals. I chose a polyclinic and a rural hospital to discuss community care, and a maternity hospital and paediatric unit to represent secondary care. A difference between Cuba and other communist countries I had visited was that nobody worried about speaking out in public at the question and answer sessions that followed. Senior colleagues and politicians also attended the talks but nobody was intimidated by their presence. Most were interested to hear about the NHS, and the majority were astounded to discover it had become law in 1948, was funded by the government and was free at the time of use. I suspect many didn't believe me.

The National Institute of Public Health was the place for two formal lectures. It was the only occasion when the audience became seriously acrimonious; a group of students became really fired up:

> "Don't you realise the severe problems related to pollution and the environment which are being caused by capitalism?"

I replied that pollution was frequently related to industrialisation and this could sometimes be in capitalist countries and sometimes in the communist world. The group were not satisfied so I gave them an account of what I had seen in the USSR and Eastern Europe. I asked if they had been to the Soviet Union, to which they replied 'No'. I then suggested they should keep an open mind until they had been there and seen for themselves. As I left, two groups remained in heated debate. All in all I think these talks and discussions were informative and worthwhile both for myself and for my Cuban hosts.

My study of the Rural Health Service was as good as I could have hoped for. Initially the discussion with the Director of Public Health at Santa Clara the capital of Las Villas Province was extremely useful – many questions I needed to ask were answered, and the director talked quite openly about the difficulties he continued to experience fifteen years after the Revolution; a refreshing atmosphere of frankness prevailed. Professor Butler's reputation helped me again as he was held in such high regard by both public health doctors and anyone connected with paediatrics and maternity work. Suggestions were then made about the next day – a visit to the area polyclinic at Gumanajague, the rural hospital at San Blas in the foothills of the Sierra del Escanbray, and another rural hospital at Topes de Calla near the summit of the Escanbray range. I readily agreed.

The night was to be spent in a sort of motel with wooden huts for sleeping. After supper the director was keen to show me the highlights of Santa Clara, the climax being the new university campus closely guarded by female students with kalashnikovs. The motel also sported a swimming pool which next morning enabled me to see the human race in all its glory. Two busloads of Czech tourists had arrived, perhaps from the cruise liner in Havana harbour, and wanted to swim. What an unattractive sight it was.

Polyclinic Gumanajagne was a success, responsible for a population of about 35,000, but it was now becoming too small as the population was growing apace. Like the majority of rural polyclinics, beds were provided for the 24-hour observation of patients – three beds for children and three for adults. Along with the usual doctors and nurses, laboratory and radiological technicians supervised their small departments. The area was divided into ten sectors and a number of micro-sectors staffed by Cuban Red Cross workers. Three small rural hospitals were an added responsibility.

The director of the polyclinic was particularly proud of the success of the immunisation programme – almost every child under fifteen had been immunised against polio in one day; the director referred repeatedly to the Federation of Cuban Women and the Committee for the Defence of the Revolution as without their enthusiastic cooperation and organising skills this couldn't have been accomplished. As I have already mentioned, these two organisations had been made responsible by law for the follow-up and supervision of health activities in the community.

We next made out way down into a valley leading to flat land between the coast and the Sierra del Escambray, to the coastal town of Trinidad. The oldest inhabited place in the region, it had been founded by the Spanish around the middle of the sixteenth century; the oldest part of the town was currently being restored. A brief walk enabled me to soak up the authentic atmosphere, which was helped by a splendid meal in a delightful bistro. My companions told me that a new law had been passed very recently which forbade any significant alterations to the architecture and layout of the old town – the picturesque nature of the place was to be retained. I couldn't quite make out if this new ruling applied to Trinidad alone or included towns throughout Cuba.

The Rural Hospital San Blas, at the foothills of the Sierra del Escambray made famous by the exploits of Che Guevara, was one of the first hospitals to be built following the Revolution; built in 1960 and opened in 1961 there was at that time no road leading to it. Trinidad was the nearest town with any medical facilities, but impossible for patients to reach and in any case too costly to use. The young doctor in charge was doing his compulsory three-year stint. He was an impressive young chap and we had a long conversation about the rural service as seen from his personal point of view. The main problem was that the area was very backward, his patients poorly educated, extremely resistant to change and suspicious of many aspects of modern medicine.

An amazing if slightly scary drive to the top of the Sierra del Escambray range came next. Sometimes there was a road, sometimes just a rutted track as we twisted our way through dense forests, impenetrable undergrowth and acute hairpin bends with great views of the hidden valleys below. This was all managed by the redoubtable Oscar with carefree nonchalance, one hand on the wheel and the other with his beloved cigarette.

Eventually Rural Hospital Topes de Callas came into view and we all tumbled out. Unlike San Blas, this hospital was now too big as the population had been steadily drifting away. It too had been built in 1960, initially as part of a TB sanatorium, but with TB now well controlled in Cuba, the sanatorium had been converted into a teacher training college, the remaining building being used as a small hospital. It didn't take long for the authorities to realise this was a hopeless place for a teacher training college so it was transferred elsewhere – I think to Trinidad. At the time of my visit the population was only 5,000 so I asked the doctor what the future held. Without hesitation and looking straight at the Director of the Health Department at St Clara, he replied:

"Nobody knows what to do."

This complete honesty was so refreshing and the Director didn't disagree; I wondered, but didn't ask, if they thought Che had been responsible for the rather hasty building of these facilities.

As we travelled through the countryside the main crops were easy to spot – predominantly sugar cane, tobacco and rice. All farms had been collectivised as in the Soviet Union and there were very strict rules regarding how much any individual worker could grow for private consumption. Every now and then huge factories involved in sugar production could be seen. Rather more picturesque were the ancient steam trains pulling six to eight wagons full of sugar cane, puffing their way across the landscape from the collective farms to the factories.

What influence did Fidel Ruz Castro and Ernesto Che Guevara have on the Cuban people and what impression did they leave behind? Their pictures and portraits were everywhere – on the streets, in all public buildings and many private homes, rather like pictures of the Pope found in many homes in Italy, Southern Ireland and Poland.

There were rather more pictures of Fidel than Che; he was admired and respected and most people believed he had lifted Cuba out of corruption, crime, inequality and the moral sewage of the Batista regime. His faults and weaknesses were tolerated – even found amusing – such as his inability to give up smoking (he finally managed this in 1985), his inability to address the nation for less than three to four hours at a time and his great liking for good food. The majority believed he had led a simple, hard-working life, that he was a private, possibly lonely man, and almost nobody thought he had been involved in any financial corruption. It was believed by all that he had put Cuba on the world stage.

Che was more difficult to assess. He was, after all, Argentinian and Cuba was only his adopted home. After travelling the world almost as a spokesman for Fidel but also as a revolutionary figure in his own right, in July 1966 he secretly returned to Cuba to train his new guerrilla army for further revolution in South Africa. Advised by Castro to use Bolivia as his base, he resigned from the posts he held in the Cuban government and gave up his Cuban citizenship. In the autumn of 1966 Che and his men left for Bolivia and almost exactly a year later on 5 October 1967 he was captured by Bolivian forces and executed the following day. He has remained a romantic hero, not only in Cuba but throughout the world – strikingly handsome and eternally young. Some in Cuba have rather wildly suggested that Che was to the revolutionary spirit what Christ had been to the Church. Seven years after his death, at the time of my visit, it was easy to understand that in spite of such misplaced hyperbole, people were still transfixed by the images and stories of this rebel who sacrificed everything for his beliefs.

One evening I had a great opportunity to listen and watch Castro addressing the nation – a number of my Cuban colleagues wanted me to see him in action. It was the United Nations Year for Women and basically what he said was that Cuban men must show less machismo, must be more respectful to women and generally help more in the home. The speech only lasted just over two hours and we half watched, half listened as we drank many homemade cocktails. I asked if the speech would have any effect – roars of laughter and a resounding 'NO!'

Although not directly connected with Castro, on another evening I had a fascinating insight into senior government ministers on an evening out in public. I had been taken to a performance by the International Ballet, one of the reasons the hotels were so full. The artistes were from the USSR, Hungary, Czechoslovakia, Romania and Cuba with Argentina and Brazil thrown in. There was no orchestra and the music was played on a gramophone using rather scratched records; only popular excerpts were danced – pas de deux and the like from the classical romantic repertoire such as *Swan Lake*, *Rite of Spring* and *Romeo and Juliet*. Utterly bizarre. Two rows directly in front of us was an official government group including Raól Castro, his wife and others I'd never heard of. No security guards could be seen and I was assured it was quite normal for official groups to sit amongst the hoi polloi without them.

The evening was spoilt for me by the audience – including the government groups – talking throughout without any embarrassment. Just before the interval Raól Castro suddenly stood up and departed without his wife. No one seemed to notice or even comment. My companions insisted it would have been just the same if it had been Fidel sitting there.

I had no idea until this performance by the International Ballet that Fidel at the very beginning of the Revolution had been concerned that art and culture should not be restricted to the wealthy or the upper echelons of society. He wanted everyone to be involved, so art colleges, drama and ballet schools would be open and free to all children, and all styles of music – jazz, classical, folk etc would be available; he had genuinely hoped to create a workers' paradise.

When Castro came to power in '59, almost his first decision was to set up a national health service, taking an even higher priority than education. One of his important pledges was to guarantee there would be a doctor at the end of every street; unsurprisingly most people saw him as their saviour. It is difficult to know whether this was just a rhetorical promise or a genuine intention. In truth, no real thought could have been given to this promise, such as whether it was necessary, whether the required number of doctors could be trained and financed, and what work they would be asked to do.

This lack of clear thinking regarding the activities of health workers had not changed since the Revolution; over the intervening fifteen years the idea that a suitably trained nurse could carry out some of the work done by doctors, and that auxiliary nurses could do tasks performed by trained nurses, was not on the agenda. The Cubans seemed unaware that advanced industrial societies were already thinking along these lines, and they were opposed to such changes happening in the developing world. They wanted to build up a doctor-dominated service and didn't support the idea of barefoot doctors in Mao's China and similar workers in Iran and other countries in the world. The *feldscher* was never mentioned during my stay; clearly Cuba agreed with the Soviet Union and considered the *feldscher* to be a poorly and inadequately trained doctor who should be removed from a modern health service.

Cynics and those opposed to Cuba politically have been astonished by the help given by Cuba over many years to non-aligned and developing countries in times of conflict or natural disasters – the help usually took the form of large numbers of doctors, sometimes a hundred at a time, being sent to the afflicted areas. These cynics and opponents of Castro believed this was the only way Fidel's doctors could be usefully occupied; there was certainly some truth in this view, so their cynicism was not entirely misplaced.

It is true that if Fidel had wanted to modify his original idea that there should be a doctor at both ends of the street and living in the community of every small town and village, then the population could justifiably say he had reneged on a serious promise. This however was not the case and throughout his long life as President his views on having a doctor-dominated health service never changed.

Regrets come in all shapes and sizes and for me Cuba was no exception – being unable for a variety of reasons to return to this fascinating country was one of them. Many years later, however, this disappointment has long since evaporated owing to five flights a day of sex tourists landing in Havana from Madrid and daily flights from all over Europe and the United States. Can it be that sadly the culture and way of life of the Batista era is returning?

Roberto had been an enormous help and had become a good friend, and as we said goodbye we knew what this meant at the height of the Cold War. But amazing things happen. Towards the end of August 1976 Roberto and a colleague spent a few days in Wells – our roles were reversed and they were able to see how my family and friends were living. They had been sent to Stockholm for a conference, the first time either of them had been out of Cuba, and surprisingly they had been given permission to stop over in England so I could show them how general practice (primary care) was organised. As far as I can remember it was the Cuban Embassy in London who contacted me to say they were coming to Wells – all very exciting.

A small party was arranged including Professor Neville Butler and another doctor from the Bristol Children's Hospital who had recently been to Cuba with the professor, someone from the BBC World Service South America Department, friends of ours and a patient who spoke Spanish.

I asked Roberto if they could make up some cocktails and he agreed with great enthusiasm. What did he need? Rum, various fruit juices, spices and lemons. Patrick, one of our kids, did the shopping, and on his return Roberto's response to the three lemons was almost hysterical – Patrick hastily beat a retreat back to the shops and returned with fifteen. About an hour and a half later two wonderful cocktails had been prepared. It was a memorable evening with the two Cubans smoking cigars continuously.

A couple of days later another goodbye, and this time we never met again.

16

REPUBLIC of CHILE

There was no direct flight from Cuba to Chile – the quickest way was via Peru with a stopover in Lima. Only Aeroflot flew from Havana to Lima and although the plane was due to leave at 9am it didn't depart until 1.15pm. Slowly I was learning the futility of asking airport officials, or any officials for that matter, about travel delays, particularly in the communist world. I remembered clearly the trouble I had had at Irkutsk airport in Eastern Siberia – I had asked one friendly-looking chap about the delay and he'd replied that the flight could be delayed until the next day, or maybe there wasn't any fuel, or even an available plane. The message was: stop asking stupid questions, just sit and wait.

Without a cloud in the sky, first the Caribbean Sea, then the Panama Canal and the coastline of Columbia, Ecuador and Peru was clear to see with the northern range of the Andes plunging into the Pacific Ocean. It was like looking at a huge map, a wonderful geography lesson.

Aeroflot made sure I didn't forget I was still under the influence of the Soviet Union. As we were coming into land in Lima an announcement was made about the time of arrival – but according to Moscow time, not local. It caused a bit of confusion amongst the less experienced passengers like myself who had never been on this flight before; needless to say, the flight attendants were in no mood to help. Mind-boggling, really, yet quite amusing on reflection.

My first enquiry about visiting Chile had been in a letter to the Embassy in London on 24 January 1973 and slow progress was made with Professor Hugo Behm, Department of Public Health and Social Medicine at the University Medical School in Santiago; eventually we agreed the visit should take place in 1974/75.

On 11 September 1973, after ten days of fruitless negotiations between the government of Salvador Allende and the Army Chief of

Staff General Augusto Pinochet, a coup d'état took place. La Monedo or Presidential Palace right in the centre of Santiago was bombed and quickly surrounded by tanks. Allende refused to surrender and broadcast his last declaration of defiance to the Chilean people around 9.30am when, at about the same time, the tanks opened fire and troops entered the palace; whether Allende was murdered or committed suicide still remains a matter of dispute. It matters little – a democratically elected coalition government had been replaced by a military dictatorship which was to remain in power for the next seventeen years.

I wrote to Professor Behm in December '73 asking if it was still in order to visit Chile. A reply came, not from Professor Behm but from Dr Bogoslav Juricic, Head of International Relations, Department of the Ministry of Health, assuring me it would still be in order.

However, horrifying reports had started to come out of Chile which gave me pause for thought about whether I should go. Two things persuaded me to say yes. First, I had visited the USSR without condoning what was going on there, although admittedly there wasn't an active civil war at the time. Second, a London-based Medical Committee for the Defence of Chilean Health Workers(MCDCHW) was encouraging me to make the visit and just before leaving had given me a list of doctors and nurses known to have been imprisoned and possibly tortured. It was hoped I might be able to find out what had happened to them and possibly get to speak to them (alas I was singularly unsuccessful in this).

On first morning at the Ministry I asked if I would be able to meet Professor Behm during my stay:

"No"
"Why not?"
"He is in prison."
"Why?"
"Because he is a communist."

By the wildest stretches of the imagination Behm could never have been described as a communist: from his articles and lectures he was regarded as an academic with left-wing views who was passionately concerned with the relationship between ill-health and poverty and the consequent need for social justice. Within the Colegio Medico de

Chile (equivalent to the British Medical Association) he was a complete outsider and his imprisonment was no surprise to the majority of members. He was judged to be a communist by the government of President Pinochet. The left wing, often referred to as the communist government of President Allende, was seen by many to have been responsible for the economic collapse of the country, and so the dictatorship of Pinochet was a price worth paying. A later request to visit him was again refused – 'it couldn't be arranged'. I learned subsequently he had been released from prison in 1977 and had fled to Costa Rica. I tried to contact him without success.

The authorities at the Ministry of Health looked at the list of doctors and nurses given to me by the MCDCHW; the little information I gleaned was – six of the doctors remained in prison, one had been freed soon after arrest, two had eventually been released and gone abroad (one of whom had had her second child whilst in prison). No further information was given about any of the others on the list.

While I had no doubt about the integrity and veracity of the information given by the Chilean doctors in exile and by Amnesty International, nor of the honest motivation of the London-based MCDCHW, by the end of my visit I was confused by what I had heard from both pro-Allende and pro-Pinochet doctors and their relatives and friends. It seemed everything was not quite as clear-cut and straightforward as I had originally thought.

Chile had been almost universally condemned since the overthrow of Allende. There had been moral outrage that a democratically elected president – the only one at that time in Latin America – and his government had been deposed with such violence. There was no dispute that trade unions and political meetings had subsequently been prohibited, the press and news media muzzled, and that the stories of illegal imprisonment and torture and the question of the disappeared, were true.

Allende's Popular Unity government was a coalition of his own Socialist Party, the Communist Party, various strands of Marxism, Social and Christian Democrats and a few independents. Allende, once he had won the election in September 1970, needed unity within the coalition to withstand the extreme right-wing parties, the rich landowners, the multinational owners of tin and copper, and most importantly those members of the armed forces who opposed him.

I never managed to discover if there was any truth in the allegations in the press and on the radio (and by physicians I met) that the communists and marxists were as bourgeois in their attitudes and behaviour as the very people who were opposing them – that they dressed in fine clothes, had expensive wives and sent their children to the best schools. I was shown some of the splendid villas of Pinochet supporters and sad disillusioned followers of Allende – the homes of the so-called socialists. I never heard anyone suggest that Allende or his family were anything but decent ordinary folk, but unfortunately he himself lacked the necessary revolutionary fervour and the charismatic leadership of Fidel Castro and Che Guevara.

Another story I was told related to the rich farmlands in the south of the country and how the communists and marxists behaved. Apparently any rich landowners who hadn't left were shot; meanwhile the poor farm labourers had to cope as best they could and then watch the crops being harvested and taken away with nothing being re-sown for the following year. Cattle were killed and eaten, food production went down and the price of food escalated. Both suppliers and opponents of Allende told me the same tale.

By chance one of the books I had with me was Mikhael Sholokov's dramatic, cruel and passionate novel *And Quiet Flows The Don.* It tells the story of the Cossacks – at peace, at war, in revolution, and finally in civil war, with descriptions of the initial arrival of the Bolsheviks to the Upper Don and their barbaric, primitive and ignorant pillaging of the rich farmland of that region – some similarities with southern Chile.

Moreover, on arriving home, what became apparent was the involvement of the United States' government, the CIA and their agents in Chile, and the American Embassy in Santiago. Their intention was simple – to undermine democracy and create social unrest, to support and help organise the assassination of Allende, and to further strangle the economy. President Nixon and Henry Kissinger have a lot to answer for.

The medical profession seemed to have been as unpopular with the Popular Unity government as with any other part of society. This had been brought about by hospital doctors supporting a countrywide lorry drivers' strike over the cost of fuel in October 1972. The doctors' support was on account of the shortage of medical supplies and drugs being delivered to the hospitals. Both groups were in fact striking against the economic mess at the time that apparently resulted from government incompetence but in reality from interference by the United States.

The second doctors' strike occurred in September 1973 just before Pinochet's coup d'état. The Colegio Medico de Chile required all physicians to sign their name and record their reasons for refusing to join the strike, both those in support of Allende and those who refused on ethical grounds. The reason for the strike was purported to be on account of low pay in hospitals and *consultarios* (primary care facilities). While this was undoubtedly a factor, eventually it became a political act against the government. Following the coup everyone on the list was arrested by the military junta. Some were killed without trial, some were released, and others were still in detention at the time of my visit.

Some doctors were angry; to suggest the whole profession should be tarred with the same brush was manifestly unfair and made bigotry the master of reason. The international medical community decided to try and exclude the Colegio Medico from international conferences and meetings; their response not surprisingly had been 'What about China? The Soviet Union? Countries in the Middle East?'

Individual doctors I spoke with couldn't understand how two different standards were being applied. The certainty of foreign armchair critics sitting in the comfort and safety of their homes – they just didn't know what they were talking about; such people should have lived through the last four to five years before daring to open their mouths.

It was unfortunate, perhaps unwise, to get myself involved in the politics of my host country, but there was little alternative since by the time of my arrival in 1974 the knowledge of the recent murders and imprisonment of health workers had spread around the world. The experience of Dr Sheila Cassidy, a British doctor who had been working in Chile since 1971, and her arrest in 1975, also received world coverage. After her release and return to the UK in 1977 her book *Audacity to Believe* recorded clearly and without drama or sensation what it had been like to live in Chile before and after the coup.

Although politics took up a lot of time, in the end the study of primary care benefitted enormously due to the help and cooperation of individual doctors with whom I had been discussing politics. The Ministry of Health had done virtually nothing except give me permission to visit the country and obtain a visa. Dr Juricic at the Ministry was formal, an old-fashioned physician who had been educated and trained as a specialist; he had organised a hospital-dominated programme for me, exactly what I had asked the Ministry not to do. I immediately realised there would be no possibility of getting anything altered. I would just have to play it from day to day. Permission had been granted to visit Santiago and its environs, but nothing farther afield. Interpreters and drivers were not provided and I just hoped some doctors would speak English and maybe help with transport.

Chile had a population of a little over 9.5 million; 3 million concentrated in Santiago, 1.5 million in Valparaiso and 1 million in Conception. The country had the familiar urban/rural split as well as *poblaciones* – working-class areas of abject poverty and poor health that occurred in urban housing estates and residential areas as well as in any village or settlement.

As I had no transport and the local buses were hopeless and taxis too expensive, I decided I would walk everywhere, making sure I carried nothing of value with me. I walked on unmade or cobbled roads, seeing block after block of flat-roofed dwellings made from crumbling stucco and collections of wood, corrugated iron, bits of tin and endless cardboard. Everywhere I looked was grey and depressing with drunks sprawled all over the place and many hungry, barking, stray dogs which actually were the only things that really frightened me. The filth was indescribable with sewage floating in the muddy ditches where children were happily playing as rats scurried around.

Since the early 1930s a modified form of health insurance had been introduced and in 1954 Chile became the first country in Latin America to introduce a state-run health service. The *Servicio Naccional de Salud* (SNS) was 75% financed from direct taxation, 10% through social security payments and 15% from a variety of smaller measures such as prescription charges and a cemetery tax. From its inception little attempt was made to provide a service for the whole population. It was accepted that about a third would continue to pay their physicians privately, and successive governments realised that a substantial portion of a doctor's income would stem from this source.

By the early '60s President Frei and his government recognised that the SNS was seriously underfunded, which was having a number of consequences. First, private practice had been steadily increasing. Second, separate services had been created for the armed forces, the police, railway workers, coal and tin miners and many white-collar workers. Third, the great majority of those living in rural areas had no service at all.

In 1970 when Allende became President he made a serious attempt to provide a comprehensive service which was to be financed by central taxation plus taxation of the oligarchy, landowners and the wealthy business community. In addition the Popular Unity government made a genuine effort to change the emphasis away from hospitals to neighbourhood health centres or *consultorios* – an entirely logical and essential step if there was to be any real prospect of improving the health of the poor and not so poor.

The effects of poor housing, sanitation and malnutrition, particularly amongst children and pregnant/nursing mothers, had been accepted by President Frei and his party as early as the late '50s, and Allende was now eager to again emphasise these public health issues and attempt to democratise the SNS. Clearly Chile had led the way in Latin America regarding democracy and social welfare policy, and Allende was keen for this to continue.

Casejo Local de Salud (local health councils) were set up in hospitals and *consultorios* with representatives from trade unions, women's organisations, schools and health workers; the aim was to provide a link between the SNS and patients/the general public.

Casejo Pantarios (executive health councils) were initiated at the same time and also at hospitals and *consultorios*. The council consisted of twelve members – six local representatives and six health workers – the chairman being the director of the hospital or *consultorio*.

Responsables de Salud (responsibility for health) was the third organisation to arrive on the scene and had been directly modelled on the Committee for the Defence of the Revolution as in Cuba. It seemed that people had accepted direct responsibility for giving advice about sanitation and other public health measures and for successfully helping to organise the distribution of food, especially milk, at the nation-wide malnutrition centres.

It is important to realise that as soon as the military junta came to power, all three organisations were immediately disbanded.

As already mentioned, President Allende was opposed by most of the medical profession (and the rest of the middle classes) who saw his intention to concentrate on the *consultorio* service along with his attempt to resolve the mal-distribution of doctors and resources as a socialist/communist threat – this was of course predictable. Such fundamental changes, however necessary, are always initially opposed by most doctors involved in clinical medicine. It is easy for hospital doctors to benefit from the kudos of specialisation and hide behind the excitement of high-tech medicine, and the general public are always fascinated by the glamour of the tv screen.

Whilst I was there a perfect example was occurring in a most luxurious hotel in the centre of Santiago close to the damaged and heavily guarded presidential palace – a five-day conference on cardiac surgery. Well-known cardiac surgeons from all over the world, including three from the UK, were taking part. Throughout the length of the conference armed troops were on the street, a strict curfew was in operation, and meanwhile the economy was collapsing. In fact from the point of view of the conference, the SNS had already collapsed and the cardiac surgeons were of no relevance to the health service. But I met less than a handful of people who considered the conference to be inappropriate.

One university hospital, two area and one emergency hospital and only one *consultorio* were the facilities the Ministry had decided I should visit. Unofficially I was also able to visit a paediatric hospital and three further *consultorios* – the doctors who helped supervise these visits were adamant the Ministry should be kept in the dark and insisted they themselves should remain anonymous in my final report or any other publication.

San Juan de Dios was an area hospital and mercifully the Director was too busy to see me in spite of having an appointment. By chance and good fortune I met Dr Kuzmanic, a nephrologist – he spoke and understood English well and listened with a puzzled expression as I explained the purpose of my visit. He had already offered to take me round the 600-bed hospital but immediately offered to take me to *consultorio* Andes instead; this was one of the seven *consultorios* for which the hospital was responsible and exactly what I wanted.

As we drove there it became clear that *consultorio* Andes was where Kuzmanic carried out his four-hour shift for the week. Hospital specialists were employed by SNS to work for six hours per day as well as the four-hour shift per week in *consultorios.* On the ready admission of every doctor I spoke to, the authorities knew they spent as little time as possible working in both hospitals and *consultorios.*

The majority of hospital doctors, particularly the more senior ones, spent as much time as possible in private practice; with regard to primary care (*consultorio* work) they frequently failed to turn up even for the meagre four hours per week. Two excuses for non-attendance had some validity; one was the almost non-existence of any equipment, and the other was the steadily declining rates of pay that were well below that of the armed forces, police, civil servants, railway workers and coalminers.

Despite my obviously limited observations it was clear the *consultorio* service had almost collapsed, although I met a number of young newly-qualified doctors and medical students who were voluntarily spending two to three hours a week in *consultorios.* How much this helped I've no idea, but it certainly raised morale within the *consultorio.*

Kuzmanic and I arrived at the *consultorio* Andes about 10am and left soon after midday, but at least he had turned up. 'You don't need to be trained for this sort of work as it is very easy' illustrated so vividly his understanding of primary care. For him primary care should be carried out either in the out-patient or emergency departments of area hospitals, and the *consultorios* were irrelevant.

Consultorio Andes covered a population of around 70,000 and theoretically was staffed by five super-specialists – cardiologist, chest physician, neurologist, nephrologist and endocrinologist – and nine specialists – five paediatricians, two obstetricians, one gynaecologist and a general surgeon. The shortage of midwives, nurses and auxiliaries was obvious and apparently the same throughout the country. Facilities were non-existent, it was literally a biro-and-stethoscope situation – no laboratory, ECG or physiotherapy and it was exactly the same in the three other *consultorios* I visited. The Andes was unique though in one respect; it had a simple x-ray unit (no contrast media), but just one problem – it had never had a radiographer.

The out-patient and emergency departments in the Jose J Aguire University hospital, the San Juan de Dios and the Barros Luco-Trudeau hospitals were much the same as found in the UK. The Emergency hospital dealt exclusively with trauma as well as surgical and medical emergencies – in the UK such a hospital does not exist. The two paediatric hospitals were basically used by mothers as their main entry into primary care, but only a small number out of the population of 70,000 lived close enough to be able to reach it.

One further point – the Jose J Aguire University hospital with 1,000 beds had no responsibility for any *consultorios* thus giving an immediate and accurate insight into the attitude of those who were responsible for medical education. Students quickly realised that those in charge of their profession considered primary care to be of no significance and was at the bottom of the educational ladder.

Only the most socially minded or those with the most enquiring minds recognised the opportunities to be found in a *consultorio* – to see at first hand the problems the poor and not-so-poor experienced, thus gaining an understanding of the direct effects of poverty on most illness and disease.

I saw nothing of the Rural Service so it was extremely difficult to decide between the conflicting reports, stories and anecdotes which couldn't be verified.

There was no doubt that compulsory 'national service' for all newly-qualified doctors à la Soviet Union had been initiated by Allende, although what was actually needed were really experienced physicians. Allende also intended to increase the numbers of midwives, nurses and auxiliaries, particularly in rural hospitals and their satellite clinics, but he never fully explained to the population how difficult this was going to be; it was estimated it would have taken at least five years to set up the necessary schools of nursing.

The 'Health Train' was one thing that had been quickly organised to tour the southern part of the country; nobody disputed this or the good it did – it was estimated that over 30,000 people, mostly women, children and the elderly had been treated.

In discussions at the Institute of Public Health and the Department of Health and Social Affairs at the university it was agreed that the attempts that had been made to rebuild urban *poblacions* (areas of serious poverty) had ceased and the concept of the *consultorio* had been virtually dismissed. My observations during the visits I had made to a number of *poblacions,* which had almost merged together to create a large area of absolute poverty, were confirmed in these discussions. However, I found the *consultorios* were still functioning within their limitations.

All my visits had been unofficial and without permission, which caused some anxiety amongst the staff, who questioned me nervously about whether I had been followed.

Paediatricians, both supporters and opponents of Allende, couldn't understand why the distribution of free milk for children and pregnant mothers had been virtually discontinued over the past year. The pro-Allende group maintained that the free distribution had been started by Allende, but those opposed to him pointed out this policy had been started as long ago as 1958/59, initially for children up to one year and then up to seven years in 1964. I managed to visit one of these centres and it was clear that both supporters and opponents of Allende were correct – Allende ensured the centres continued and had also been responsible for the addition of other foods.

Paediatricians and nurses went to far as to say that in their opinion more good would be done by improving sanitation and general hygiene and providing better housing with less overcrowding than by the distribution of food. All that happened was the valuable protein just disappeared into the sewers due to the widespread epidemics of diarrhoea and vomiting among the under-fives. I have to say I didn't agree with that conclusion.

One meeting at the Ministry of Health I especially remember; the director and deputy director of the maternal and child health services, plus a young female doctor who had recently returned to Santiago after working for five years in the rural service, were present – all three women were anxious to talk, all three were completely focused on trying to improve mother and child care and to highlight the effects of poverty on health. Their main frustration and disappointment concerned the mismanagement of the SNS; a number of examples were talked about but I remember the experience of the young doctor. The two-year stint had been extended to five years as a punishment for her enthusiasm in supporting primary care, thus making her an automatic supporter of Allende. 'What a mess we are in' they said. In fact none of them had been great supporters of Allende, rather they had been against and continued to be against the philosophy of their own profession.

Apart from the MCDCHW another request came my way. A friend heard I was visiting Chile and would I take some personal stuff to their friend Robin working at the British Embassy in Santiago – I think he was the military attaché. Anyway I duly phoned him and explained what I was doing.

> " Yes of course let's meet .... I would like you to meet a missionary doctor I know, I think you'd find her rather interesting."

And so one Sunday morning I found myself walking to the English church for a meeting with Robin and his wife and the missionary doctor.

She had qualified in the UK in 1967/68 and went straight out to Chile after completing her pre-registration year. On arrival she undertook a further eighteen months' training in hospital – this was required before she could take the Chilean exams which would enable her to practise. She described the utter chaos and near anarchy of the last two years of Allende's government. She recalled that when she returned to the UK for a holiday, the Chilean Embassy in London refused to give her a re-entry visa as they had no record of her having a Chilean medical degree or evidence she had worked in the country as a doctor. As she explained, she had been one of the very few doctors who had obeyed the regulations and taken the exam.

"I smile about it now but I wasn't smiling then."

She described the current Pinochet regime as a grim dictatorship with all the implications of the secret police, of armed troops in the street and a curfew still in place. She believed the coup d'état had been the only possible course if outright civil war was to be avoided. She spoke calmly, supporting neither Allende nor Pinochet, but she admitted the future was bleak. After church, as we wandered back to Robin's home, we unexpectedly came across a situation that reminded me of Cuba. A largish crowd was gathering outside a Roman Catholic church and on getting closer we could see it was the congregation coming out of church, mainly young families with girls dressed in white, some with veils, and the boys in smart shorts and white shirts. It was the occasion of their first communion and nothing but joy and happiness and pride on the faces of the parents and grandparents. Whether you are a 'Young Pioneer of Cuba' or a 'First Communicant of Chile' the response of the family is just the same: all very reassuring.

Santiago is dominated by the Andes mountain peaks. The city itself is rather unremarkable apart from San Cristóbal on the edge of the city with its cable railway, and Santa Lucia on a small hill nearer the centre with a park and gardens. From both hills you get a complete view of the vast dusty *Barrancas,* a working-class district spreading in all directions.

Robin lived in the Barrio Alto, the 'high neighbourhood' or expensive part of the city, lying close to the foothills of the Andes. The house was surrounded by enormous affluence with numerous spectacular mansions of lawyers, architects and physicians as well as the hereditary wealth of aristocrats and the ruling class. Robin's home was a splendid bungalow with a beautiful garden and swimming pool – all owned of course by the British Embassy – with servants, gardeners and housemaids to boot.

After sherry and much chatter we moved to a friend's place – he was the Commercial Secretary – for lunch in an equally enchanting setting. My goodness, diplomats know how to look after themselves! What the ambassador's house must have been like I couldn't imagine. We ate a superb lunch in the garden with wine, liqueurs and brandy flowing and the servants doing their stuff. Ex-pats as well as foreign guests were milling around – I couldn't work out how they all fitted in.

I had barely got back to the hotel before Dr Kuzmanic, who had kept in contact since our first meeting, arrived. His home was in another beautiful area on the opposite side of the river from where I had just had lunch. Similar imposing houses and lovely gardens were scattered throughout the wooded hillside, again leading to the foothills of the Andes overlooking Santiago. Kuzmanic's wife and three daughters completed the family. There was great excitement as the middle daughter had just graduated top of her class at her private school and the following week she was going to enrol in the Medical Faculty. I thoroughly enjoyed an evening of Chilean music, Chilean wine and Chilean friends – mostly medics plus a couple of lawyers – who had come to join us. Conversation never flagged – everyone spoke some English. Initially the conversation was about the SNS and the NHS in the UK, but soon the politics of Chile took over with overwhelming support for the coup d'état, even if most found Pinochet to be a threatening and pitiless dictator. Europe and our place in Europe ended the evening.

The English philosopher and social reformer Jeremy Bentham at the end of the eighteenth century became a pioneer of Utilitarianism which argued that the aim of all legislation should be 'the greatest happiness for the greatest number' – this was long before Marx, Engels and Lenin.

If primary care depended solely on original and independent thought, on stimulating and unconventional ideas, on general disdain for orthodoxy, on flexibility and experimentation, on distrust and fear of bureaucratic inertia, on hard work and boundless energy and a desire to get things done, then the United States and countries that go along with the States would be leading the world. But health care, particularly primary care, is a product of the social, economic and political environment of any country. It is constrained and influenced by the mentality and philosophy of both patients and doctors. If most of the doctors and some patients believe that Bentham, judging by what he stood for, was a socialist, perhaps even a communist, therein lies the basic problem for the United States – and for Chile.

*

In comparing the health services of Chile and Cuba, the effect of each on children was significant. In Cuba between 1959 and 1974 neo-natal, peri-natal and the death rate for under-fives had changed from those of the developing world to those found in some industrialised countries. In contrast Chile, in spite of having some form of national health service since 1954, had not managed to improve children's health to anything like the same extent. It seems that the country which has followed the more equitable path had reaped the greatest benefits for children, and *pari passu* for women as well. Likewise the rationing of meat, poultry and eggs and the provision of ration cards for basic food which was still in operation in Cuba, had contributed to the improvement in the general health of the population.

A further comparison highlights another significant difference. Cuba had endeavoured to train and educate doctors to understand and tackle the problems of primary care and to make all health workers feel their work was essential and worthwhile. Chile on the other hand, with its specialist-oriented, hospital-dominated education and training, had ensured primary care was carried out by reluctant physicians with neither the desire nor the training to deal with its problems.

17

JAPAN

A Nuffield Foundation Travelling Fellowship enabled me to visit Japan to study how primary care was organised within their health service and the extent to which general practitioners were involved in hospital work.

I was to be away for two months, which would have been impossible without the help given by the Nuffield Foundation towards the cost of a locum. A letter dated 3 December 1971 informing me that my application had been successful also stated:

> '. . . the funds available are somewhat restricted this year and I am afraid I cannot tell you precisely how much your award will be . . .'

Obviously everything including travel to and from Japan and my accommodation, would have to be organised as cheaply as possible.

Six days after arriving in the country the English pound was devalued from 735 yen to 700 yen with a further devaluation to follow. Nothing much seems to change.

Following correspondence with the Japanese Medical Association (JMA) and a number of doctors working in public health, general practice and the hospital service, I had the enormous good fortune to be directed to Professor Tei Seki at the Department of Public Health and Dean of Osaka University Medical School (which competed with Tokyo to be the top State medical school). At the time I had no idea that over 70% of medical schools were private.

Unknown to me, Professor Seki was viewed by clinicians with suspicion; it was rumoured that in his younger days he had been a member of the communist party – certainly he had left-wing views. It is vital to understand that the majority of doctors were staunch supporters of the Liberal Democratic party (conservative) which had been in power almost continuously since the early 1950s. The close link between the medical profession and the Liberal Democrats was related to tax benefits and favourable planning decisions regarding the building of private hospitals and clinics, in return for a one billion yen contribution from the JMA to the party; the amount donated increased roughly in line with inflation.

This relationship was the direct result of Taro Takemi's twenty-five year presidency of the JMA from 1957 to 1982. Takemi's uncle-in-law Shigero Yoshida was Japan's first post-war prime minister thus giving Takemi unrivalled access to Yoshida and his successors, and to officials at the Ministry of Health, Labour and Welfare.

> 'The successful formula that Takemi created – linking the JMA, the ruling party and the bureaucrats into an iron triangle – worked well for the Association until the Koizumi cabinet was formed in 2001.'

– so wrote one of the editors of the *British Medical Journal* on 8 January 2005, vol 330.

Professor Seki and the team he had built up were enthusiastic followers of the NHS and believed Japan had much to learn from Britain. They were strongly opposed to the policies and behaviour of the JMA, while at the same time doctors working in private hospitals and private clinics were equally opposed to the Department of Public Health in Osaka.

I had been warned not to visit in the hot, humid summer and if possible delay to late September; this suited me well as I had been planning to return home overland through Siberia. My flight left on 17 October 1972, stopping at Bahrain for refuelling, then continuing on to Singapore, arriving about twenty-four hours after leaving London. As I climbed down from the plane in the late evening the temperature was still 80°F; how I wished I didn't have two large suitcases, a hefty travelling bag and a briefcase as well as a heavy overcoat for the return through the Soviet Union. I felt rather self-conscious as most of the other travellers were ready for Bondi Beach or its equivalent.

The drive back to the airport in the morning couldn't conceal the extremes of wealth and poverty that made up Singapore.

Cathay Pacific Airlines flew up the east coast of Malaya and across to Vietnam with its beautiful coastline of long narrow stretches of golden sand and an ongoing, unremitting war that, had I but known, still had three more years to run. We then turned quite sharply away from the coast over the South China Sea to Hong Kong for refuelling. Next came Taiwan for a brief stop before finally reaching Osaka, about 48 hours after leaving London. It was a wonderful sight, thousands of twinkling coloured lights almost as far as the eye could see. In my diary I wrote:

'I imagine Osaka looks better at night.' How right I was.

Japan lies on the edge of the Asian continent and is composed of four large islands stretching from Hokkaido in the north across the narrow Tsugaru Channel to the main island of Honshu (which is about the size of the UK although only 20% is habitable) then down to Kyushu in the south. The thousand miles of coastline is separated from China by the Sea of Japan. From the tip of Kyushu many small islands stretch out into the East China Sea towards Taiwan; in the closing months of the Second World War, as the Americans fought their way towards the mainland of Japan, these small islands such as Okinawa became household names.

The United Kingdom and Japan have a number of things in common, though more apparent forty years ago than today. Both were over-populated industrialised islands, both had royal families and neither was willing to speak any language other than their own. They were also unpopular with their continental neighbours, but for different reasons. In the case of Japan it was mainly because of its military aggression over many years and the cruel and inhuman behaviour of its armed forces. Britain, with its close ties to the United States and its record as a powerful global empire, has always been a reluctant part of Europe and is still known as perfidious Albion.

Health services evolve because of the diverse historical, political and cultural backgrounds of each country, and I believe this applies particularly to Japan. Until the middle of the nineteenth century there was almost no exchange of ideas or people with the outside world, certainly with the western world. Japan had remained isolated, independent and remote for over a thousand years and rigidly maintained its own customs, traditions and language. Buddhism was an exception and in 550 AD it had spread from India via China and

Korea. The language developed from China, and about this time too the Chinese writing system was adopted (before this Japanese was strictly a spoken language), but there is much debate about its origins.

Medicine had been involved in this isolation; traditional medicine arrived from India, China and Korea, and bar a number of exceptions remained the only medicine to be practised until the middle of the nineteenth century. In 1593 Portuguese catholic missionaries reached the southern tip of the mainland and over a period of about forty years had tried to convert and introduce some features of western medicine. A further exception occurred at roughly the same time when in the early seventeenth century Dutch traders arrived in Nagasaki and were permitted to trade locally. Dutch medicine quickly followed and was practised in a small area around Nagasaki. But from around 1630/40, for the next 250 years absolute isolation returned and the country was again closed to foreigners. Thus by the time of the Meiji Restoration or Revolution in 1867, knowledge of western medicine was almost non-existent, although again there were exceptions. In 1849 a Dutch physician named Mohnike imported smallpox vaccine via Nagasaki; by 1858 a vaccination centre had been set up by a small number of Japanese physicians who had received some training in Dutch practices. In the same year a Dutch naval surgeon, Pompe van Meerdervoort, arrived in Nagasaki and started to teach European medicine to any student who chose to attend his lectures. It is interesting to realise that vaccination with human smallpox had been introduced from China as early as 1744, fifty years before the work of Edward Jenner with cowpox in rural Gloucestershire. However, the imported Chinese human smallpox caused thousands of deaths and never found favour with the Japanese.

The object of the Meiji Restoration was to modernise by throwing off the old feudal yoke and eliminating isolation. Medicine was given a high priority and became an important element of this new image; traditional medicine had long been found wanting, first clinically, and second because it was disorganised, with each practitioner working independently and with no defined education or training. Western medicine was therefore adopted in 1868, and by 1874 a new law had been passed to prohibit the practice of traditional medicine. State medical schools were soon set up, Nagasaki not surprisingly leading the way in 1868, followed in 1869 by Tokyo, and Osaka in 1870. In addition, in most prefectures (similar to counties in the UK) public hospitals were built.

By 1887 serious financial problems led to the closure of most of the prefecture hospitals so doctors were then forced to set up their own private hospitals, often called clinics, with virtually no regulation or planning. The problems facing the hospital service when I arrived in Japan undoubtedly originated from this situation.

Bismarck, the Iron Chancellor, had enabled Germany to pioneer the introduction of health insurance in 1889 – this appealed to Emperor Meiji and Japan discarded the influence of the Netherlands and turned to Germany. In 1910 the Emperor introduced health insurance, although sixty years later at the time of my visit much still remained to be done. It was claimed that 88% of patients attending hospitals or GP clinics had their medical expenses covered by some form of insurance. In reality there were great variations both in contributions and benefits and at most only a third of the population was adequately covered.

The Second World War had literally reduced Japan to ashes, both physically and politically, so that sixty years after the Meiji Restoration with its high hopes of modernisation, the Japanese people had to start all over again, and this applied to medicine along with everything else. For obvious reasons German influence was discarded and the new dynamic foreign influence, the United States of America, which occupied the country, took over. With regard to medicine this proved to have been a mixed blessing and had been mainly responsible for the incomplete and inadequate health insurance that existed at the time of my visit. If Bismarck's scheme had been kept to, health insurance would have covered the entire population as it had in Germany for many years. The consequences of following the USA is clear to see – even in 2015 well under 50% of the population are covered by health insurance and President Obama's endeavours to introduce a Health Care bill has been opposed at every opportunity.

In the early 1970s travel to Japan, at least from Europe, had barely started and my knowledge of the country was no greater than that of the average man in the street. A land of *geishas* and *samurai* warriors, tea ceremonies, flower arrangements, strange gardens, the utter simplicity of a Japanese home and the Japanese ability to find beauty in the smallest thing, even amidst an urban sprawl of flyovers – this was the extent of my understanding. Traditional and conformist, individualism was not highly prized, along with distrust of the unconventional, and there was an acceptance of obedience and hard work. Disasters and misfortunes were endured without complaint, and politeness, good manners and harmony were an essential part of living. Respect for the elderly and the family was innate as was loyalty to the Emperor, although this was just beginning to be transferred to the place of work, or even the government department in which one was employed. Juxtaposed to this ethos was pollution on a grand scale, aggression as displayed on the crowded underground, shopping ingrained in a society of unashamed materialism, the subordinate position of women, and political corruption.

Most people in the UK were probably either totally indifferent to Japan or just vaguely aware of disgraced businessmen and politicians unbelievably falling on their swords, or were obsessed by kamikaze pilots and accounts of the unbelievable cruelty and inhuman behaviour of their armed forces, all encapsulated in the popular film *The Bridge on the River Kwai.*

A close friend of my in-laws was a GP in Bristol who, along with a hundred fellow medics, had been dumped in Singapore just a week before its surrender to the Japanese, and spent the rest of the war on the infamous Burma-Siam railway. When I told him of my intention to visit Japan he was shocked and couldn't understand how I could possibly contemplate such a thing. I listened to what he had to say, but there was no point in trying to explain as he simply couldn't understand; his thoughts were representative of his generation and it has taken at least another generation to move on from these views.

The first letter I received from Professor Seki was dated 22 June 1971:

> 'I am very glad to hear you are planning to come to Japan and I want to assure you that I would do my best to make your trip a profitable one (not in the financial sense). As far as I know there are very few publications on Japanese medical care services and

> general practice in particular which are written in foreign languages and it is my hope that you would make a good contribution in this area. Also I am sure we should be able to learn from your opinion about Japanese service systems when we meet each other.'

He then made a number of suggestions regarding what facilities and organisations I should visit, and continued:

> '. . . All these are available in our Osaka area but, if you like it, we are glad to arrange for your visit to home doctors and hospitals in other areas than Osaka and also visit with the Ministry of Health in Tokyo.'

Naturally this letter and further correspondence gave me a feeling of confidence that I was in good hands, and a worthwhile programme would be organised; in addition Professor Seki supported my view that the Japanese Health Service had been neglected by foreigners, certainly with regard to any publications in English.

Dr Suzuki had met me at the airport so at least I knew one Japanese by sight. Nevertheless I was anxious while waiting for him at the YMCA hostel. As we walked the half mile to the medical school I became increasingly nervous about the actual meeting. How would I know how to behave? Might I unwittingly break some custom or tradition? What about bowing? Who would tell me if I spoke out of turn or dealt with any disagreements in an inappropriate manner? Would it be alright to argue, and how direct could I be?

There was no need to worry. Tei Seki and his team were initially formal, polite, and spoke quietly and carefully. We then shook hands and all bowed to me, some more deeply than others – it seemed the more senior they were the smaller the bow – just an inclination of the head and shoulders. A number bowed to each other. We sat round a circular table, which was always used when a meeting involved discussion. Everyone smoked, the majority heavily, including Professor Seki. He was in charge and nobody spoke spontaneously without receiving a nod from him. As a guest I was always deferred to first even when it seemed inappropriate; gradually we relaxed, but the meeting remained strictly hierarchical.

By the end of the morning I was conscious I might have appeared to be impatient. Had I been too direct in my observations and had I always expected a direct answer to any question? It took me a little time to understand how different our thought processes were – I found the Japanese to be more polite, more patient and often repetitive in discussion, but this was simply due to the way they viewed any subject or argument. By the time I left Japan my experience had been that meetings requiring discussion were always conducted at a round table; discussion might seem oblique and was in fact rarely direct; what appeared repetitive was more often the need to approach every topic or idea or opinion from as many points of view as possible; all was confined within the boundaries of a triangle, at the centre of which might be the final decision, conclusion or answer – but not always – and sometimes I felt my colleagues were literally twisting and turning in search of the harmony that is so cherished by them.

Tea was drunk throughout the day and lunch was brought in from a neighbouring shop in small, rigid paper containers – rice, bits of fish and chopped vegetables; I was transfixed by their expertise with chopsticks. I learned that to remain healthy it was necessary to eat a number of different foods each the day – one pea, a grain of salt or pepper, rice, a bladder of seaweed – virtually anything was acceptable. I think the recommended number was either 29 or 33. However, I was pretty certain I was not going to find Japanese food to my liking.

The meeting finished in late afternoon; I couldn't believe the planning and attention to detail that Professor Seki and his team had put into my proposed schedule and their insistence I should say if there was anything I was unhappy about. In fact almost no alterations were needed.

A decision had been quickly agreed about my itinerary: five weeks or so in and around Osaka and visits to Nara and Kyoto; five days in Matsuyama on Shikoku Island on the Inland Sea, getting there by boat from Kobe, returning by ferry to the mainland, and finally back to Osaka by train; a weekend in the concrete urban sprawl of Yokohama for a meeting concerned with medical education/teaching hospitals; five days to be spent with Professor Seki on the Izu Peninsular that juts out into the Pacific Ocean to study the rural health service and stay in a Buddhist temple; and the last ten days to be in Tokyo to include a meeting with the President of the Japanese Medical Association and other officials who might be interested to hear my views. Apart from seeing a wide variety of facilities, discussion on systems of medical care, on medical insurance and doctors' remuneration were to be included, whilst I was expected to give formal lectures on the NHS at medical schools, prefecture and local medical associations followed by questions and answers.

As the day ended I wanted to ask if a visit to either Hiroshima or Nagasaki would be possible. Such a request would have nothing to do with health services and I wondered what my hosts would think. How did the Japanese really feel about the end of the war? I didn't want to put them or myself in an awkward position so it was a relief to learn that Hiroshima had been included after the visit to Shikoku Island with Dr Dodo.

Clinics were usually run by a single doctor although partnerships of two were just beginning; there was total opposition to group practice as developed in the UK. Any doctor working in a clinic would be a specialist, most commonly in general medicine, but there were also a significant number of surgeons – general surgery, obstetrics, gynaecology, ENT, orthopaedics and ophthalmology. Cardiac and neurosurgery was exclusively restricted to hospitals. The majority did not consider themselves to be general practitioners although they regularly advertised themselves as family doctors, cynically appreciating that this was what patients were looking for.

In 1970, 44% of clinics had beds and this percentage had increased by 1972. Only clinics with twenty beds or more were registered as hospitals in Japanese health statistics – what percentage of the 44% had more than twenty beds was not recorded.

All the clinics I visited were in the doctor's private residence and those with beds had an operating theatre and post-op beds on the top floor, or in a single-storey building attached to the residence, or as a separate building in the garden. A wide variety of procedures were carried out – gastrectomy, cholecystectomy, colectomy, hysterectomy, and caesarian section, and an assortment of minor orthopaedic operations as well as hernias and varicose veins.

The standard of post-op care was poor, in part due to a shortage of nurses and in part to the quality of their training. Patients were frequently left in the charge of a practical nurse or nursing aid, very rarely a trained nurse. The absence of midwives was even more noticeable. I didn't attend any operations, but while talking to clinic doctors I quickly realised how poor the service was – including no anaesthetic room and frequently no anaesthetist – and how anxious patients would be if they knew the truth. These serious defects were recognised by many looking in from the outside but rarely by those working in the clinics.

The diagnostic and therapeutic facilities and equipment were far more impressive than anything in the UK; over 70% had x-ray units including contrast media for barium meals, enemas and IVPs; 10% had gastroscopes and cameras in the hope of diagnosing cancer of the stomach at an early stage, Japan having the highest incidence of the disease in the industrialised world; 70% used ECGs.

It is important for doctors working in primary care to have easy access to diagnostic and therapeutic facilities and Japanese physicians certainly had that. Nonetheless doctors involved in future planning had decided that the current arrangements were an inappropriate way of utilising x-ray equipment and that it was likely that x-ray reports by clinic doctors were poor and often inaccurate. As a result Diagnostic Centres were being set up by groups of clinic doctors with the aim of centralising the use of radiological equipment, and at the same time raising the diagnostic standards by employing radiologists. With a similar intent a centralised pathology service had been initiated with the employment of bacteriologists, biochemists and haematologists so as to provide a far better service for both patients and doctors.

One drawback with these two initiatives had been the difficulty in finding the best location for patients, who had always been accustomed to having their consultation and investigative procedures carried out at the clinic. But I had little doubt that within the next ten years Diagnostic Centres would include both radiological and pathology services with the necessary specialists being employed by clinic doctors.

All clinics had their own dispensaries. It had been deeply ingrained into Japanese culture over hundreds of years by traditional healers that following every consultation the patient would expect to be prescribed something – creams, ointments, herbs, potions or whatever. Since the end of the Second World War this expectation has exploded and become almost insatiable so that a huge increase has been seen in the use of pharmaceutical drugs, so much so that at the beginning of the twenty-first century Japan heads the industrialised world in the per capita consumption of drugs.

Interestingly *kuzuski* is the old name for a traditional healer and *kusuri* is the modern name for a medicine or drug.

The problem of dispensing drugs cannot be over-emphasised; in 1972 over 20,000 prescription drugs and medicines were available, all of which cost different amounts which the doctor could claim for. According to Professor Seki, for every 100 consultations 220 prescribable items were dispensed and 49 injections administered. And as long as a doctor's remuneration continues to be related to the number of drugs and medicines dispensed, and remains unconnected with a consultation fee, there will be no end to this situation. A financial nightmare.

To reform and change the habits of patients has also proved difficult. Both intravenous and intramuscular injections have long been seen by patients as the best treatment a doctor can give – by law it is illegal for injections to be given by anyone other than a doctor, or a nurse working under his supervision, and patients were strongly encouraged to attend for common often self-limiting conditions for unnecessary injections, and at the same time be prescribed iron and vitamin tablets. In fact the injection could be as innocuous as sterile water or saline!

Health care in most countries comes about through political decisions, but in Japan decisions were influenced much more by culture and tradition. As I sat in a clinic or hospital waiting room, patients seemed to be enjoying their visit to the doctor and the inevitable prescription of drugs – it was a sort of ritual, a way of life and was undoubtedly largely responsible for the high consultation rate of fifteen per year, the highest in any country in the industrialised world. Interestingly there is no evidence that Japanese patients might have been suffering greater morbidity, which could have been a factor in the consultation rates. Over thirty years later in the first decade of the twenty-first century there has been no let up in their love of going to the doctor. I can imagine that in another thirty years the same orderly attendance at the doctor's won't have changed. Why should it?

Such behaviour is just deeply embedded in the character of this extraordinary nation.

Clinic doctors proved to be extremely hard-working and fiercely independent. Consultations were usually between 9am and 12.30, home visits between 3pm and 5pm and a further consultation session between 6pm and 8pm. The number of consultations per day varied considerably between 60 and 180, with home visits kept to a minimum of 6 to 10 per day.

A lasting memory of visiting clinics, whether in a village or town, was the apparent chaos in the numbering of houses. I didn't like to ask in case I was just being dim, and it was only towards the end of my stay I uncovered half the mystery. We were always on foot and on the second day I realised that consecutive numbers didn't exist; odd and even numbers were on both sides of the road and it didn't matter if it was a main street or a long twisting lane, we just wandered up and down – rather aimlessly as I thought – sometimes not even a street name – and numbers 135, 3 and 74 could be next to each other. It transpired that the lowest numbers represented the oldest buildings or the families that had been there the longest – but not quite, because just as I can buy a personal number plate for my car so the Japanese can buy or organise a bribe for a particular number for their house. Many years later a Japanese visitor 'explained' the second half of the mystery – police boxes.

> "What do you mean by a police box?"
> "Well, they're obvious in every town or village and are scattered in every district throughout a city. You tell the officer the name of the person or family and he will look at his map and show you how to get there. Often he won't even have to look at the map."

To my knowledge I never saw a police box and neither did any of my colleagues, as far as I remember, ever speak to a policeman or mention a police box. All very Japanese.

The question of who was responsible for providing out of hours care at night and on Sundays was giving rise to debate within the profession and in society. The problem started in the early '60s – until then the majority of clinic doctors provided emergency cover, believing it to be their moral responsibility. But like every other country in the world, the way of life began to change, so that by 1972 most single-handed clinic doctors were reluctant to be on duty seven nights a week, particularly as payment was poor. In the past, patients could consult any doctor although usually they preferred to see the one they knew; however, since the mid-'60s the doctor/patient relationship had been gradually changing and there was a tendency for patients to go from one doctor to another even during a short illness – they no longer considered the clinic doctor to be their personal family doctor. Yet, paradoxically, in survey after survey, the 'family doctor' was still what patients were seeking. A further complication arose from patients no longer being registered to an individual physician, so increasingly doctors felt they were only under nominal legal responsibility and diminishing moral responsibility.

The response of doctors to out of hours calls was understandably pragmatic; if the doctor knew the patient and the family and believed he was their doctor he would provide treatment, or help arrange admission to hospital. If not, the patient had to dial 119 and it then became the responsibility of the ambulance service to arrange hospital admission. In a nutshell, if the patient was loyal to the doctor, he would be loyal to the patient: quid pro quo.

In typically Japanese fashion the ambulance service was organised by the fire service, which wasn't connected in any way to the health service; in theory at least, all fire stations had ambulances as well as fire engines, but the ration of one ambulance per 100,000 population was inadequate by any standards. A report on 6 December 1972 in the Japanese *Times* (English language) showed that ambulances were being used at least five times more frequently in 1971 than in 1962, partly owing to more road accidents but mainly due to the unwillingness of clinic doctors to do out of hours work. Furthermore, ambulance cover was only provided in 50% of cities, towns and villages; in large cities like Osaka, Emergency Medical Service Information Centres were currently being set up by prefecture governments to deal with emergency calls when ambulance crews were unable to find hospital beds. If such centres proved to be a success it would reduce – even stop – the scandal of ambulances driving from hospital to hospital before the patient, often seriously ill, could finally be admitted.

Information from Japan has confirmed that these Emergency Centres have been a great success over the past forty years.

As the visit to the Uzu peninsular drew nearer so it was impressed on me how privileged I was to be going there with the Professor. It was a special place which Seki later told me he had been visiting for thirty years, usually for a week twice a year – always on his own, never with his wife or children, and he always stayed in an annexe attached to the local Buddhist temple close by the harbour in the small fishing village of Koura. He had known one of the priests for many years and this friend was now the senior monk. He explained he was not a believer, but these two visits each year acted as a 'spiritual blood transfusion' without which he felt he would not exist. I felt deeply honoured.

He and I caught the Hokkaido Express to Tokyo; it was a day of bright sun with clear views of the hills and mountains including a breath-taking view of Mount Fiji as we sped past. Soon afterwards we left the train at Atami to catch a local one to Izuki Shimoda at the far end of the peninsular. We passed along a rugged coastline through deep valleys and many tunnels, the hills covered with trees in their autumn splendour, the maples a brilliant red. At last, deep in the countryside we stopped at a small station for the final stage of our journey by bus to Koura.

At the guest house a monk arrived almost immediately to take away my luggage, remove my shoes and provide me with slippers. He also showed me where to bathe and handed me a kimono – this was to be my second experience of bathing in the Japanese tradition.

Supper followed with Seki and his friend, the senior monk, an old man who spoke no English. The food was almost uneatable – raw fish still twitching as it had been collected only a few minutes earlier from a trawler in the harbour. The eyes of the fish were a delicacy for the honoured guest: absolutely unreal. Seki came to my rescue, realising I couldn't eat the fish, and kindly asked what I would like instead. Eggs were the first thing I could think of as long as they weren't raw. We finished with green tea and a biscuit before bed. For the rest of my stay I had little else except great helpings of scrambled eggs or huge omelettes.

On returning to my room a monk had already closed the outside shutters, which was just as well as a storm was starting to rage. How on earth will my room with its walls of paper and windows of sliding wooden slats on the inside, survive? It was an unbelievable experience being in this traditional Japanese room. The floor was covered with *tatami* mats made from straw rice, each mat about six by eight foot. A room size was measured in terms of four, six or twelve mats. Rich and poor alike, as I was to see on home visits, used the same matting. Shoes must never be worn while on a mat – a terrible faux pas – slippers were always provided. Likewise on entering a toilet a different pair of slippers had to be worn.

The main room of every house, however small, had a recessed alcove, a *tokonama,* which was set in the wall facing the entrance. Placed in the alcove would be a precious object or a single flower or a beautiful autumn leaf. (My room was only for sleeping so had no *tokonama.*) The furniture would consist of a low lacquered table with small hard cushions made of straw rice spread over the *tatami* mats; as an honoured guest I would always sit with my back to the *tokonama.* The room contained nothing else other than low wooden cupboards along one or two walls.

The Japanese in 1972 were still a small people. I never saw anyone who was overweight and the elderly were surprisingly agile. When a smallish person came into a room everything changed once they were sitting cross-legged on the floor – they looked the same height as any westerner. The reason for this is that the femur is very short compared with the rest of the body. Both old men and old women could sit cross-legged for hours and hours while most westerners would find even an hour problematic and would be fidgeting from buttock to buttock. At this time osteoarthritis was extremely rare, in part due to the absence of obesity, and this was another reason sitting cross-legged was so relaxed and easy.

One of the bonuses of Seki's devotion to the temple was that he had come to know a number of clinic doctors both in the area and at the local district hospital. We caught the 9am bus to Dr Hamanaka's clinic in Minami-Izu, a village with a population of around 14,000 and three clinic doctors covering the area. Originally his clinic had included nine beds (not having the necessary ten beds to be referred to as a hospital) for simple general surgery such as hernias, haemorrhoids and varicose veins, but he had given up surgery some years before on account of ill-health. His wife was a trained nurse and it was she who had administered the anaesthetics under his surveillance. During the day we visited one of the other doctors and his wife who both spoke good English and gave us a good lunch – un-Japanese and cooked. They lived in an old wooden house with a delightful garden that looked towards tree-covered hills beyond; stepping stones in the grass led to small shrubs and ferns, no flowers.

It was interesting that both clinics had large pharmacies and a small x-ray unit for chests and simple fractures. We returned to Dr Hamanaka's clinic where a man was waiting for an extensive dog bite on his arm to be sutured. Seki and I were then invited into their home where he and his wife proudly showed us one or two of their daughter's engagement presents carefully laid out on the *tokonoma,* where his own collection of traditional swords was also displayed. In the late afternoon the telephone rang and we set off in the Hamanaka's car on a home visit to a remote fishing village nestling picturesquely in the hills on the edge of the sea. The patient's family were happy to ask Professor Seki and myself into their home and we sat around on the floor while Dr Hamanaka examined his patient behind paper screens; acute tonsillitis was the diagnosis and the doctor's wife made up and gave the injection of penicillin. The patient was a fisherman with a wife and two children – their home was modest, four to six *tatami* in size I would guess. After green tea and quiet conversation Seki and I returned to Koura where we all joined the old priest for more green tea and a chat: a very good day.

The 7.30am bus took us the following day to Shimoda, the nearest small town, with men and women already hard at work in the small rice fields. Here we changed buses for the National Hospital at Minato where I had a useful and interesting discussion with the director. Most of the time we found we had the same opinions and attitudes and Seki, bless him, kept in the background and only intervened if something needed explaining: another good day. Further visits to three clinics occupied another day and Seki insisted we spent some time talking about the history of Japanese medicine and its continuing influence in the late twentieth century. This took place in a quiet room in the temple, sipping green tea. On the day of our arrival Seki had told me he would like to call me John and I could call him Teish; this was a surprise and quite unexpected and we certainly became quite relaxed in each other's company.

At his instigation we had two long walks – 'we must think about nature and other things than medicine' – and enjoyed superb views of rocky headlands, crashing waves where the spray reached us high up on the cliffs with white horses as far as the eye could see. I could easily have been walking the South Devon Coastal Path and found it difficult to believe I was looking at the Pacific Ocean. The difference was that the three villages we looked down on were still thriving, fishing boats being busily unloaded onto the harbour wall. Every available bit of land was cultivated – very small fields with carefully-built dry-stone walls climbing up the steep slopes, protected by long grass. Everywhere was neat and tidy and small, just like the paddy fields we had seen the day before. Throughout our time on the Izu a strong wind made keeping upright difficult. Teish was extraordinarily fit considering his age and the amount he smoked (he always seemed to have a cigarette in his mouth).

On one occasion whilst we were resting, Teish told me he was puzzled by certain aspects of Christianity and he was sure many Japanese were equally puzzled. He couldn't understand how the crucifixion of Christ could save mankind and was mystified that in the Eucharist the bread and wine represented the body and blood of Christ. He was especially perplexed that believers are then instructed to eat the body of Christ and to drink his blood. I did my best but it was going to take more than half an hour.

Finally he was keen to take me to a Zen Buddhist temple so that I could experience one of their special ceremonies. We were up at 6am to catch the 7.30am bus for Shimoda, and then by taxi to Yokokawa village where we walked for a short distance up an open valley, wooded on both sides, to the Taibaiji temple. The special ceremony was actually a memorial service for the chief priest who had recently died. The whole village seemed to be out and about, the women busily preparing food and drink, which was laid out on long trestle tables. Many of the villagers had already started eating and drinking. The service lasted about two hours with an unaccountable interval of about twenty minutes. It was of course quite incomprehensible, sung in Chinese and Tibetan but mostly Japanese, and I found it a dreadful dirge with no tune or harmony (at least to my western ear). I don't think Teish understood much of it either. A fat little priest tried to organise the congregation going into the temple and keep those outside in some order, but he became more of a distraction than a help.

On our way home in the bus Teish began to talk about Buddhism and I asked him about Shintoism; Shinto was the religion that predated Buddhism but no one seemed able to explain its beliefs and ceremonies. I was astonished when Teish explained there was no Japanese word for Shinto – two Chinese characters meaning 'way' and 'god' had been used, hence the nearest one can get to an understanding is 'the way of the gods'. A clearer explanation came many years later when a young female doctor was visiting the UK and staying with us in Wells:

> "It is similar to the stories of the gods of ancient Greece and to a lesser extent Rome – fire and water, sun and moon, wind and rain, day and night, peace and war, the sky and stars, this world and the next. Spirits and gods can only be found through nature."

Apparently Buddhism had originally been thought to be too difficult for ordinary people to comprehend so it remained the religion of the aristocracy over centuries. It had even been suggested that the difficulties had been so great that Buddhism should be a religion for priests only. Many sects developed and at one stage the *Jodo* sect simplified everything:

> 'Put your trust in Buddha. What is to be will be. Buddha will take care of you in the next world whatever you do in this one.'

This was an English translation because it freely uses the future tense, which is unknown in the Japanese language.

The Japanese had no difficulty in subscribing to both religions as it depended on the occasion. Shinto has no answers to death but is very good at cheerful celebrations and festivals, so virtually all marriages are conducted in Shinto shrines or at least by Shinto priests. In death and bereavement the majority seek consolation and turn to a Buddhist funeral.

In spite of the insistence of almost every Japanese I met that they were non-religious secular people, what I observed was something different. Both shrines and temples were packed with family groups both large and small, with many school parties in neat uniforms, and busloads of aged Japanese tourists all queuing obediently and quietly and with great patience. Once word got round that it was permitted to enter the shrine or temple, the queue moved forward at a gentle pace, all eager to enter the sacred building.

The two old capital cities of Nara and Kyoto contained the most important and impressive architecture, but I wouldn't use the word 'beautiful' in relation to most Buddhist statues or temples – in fact I found the majority of them to be ugly and alien, providing no sense of spirituality and, within the temple, little opportunity for contemplation or any sense of another world. The *Diabutsu* or Great Buddha in Nara was the most glaring example, 82 foot high and weighing 551 tons: just grotesquely huge. The *Kondo* or *Daibutsuden* and its environs was literally filled with hundreds of Japanese, which my friends assured me happened every day – mystifying and curious in a supposedly non-religious society. A feature of every Shinto shrine and its surrounding area is the gateway known as *torii* through which every visitor must pass. These *torri* are instantly recognisable and are as common as minarets in the Arab world. According to Teish nobody has any idea about their origins.

The differing attitudes between Japan and the West regarding death and sex were interesting. For thousands of years suicide was considered a noble act in certain circumstances: kamikaze pilots and the armed forces in the Second World War who would rather kill themselves than live with the dishonour of surrendering to the enemy; politicians, bankers, businessmen who have disgraced themselves or their organisations, are held in the highest esteem for making the supreme sacrifice. With the appearance of Christianity 450 years ago, the Japanese have been unable to understand its opposition to these honourable deeds. And yet some western nations – Netherlands, Belgium, Switzerland and some states in the USA – have legalised suicide/assisted dying for the terminally ill, and other countries are striving to change their own laws. In Japan there is total opposition!

Likewise why did Christians think so differently about sex? After the end of the Second World War it came as a great surprise to the Japanese that American GIs equated nudity with sex and prostitution, which was completely alien to their own culture. Both Americans and Australians seemed unable to understand or believe that *geishas* were hostesses and not prostitutes. Their prime function was to entertain through their beauty, intelligence, charm and skills in dancing, music and conversation.

Just as we in the West have been largely unaware of much Japanese (and Oriental) history, so have they been unaware of much European history such as the Renaissance and the Reformation. Owing to the decline of religion throughout most of Europe over the second half of the 20th century and this first decade of the 21st, along with the spread of secularism, it has been forgotten that many institutions, ideas and attitudes are historically bound to Judaism and Christianity. When visiting their hospitals, both large and small, my attention was quickly drawn to the way the hospital was run. St Luke's hospital in Tokyo was founded by a group of Christians just after the war; in 1972 nuns were still in charge of the wards and the matron was also a nun. The atmosphere was unique, quite different from any other hospital I had visited – it was the only one which was not run as a for-profit business.

It is pertinent to mention the Hospice Movement founded in England by Dame Cicely Saunders in 1967 with the opening of St Christopher's. In Japan in 2012 no hospice movement existed. A Japanese colleague and a good friend for over 30 years has two sons, one a geriatrician and the other a paediatrician; both are endeavouring to set up a hospice for their own specialty, yet they have found it almost impossible to interest the general public in the voluntary aspect of the movement; the public still strongly believe it is the responsibility of the Ministry of Health to provide the money and pay the staff. The latest information is the involvement of the Crown Prince and his wife who have recently made two visits to a number of hospices in England. If the royal family were to get involved then society's attitude could well change; the two sons are living in hope.

*

The guide book didn't exaggerate in its description of the hundreds of islands in the Inland Sea nor the charm of Shikoku Island. After landing at Matsuyama, the prefecture capital, a long bus ride to Dogo Spa to stay in a traditional Japanese inn gave me an opportunity to see the gentle countryside as we travelled through wooded hills surrounding flat rice-fields with brightly-clad workers hard at work. Simple wooden houses in small quiet villages completed the scene.

My stay in the inn was certainly an experience, with sweet-scented unrecognisable food plus raw fish – the head of a fish especially for me – but Dodo, my colleague and interpreter, helped me out on this. Waitresses came to the tables on their knees, always smiling, and served the food with endless bowing and nodding.

Meetings with the local Medical Association, visits to a private hospital and an internal medicine clinic, and a question and answer session about the NHS completed the medical side of the visit.

We went by ferry from Matsuyama to Hiroshima; I presumed Dodo had been chosen intentionally as he had been living on the outskirts of the city on 6 August 1945 – he would have been about four years old. Neither of us asked the other what we were thinking. What was in *my* mind was that I was in the city which would be remembered for all time as one of the most infamous places in the history of mankind. Eight years later I would feel much the same about Sarajevo, a city that had also changed the course of history.

We walked silently to the Peace Arch, sometimes called the Cenotaph, a simple concrete memorial to the dead erected at the epicentre of the explosion. Looking in one direction is the familiar sight of the gutted building of the former Institute of Industrial Development known as the Dome, the only standing relic of the explosion and one that has come to symbolise the horror of the atomic age. In the opposite direction is the Peace Memorial Hall, a modern building supported on concrete stilts, which to me looked strangely out of place.

The Park of Peace, that includes all three buildings, is a large area, particularly by Japanese standards, with the 330-foot-wide Peace Boulevard running through it. The Park was part of the roughly seven square miles of flat wasteland of total destruction known as the Hiroshima Desert. It was difficult to absorb everything, but the enormity of the horror was beginning to register and we walked in silence; Dodo remained inscrutable.

Within the Park of Peace on a now pleasant hilly woodland stood the Atomic Bomb Casualty Commission (ABCC) established in 1946 by President Truman to study the survivors of Hiroshima and Nagasaki. With financial difficulties and often under threat of closure, it struggled on until 1975 when it was replaced by the Radiation Effects Research Foundation (RERF), a Japanese/American private foundation which continued research for the next thirty-five years with some unexpected findings that have been little talked about or reported.

In the *BMJ* on 15 July 2006 Geoff Watts, a respected independent science journalist wrote:

> 'In referring to the events at Hiroshima and Nagasaki, the programme could also have pointed out, though for some reason it didn't, how studies of A bomb survivors and their children have already revealed that the long-term effects of radiation are much less than expected . . . RERF has had this to say on the health of children of adults who survived the blast: . . . *to date there has been no evidence of increased risk of death from cancer or other causes nor of the incidence of cancer. In particular, mortality during childhood . . . has not been related to parental radiation.* Despite the importance of understanding the effects of radiation, especially since the disaster of Chernobyl, the painstaking work of RERF must be amongst the least publicised of all long-term scientific endeavours. Indeed in the last decade of the twentieth century the project was nearly abandoned for lack of funding. Its problem may have stemmed from its failure to say what people expected to hear. Maybe even what they wanted to hear.'

– a serious charge which has since been substantiated by continuing research. The suspicions of Geoff Watt remain unanswered. How I wish I could talk now to Dodo – I know he had two young children.

My first few days in Japan made me realise what it must be like to be disabled – apart from Libya it was the first time I'd been unable to understand any street signs or directions, any advertisements, the names of shops, in fact anything. Coca-Cola was the only non-Japanese word to be seen. I remember the first time I came back from

Tokyo to Osaka on the Bullet Express and either Cho or Suzuki had offered to come and meet me. Confidently I had declined their offer and it took me nearly twice as long to get from the railway station to the medical school as the train had taken from Tokyo to Osaka.

At the weekend Cho and I went to Yokohama to attend a conference concerned with changes to be brought about in medical education. Quite by chance a conference on the Japanese language was also in town. I can't remember how, but one evening we got mixed up with some of their delegates and it turned into a most illuminating evening. The first thing they agreed about was that there was no other language where there were so many ways of saying nothing. Next it was decided there are no words to express 'I love you' and great debate followed about alternatives, the conclusion being 'the moon is beautiful'. I really couldn't decide if there were literally no words or whether 'I love you' was just too vulgar to be acceptable. A further mystery about the language was also referred to: in old Japanese the past and future tenses did not exist and even today there is still no future tense. I had personal experience of this when one afternoon Cho's youngest son was carefully trying to make a toy boat out of an old newspaper and I asked his mother if he would be able to finish it the next day. She replied:

"He uses tomorrow's newspaper."

As the saki flowed, the richness of the language was analysed – the power of nuance in describing things, the reluctance to be confrontational, and the need and ability to view new ideas, thoughts and discussions from every angle that could sometimes leave a non-Japanese uncertain and nonplussed. Comparisons were made with the beauty and poetry and ambiguity of the Arab language plus the fact that many Arabs cannot read, speak or understand classical Arabic – just as many Japanese have the same problem with the language of the Emperor or the aristocracy.

Some credence has been given to the idea that the second atomic bomb was dropped on Nagasaki only because the Emperor's reply to President Truman's ultimatum following Hiroshima was subtle, ambiguous and misunderstood. Certainly support has been given to this notion by Fosco Maraini, an Italian who was interned along with his Japanese wife throughout the war. In his book *Meeting with Japan,* first translated and published in English in 1959, he describes his memories and those of his wife. At the end of the war he wrote:

> 'August came and it was clear that the end was near. The police hardly showed themselves and we even went down into the village where everyone knew us and greeted us as friends . . . I do not know whether it was the 7th or 8th of August that we read about Hiroshima, but for a few days the newspapers were unable to give a satisfactory explanation of the disaster. Nagasaki followed. Some aircraft passed low overhead and machine-gunned people in the fields. On the 15th a boy came running along to tell us the Emperor was going to broadcast: this was the first time in history that such a thing had happened and it caused a great sensation. "Perhaps he will tell us to fight to the death", one policeman suggested half-heartedly. Then a curious thing happened. The Emperor delivered his broadcast in which he announced the surrender but none of the Japanese around us were able to understand him. The speech was written in court language so remote from ordinary speech that you needed to be a philologist to grasp its meaning. The result was that until the evening when the newspaper arrived with explanations, the police refused to allow us to go out. By then, by moonlight, we at last heard we were free.'

And so this further complication could quite easily have been significant; the Emperor communicated with President Truman in 'court language', the language of aristocrats and *samurais* based largely on old Japanese. It is easy to see how such a misunderstanding might have occurred.

Another mystery for foreigners is the Japanese bath, which is held up as some sort of spiritual experience – I was intrigued by the whole idea. A friend in the UK had had contact with a Japanese Christian priest living in Kyoto – an unusual man as less than 1% of the population are Christian. I was invited over to stay with him and his family for a couple of days. I was nervous and had no idea what to expect – but I couldn't wait for the bath!

It was early evening just before the evening meal when my host informed me it was time to bath. He took me to the bath in a screened-off area of the main room and gave me a kimono and slippers to wear afterwards. The honoured guest must bath first, then the males in order of age followed by the women, then daughters, and finally servants if there were any. It was explained I must soap myself before getting into the bath but all soapsuds must be cleared from my body before getting in. Soap was provided in a small metal container and another container was filled with water to clean myself. It doesn't take much imagination to realise how difficult it was to clean my body in this way. The bath was a deep wooden square tub with a wooden seat in one corner where I eventually sat with the water covering my shoulders. I became obsessed with the soapsuds as everyone would know who was the culprit if any were floating on the surface. After all, seven of us were going to be using the same water. The screened-off area was steaming, like a sauna, but I had no idea how hot the water would be or how long I was meant to sit in the bath. Finally I ventured in by climbing up small wooden steps attached to the bath. Sadly I had no spiritual experience or sense of mystery – just wondering when I should get out! When I eventually returned to the main room in my kimono and slippers I couldn't help thinking of *The Mikado* and how absurd I must have looked to my Japanese hosts. At any rate I felt truly embarrassed.

It was only when visitors started coming to stay with us in Wells that we learned how shocked they were by having a bath and a lavatory in the same room; the function of washing and the act of defecation were kept totally separate in Japan. Almost all declared that this was the worst aspect of coming to the West. Another thing my wife and I immediately discovered was that all the hot water in the tanks would be used in one bath and the bathroom floor would be awash. Finally we learned that Europeans (I can't remember if it included Australians and Americans) have an odour about them which they found unpleasant.

They needed little encouragement to wax lyrical about having a bath; it seems the original rituals were religious and stemmed from Shintoism which had in some way created a feeling of moral purity being associated with cleanliness.

At a personal level, as well as Teish, his colleagues at the university had shown courtesy and patience, but two in particular, Cho and Suzuki, had gone way beyond this, giving me unfailing help, advice and comradeship both professional and personal. Additionally they were really keen I should experience and see as much as possible of everyday life and customs. I never tired of seeing primary school children sitting in groups, twittering away like a collection of sparrows or walking in straight lines in their cute uniforms with their teachers. Children were certainly Suzuki's forte.

Like most Japanese, traditional gardens were Suzuki and Cho's pride and joy; they loved to show me the famous gravel garden with the five rocks representing the continents of the world, or gardens with a different intent where one walked without hurrying along *tobiishi* (footpaths) seeking perfectly proportioned bridges, or meandering amongst carefully positioned rocks and stones or raked ground where hopefully one could find a moment for contemplation and solitude. There was no symmetry. Flowers were rare, and beauty was in a single shrub or a bonsai tree amongst wild grasses leading to absolute silence – everything designed to give a sense of the unspoilt beauty of nature.

At the other extreme was the countless number of times my companions would tell me how meaning could be found in the most unlikely spots – a small Japanese house with minute garden, or an elderly couple sitting on their doorstep under a criss-cross of motorways in Osaka or Kobe – the noise was deafening. In the grim wild overgrown tangle of brambles and willow-herb found in small areas of this concrete jungle called Yokohama a similar situation was pointed out where again two old people were happily surviving the madness of the surrounding traffic.

Mixing with physicians involved in both clinical work and in public health, the difference in income was obvious and particularly demonstrated by the make of car they possessed – or more accurately whether they even possessed a car. In Professor Seki's department Suzuki was the only doctor to own a car – nothing special, just an old VW Beetle that he would proudly take out whenever it was appropriate. In 1994, twenty-two years later, he still had the same vehicle, and when my wife and I visited Osaka he gave us a quick jaunt. Even in the mid-'90s only a couple of other doctors in the department possessed a car.

What did I learn about the way Cho and Suzuki lived? Both had their favourite pub – exclusively male, and neither Suzuki's girlfriend nor Cho's wife were ever invited to join us. In fact I rarely saw a woman out at night. I remember Cho's pub best as it was an exact replica of a small country pub in rural England, right down to the open log fire! This exclusively male environment extended well beyond the pub. But what about their domestic lives?

I never met Suzuki's girlfriend or went to his flat and I knew nothing of his private life. Tomoo Cho on the other hand told me his story; he was of Chinese extraction (Cho is a Chinese name), married with two sons, Jun and Piero, who were both at primary school. His wife Utako was delightful and spoke English well. Before their marriage she had been an airline hostess with Japan Airlines for three or four years and was considered to be very well travelled. Cho's father, a widower, was a charming old man who had been Professor of Music Appreciation at Kansaigokim University in Kyoto, a foundation concerned mainly with Japanese civilisation, history and culture – not the professorial chair that is found in the UK or in Europe. Tomoo was an accomplished pianist and enjoyed watercolour painting and Japanese calligraphy.

Their home was a modern bungalow in a wooded area of Nishinomija; the interior was plain and simple with a grand piano nearly filling one room. One afternoon Utako, Tomoo and I picked up the boys from their school and wandered home, the boys running ahead, playing and shouting, but not fighting. Cho and I talked to each other whilst Utako walked quietly behind. This was normal, women always following discreetly behind the men, but as soon as we reached home it all changed as Utako took over; within the home she made the decisions about everything.

A few days before leaving Osaka, the Saltzburg Mozarten Orchestra was performing its final concert. I asked Cho if he and Utako and his father would join me; his immediate reaction was that he didn't think Utako would be able to come as she couldn't leave the boys. I explained I very much wanted his wife and father to be my guests and hinted that I would consider it rude for Utako not to come and my invitation could not be limited just to him and his father. The concert was superb and much enjoyed by the four of us. As

I walked out of the hall with Utako she stopped for a moment:

> "It is very good you come to Japan. You see, this is the first time I have been out with Tomoo in the evening since we married."

I found this very hard to believe as they were a highly educated, civilised couple.

I then told her I was planning to take them to a restaurant, and a wide smile demonstrated Utako's pleasure. As we wandered to the restaurant I chatted with the old father and left Cho to escort his wife: a very happy evening.

Cho and I kept in contact and he visited us a couple of times in Wells; subsequently Rachel and I met Utako and Cho (as I always called him) when I was asked to revisit Japan by the medical schools of the University of Osaka and Sapparo. By this time Utako had been successfully treated for breast cancer and some years later for cancer of the rectum. Remarkably her charm and elegance remained. Cho was unchanged and still smoking heavily whilst mannerisms and characteristics I had long forgotten took me back to those memorable bygone days.

The final postscript was both sad and a complete surprise; in the late '90s I received a letter from a colleague in Japan telling me that Cho had died. I wrote to Utako and she replied:

> 'His death was due to cancer of the lung. He had been a very heavy smoker and sadly I had been unable to change his ways. He refused all treatment and died bravely at home. Perhaps I knew he was a Christian, perhaps I didn't, but anyway he had a Christian burial at the R C church between Osaka and Kobe.'

An unusual, unique man of many talents whose inner spiritual life remained a secret to the end. I didn't know he was a Christian.

From a medical point of view the essential difference between Japan and the majority of countries in the industrialised world was their view that primary care or general practice was best provided by doctors working in isolation without making use or working alongside nurses, midwives, health visitors and social workers.

The reactions to my report in Japan were interesting; some felt I had been too hard on the Ministry of Health and the Japanese Medical Association, and some that I should have been more diplomatic and less direct in my criticisms. Others suggested that my description of the inception of the NHS and the part played by Aneurin Bevan might lead to Japanese readers thinking I was opposed to the NHS and Bevan himself. Certainly nothing I had written could have given this impression and I was totally mystified – as 90% of physicians belonged to the Liberal Democratic party (Conservative) maybe they would assume I was politically Conservative as well.

There was a quite different response from Professor Seki who wrote:

> 'Every time when I am requested to write something about Japanese medical services I used to find difficult to make clear why the affairs of Japan – not only medical but more general rooted deep in the way of thinking of this country – are so different from that in European countries. More than that difficulty, to describe the outline of the complicated system is hardly possible in a short article. . . . . . . Almost all the difficulties were dissolved by your report . . . . as far as is known to me it is the only report yet to appear on Japanese medical care which is notable both for its accurate and informative descriptions.'

Clearly Professor Seki did not object to my straightforward and unambiguous writing, but over the years I have come to realise that his views and those of his colleagues in the Department of Public Health (and other public health workers as well) were uncommon and not subscribed to by the great majority of Japanese clinicians.

18

THE ARAB WORLD

The International Conference on Primary Health Care sponsored by the World Health Organisation (WHO) and the United Nations International Children's Emergency Fund was held in Alma Ata in the USSR in 1978. The meeting declared that primary health care was the key to achieving an acceptable level of health for the whole population in any country. From this conference emerged the slogan 'Health for All by the Year 2000' and the message spread around the world, being overwhelmingly accepted by the majority of member states of the WHO.

> 'A phenomenon that has attracted many observers of health development in the Third World is the exceptional progress made by a few countries well beyond what might have been expected from their levels of economic development.[5]

Low mortality in poor countries depends on the acceptance of a number of important principles before the health of a nation or a selected group of the population will begin to improve. These principles apply equally to rich countries which, if they use their resources inappropriately, will end up as a poor health achiever – the United States being the most obvious example.

Arab countries are in an interesting position; they are neither exclusively developing nor developed but are uniquely in between, with huge variations of wealth – the United Arab Emirates and the People's Democratic Republic of Yemen; of size – the State of Qatar and the Democratic and Popular Republic of Algeria; of political outlook – the Kingdom of Saudi Arabia and the Libyan Arab *Jamahiriya*: of population – the State of Bahrain and the Arab Republic of Egypt.

The Arab Spring has now radically complicated the situation as the

---

[5] Bryant J 1988 *Health for All: the Dream and the Reality*. World Health Forum 9(iii) pp 291-302

old order of the Middle East finally collapses. The Sunni and Shii schism remains the same as it was after the death of the Prophet, except it is more complicated with the voice of religious, political and secular Islam being shouted from the rooftops and the front line of the barricades; the same has happened to religious, political and secular Zionism and Jewry. Finally the extremism of al-Qaeda as well as separate groups of Jihadists (followers of holy war to defend Islam or spread the religion among non-believers), have now been joined by the horror of Isis and its intention to create a caliphate or Islamic State of Sunni extremism in northern Syria, northern and western Iraq, and large areas of Kurdistan.

I quickly became aware of the antagonism and resentments, sometimes anger, that the majority of Arabs felt about the peace settlement at the end of the First World War, in particular the Sykes-Picot Agreement between Britain and France in 1916, and it was not only Syrians who objected to this disgraceful document which initiated the carve-up of the collapsing Ottoman Empire. In 1917 the British government announced the Balfour Declaration which succeeded in promising the impossible to the Zionist Jews and the Palestinian population – the same piece of land.

By the time of the Paris Peace Conference and the Treaty of Lausanne in 1923 it was obvious to the whole world that the action of Britain and France in occupying the Levant was to satisfy their own political and imperial ambitions. Historians frequently refer to the duplicity of Anglo-French diplomacy as shameful – the Arabs I met preferred the word treacherous.

The United Nations' plan to create the state of Israel was adopted on 29 November 1947. This allocated 55% of the land of Palestine to Israel; the non-Jewish Palestinians and their neighbours were barely consulted, so not surprisingly this was rejected by the Arab world.

The first Arab-Israeli war started in 1948 and the armies of Syria, Transjordan, Iraq and Egypt entered Palestine in support of the Palestinian Arabs – within days they had been completely defeated by Israel. The result was that the Zionists ended up with 78% of the land of Palestine. The dispute continues to this day.

*

By the early 1950s the United States had taken on the mantle of being the most unpopular of all the western nations, largely on account of the power and influence of the Jewish/Zionist lobby in the States. This reputation was not however altogether fair – if they interfered they were criticised and if they didn't they were also criticised, and this continues to the present day. Ironically every Arab country accepts any help offered, particularly financial, and of course any military help it might be able to get from America. The United States' main allies remain Israel, Egypt, Saudi Arabia and the UAE and they have few scruples about which form of dictatorship they become involved with – what they are seeking is oil and stability.

In the 1950s and '60s and most of the '70s a number of Arab countries cleverly played the Soviet Union and the United States one against the other as they strived to get influence in the Middle East. But since the collapse of the Soviet Union and the end of the Cold War, the conflict between capitalism and communism has virtually disappeared. Perhaps China will take their place.

> 'Any writer who embarks on an attempt to describe and interpret the contemporary Arab world to western readers is confronted by a set of formidable difficulties. At a superficial level he encounters a stereotyped vision of the Arab, and of the Islamic religion which is closely associated with them in the mind. A more complex problem is that the average educated westerner is unaware he suffers from a prejudice about the Arabs. The New England or Hampstead liberal would be alarmed to find himself making a derogatory generalisation of the Blacks, the Chinese or still more the Jews. He feels no such compunction in his thoughts about the Arabs.'

Although this was written in 1978[6] it still applies today and is much worse since 9/11.

Or consider the words of Gerald Butt, written almost ten years later, a man who had spent some years living and then reporting in the Middle East for the BBC.

> 'The connotations of the word 'Arab' in the English language are numerous. They relate to various stereotype visions fixed in western minds as to what the Arabs are, what their lifestyle is like

[6] Peter Mansfield, *The Arabs,* Pelican Books, 1978, p 491

and where they live. If all the various epithets that have been in use from time to time are looked at closely, it is not hard to see that the Arabs have had a pretty raw deal at the hand of the English language.'[7]

Islam and Christianity have a long, bitter history of conflict stemming from the Crusades, and this has reasserted itself over the past hundred years. Within the increasingly secular societies of Western Europe and the religious extremists of Islam, the prejudice, ignorance, distrust, misunderstanding and fear on both sides have brought back the conflict once again. In addition, the oldest of the Abrahamic faiths, Judaism, is now embroiled in arguments of its own – secular Jews, religious Jews, and ultra-orthodox religious Zionists are in serious, sometimes violent clashes against each other as well as the now endless fighting in Gaza and in the occupied territories of the West Bank.

And now yet another complication has entered the history books; the turmoil over the past eighteen years in Iraq and Syria has been overtaken by the presence of ISIS endeavouring to create an Islamic state, a caliphate of extremist, conservative Sunnis in northern Syria and the north west of Iraq.

Into this maelstrom has been added the belief in the minds of many westerners that the Arabs and Islam/Muslims are synonymous and only since 9/11 has the world come to understand that Muslim fundamentalists may come from anywhere – Pakistan, India, Bangladesh, Afghanistan, Iran, Indonesia, many countries in Africa as well as in Europe, the Caucasus and even the United States.

Most of the world is agreed it will be many years before future generations in the Middle East will be free of civil unrest.

---

[7] Gerald Butt, *The Arab World: a Recent View,* BBC Books, 1987, p 9

19

REPUBLIC of IRAQ

Whilst rummaging through old correspondence it was brought home to me how fickle and unreliable memory can be; I had forgotten that the Arab world had been at the back of my mind since 1975, four years before I finished writing *An Analysis of Primary Medical Care,* and its publication in 1979.

An article in the *BMJ* in a series of *Personal View,* had appeared in April 1975 written by a consultant physician from Birmingham who had spent six months teaching in the Medical City in Baghdad, with spells in Mosul in the north and Basra in the south. Dr Alec Paton had been surprised to find the pattern of disease was remarkably similar to that in the industrialised world though the pathology was grosser and tropical diseases were quite unusual. In the main hospitals treatment was surprisingly up to date and en passant he mentioned that general practice as known in the West was non-existent.

Dr Paton had been captivated by the distinct culture, history and in particular the archaeology of this ancient land. He had been brought up on books such as *The Bible as History* and he ended his article by writing:

'I longed to abandon medicine and start digging.'

For various reasons I had been unable to include Yugoslavia in the *Analysis of Primary Medical Care* and at the time it was the country within the communist bloc which most fascinated the West, in part due to the comparative ease with which tourists were able to visit and also because of the country's independence from the Soviet Union. The incompleteness of my studies was painfully obvious and would provide an easy opportunity for those who wished to criticise the book. Therefore Yugoslavia had to be dealt with before I could move on to the Arab world.

*

What did I know of the 'Cradle of Civilisation'? Virtually nothing. Old Testament studies had been a compulsory subject at school and I vaguely remembered Mesopotamia being the land between the Tigris and the Euphrates; that Babylon and its hanging gardens were near the Euphrates, and Nineveh was near the Tigris – and yes, King Nebuchadnezzar was connected with Babylon which was one of the many sites that have laid claim to being the Garden of Eden. Over the last three thousand years religious leaders, scholars, historians and archaeologists have argued about accounts from Genesis and speculated about this mythical garden until finally, at the end of the 20th century and the beginning of the 21st, the Ministries of Culture and Tourism in every country in the Eastern Mediterranean have flourished on the argument and speculation.

As far as present day Iraqis were concerned, the most important date in their history seemed to be 637AD when an army swept north to defeat the Persians at the battle of Al-Quadissiya about thirty-five miles south-east of Baghdad. An Antique and Heritage Museum had recently been completed and on the second day of my visit Al-Quadissiya had been included in my studies. My companions were determined I should fully understand that it was not an Arab army which had dealt the fatal blow to the Persians, but an Islamic army spreading the good news of the teaching of Mohammed who had just died in 632 AD. I learned gradually that followers of Islam regarded Al-Quadissiya as one of the most important events in the history of Islam apart from the Prophet's birth and death – in fact amongst Iraqis it was referred to as the First Battle and the on-going Iraq/Iran war as the Second Battle.

At Dr Paton's suggestion I wrote to one of his contacts, Dr Salem F Damluji MD, FRCP, who was head of the Department of Medicine at the University of Baghdad. Within a few weeks I received a reply written on notepaper from the Ministry of Health, Medical City, and immediately the well-known influence of the UK's post-graduate education was apparent; he was a Fellow of the Royal College of Physicians and a Doctor of Medicine in the UK.

The British influence in medicine had developed over many years – just how and when it came about I never discovered. To many it had come as a great surprise because following the end of the First World War the British were intensely disliked and were not trusted. However, at the time of my visit, relations between the British and the Iraqi medical professions couldn't have been stronger, and the support then given at both undergraduate and graduate levels concentrated on hospital education and training and on public health. Interestingly general practice was not involved.

Dr Damluji wasted no time and quickly replied to let me know he had referred my request to visit Iraq to the Director-General of Preventive Medicine at the Ministry of Health, and it had then been passed to Dr Alleen Hassan, the Director-General at the Department of International Relations. I was truly impressed by the straightforward and speedy way my request had been dealt with, but noted with a little apprehension that primary care had not been mentioned.

My first contact with the Iraq Embassy was in April 1980; as I write now it is difficult to remember that our two countries had relatively good relations at that time. Three inter-connecting events had taken place in 1979 – Margaret Thatcher and Saddam Hussein both came to power and after the Shah's government in Iran had been overthrown by a popular uprising, in the same year the exiled Ayatollah Khomeini returned to his homeland from Paris, leading to the establishment of an Islamic Republic amidst enthusiastic acclaim and support.

The Iraq invasion of Iran did not take place until September 1980 and it was not until 1988 with both countries exhausted and economically ruined that the war came to an inconclusive end and the involvement/support that the UK had given Saddam Hussein became fully understood.

As I walked into the embassy it seemed almost unreal, as though happenstance was to play a major part in the success of my meeting with Dr A S al-Hashami, the Medical Councillor. He had previously been attached to the Iraqi Embassy in Prague and he was most interested to discover I had visited Czechoslovakia on a number of occasions. We had similar views on the strengths and weaknesses of the Czech health service and surprisingly he pointed out a serious problem with the Iraq service – the domination of hospitals over primary care and the virtual absence of general practice. Yes, he would be happy to support my application and would contact the Department of International Relations in Baghdad.

Over the next year much correspondence took place between the Embassy and the Department of International Relations as well as between myself and these two organisations. To my great surprise I found I was still corresponding with Dr Alleen Hassan after a period of six years – looking back I don't remember I ever encountered such continuity.

Towards the end of September '81 Dr al-Hashami wrote:

> 'I am pleased to send you back by recorded mail your passport after getting the required visa for you to visit Iraq along with 1st class return air ticket by Iraqi Airways. As you may see in the ticket you are leaving London on Flight No. 238 IA on Friday October 16th 1981. I have sent a telex to the Ministry of Health concerning your arrival in Baghdad and requested them to receive you at the airport and notify Dr Alleen Hassan of that. They will accompany you to your accommodation . . . I wish you a nice journey and a pleasant and useful stay in Iraq and I hope to hear from you when you return home. With the kindest of my regards and the best of wishes . . .'

What a send off! Perhaps this generation of Iraqis had forgotten the promise the British had given in March 1917 that the three provinces of the Ottoman Empire – Baghdad, Basra and Mosul – which the British had already occupied, were to be liberated. In reality the British installed King Faysal in 1921 (the son of Sharif Husayn of Mecca, now Saudi Arabia), with control remaining totally with the British High Commissioner. The continuing presence of the British did nothing more than unite these three essentially disparate provinces of the old Ottoman Empire in their hatred of Britain.

Baghdad airport 11.30pm local time – as promised I was met by an official from the Ministry of Health; a few others were hanging around hoping to get a lift in the Ministry van. We had to wait however for an Iraqi colleague who had been on a visit to Bulgaria. The flight from Sofia finally arrived and there were introductions all round. The traveller from Sofia turned to me:

"Are you Dr Stephen?"
"Yes," I replied somewhat confused.
"Are you Dr Stephen who has written a medical book about different countries?"
"Yes," I replied.
"I have it with me in my luggage. I take it every time I go abroad."

It was totally unexpected. I just smiled in reply – secretly I was rather pleased.

It was exactly one year and one month since Iraq had invaded Iran and I was immediately reminded of this by the almost non-existent lighting within the airport, just a few strategically-placed, paint-covered light bulbs. During the drive into Baghdad I was surprised by the half-hearted attempts at blackout and the undimmed lights of cars – a far cry from what I remember of Bristol during the war.

Our destination proved to be a military hospital surrounded by barbed-wire, the perimeter gate locked. After much hooting and shouting the gate was opened by two armed soldiers. My room in the resident quarters for the junior doctors was sparsely furnished with a small adjacent bathroom smelling like a sewer, the floor alive with large (by UK standards) multi-coloured cockroaches. An elderly nurse arrived with a jug of water and some fruit, and finally a young doctor turned up apologising that things were not more organised, explaining that the Ministry had only notified him the day before about my arrival. By this time it was about 2.30am and still 80°. There was no fan and the cockroaches were starting to climb over my luggage – most of them were coming in through a crack in the floor which I finally covered with a metal waste-paper basket weighed down with books. To my delight this strategy proved quite successful for the rest of my stay. Lights out was just after 3am and the alarm clock was set ready for breakfast and collection at 9am. Phew!

The morning started at the Department of Human Environment with a geography lesson explaining Iraq's borders, the flow of the Tigris and Euphrates from the Turkish and Syrian borders to form a confluence south of Baghdad to become the Shattal-Arab river leading to the famous wetland of lakes and reed beds inhabited by the Marsh Arabs. At the time of my visit, Saddam Hussein had not yet carried out his heinous decision to drain the marshes and simultaneously destroy the tradition and culture and lives of people who had lived there for thousands of years. The central region between the two rivers is very fertile and at the time employed around 40% of the population. Curiously there was no mention of oil!

I then moved to the Department of State Enterprise/Health Insurance and was given a superficial introduction to the financing of the health service and to how complicated it was for patients; in theory all hospital treatment was free, but payments for board and lodging were required in all government hospitals in urban areas: private medicine flourished in primary care.

My final move was to the Department of Primary Health Care for a quick outline of the situation in both urban and rural areas and an explanation that, following the Declaration of Alma Ata in 1978, changes were on the way. Most of the discussion centred on the inadequate number of both medical and nursing schools, the training of doctors and nurses, and finally on the great shortage of nurses and midwives which had necessitated recruitment from the Philippines, India, Pakistan, Tunisia and Cuba.

At the airport I had been given my schedule and itinerary so as twelve noon drew nearer I became fidgety and glanced repeatedly at my watch – the next meeting with Dr Ali al-Sabaunchi was extremely important as he was the Director of PHC of the Baghdad Rural Governorate or *Mohafadha*. My anxiety was unnecessary as just before midday he arrived, and with the briefest of greetings to his colleagues extricated me from the meeting. A quick drive and we were at the Directorate of PHC. He spoke and understood English well, had spent six months at the Department of Tropical Medicine at Liverpool University and was to be my guide/interpreter/mentor for my visit. We struck up an immediate rapport and he and his wife Valentina became friends with Rachel and myself and have remained so for the past thirty years.

He gave me a broad outline of how Iraq wanted to develop primary care and then, by visiting facilities and talking to health personnel I would be able to get an idea of the difference between hopes and reality. A PHC Council had been set up by the time of my arrival in response to the Alma Ata Declaration, and in 1983 a new

PHC Law had been passed to provide a new strategy away from hospital and high-tech medicine in the hope of fulfilling the slogan 'Health For All by the Year 2000'. It has been tragic to witness what has happened to the health service and everything else as well over the last thirty years, brought about by the Iraq/Iran War, the First and Second Iraqi wars and the resulting sectarian divide between Shii, Sunni and Kurd, quickly followed by the presence of al-Qaeda, local and global Jihadists and extreme fundamentalism everywhere.

In 1981 health care was available to the entire urban population and provided polyclinics, MCH units separate from polyclinics, hospital out-patient and A&E departments, and of course private practice. During the last few years Popular Clinics had also been set up.

In rural areas it was estimated that between 70% and 80% of the population had access to health centres covering populations of 5,000 to 20,000 with two or three beds for confinements and a small laboratory; really isolated areas had a simple x-ray unit, and all centres had an ambulance. Sub-centres or peripheral clinics were responsible for populations of up to 5,000 and were staffed by doctors' assistants, trained midwives and both trained and assistant nurses. The main emphasis was on ante-natal care, immunisation, health education and the supervision of clean water supplies and sewage disposal. The fourteen rural *Mohafadhas* (governorates) each had a rural hospital covering populations of 20-100,000 with between 20 and 60 beds for simple surgical, medical, paediatric, obstetric and gynaecological problems plus an out-patient department focusing mainly on MCH services. The Director of the hospital was responsible for the health centres, sub-centres and a mobile unit attached to the hospital.

Ali managed to combine medicine with aspects of Iraqi culture which interested him or he thought would interest me. He was a secular Shii so our journey to Samarra City eighty miles north of Baghdad in the Salah al Diem Governorate, nicely combined the purpose of my visit re PHC with culture. The regional hospital in the city was responsible for the main health centre in al-Tarmia village and the sub-centres covering neighbouring hamlets, all of which we were able to visit; we were also able to talk to the health workers. Ali seemed to give confidence to even the lowest grade of worker so they felt able to take part in discussions with doctors and nurses. At the main centre the chief physician spoke freely about a number of the problems he encountered. He had been working in the rural service for the past ten years and was totally committed to the work; unlike many doctors he wasn't disturbed by a limited cultural life. Undoubtedly this was related to the fact that his wife and her family lived locally so socially there was no problem.

Ali El Hadi, sometimes called Al Rawdha Al-Askariyah mosque is in the centre of Samarra and is a place of pilgrimage for Shiis, dominating the town with its magnificent golden domes. About fifteen miles north is one of Iraq's architectural treasures, the vast walled courtyard of a mosque large enough to hold 10,000 people. The mosque is a semi-ruin but many of the walls and some of the building are still in an amazing state of repair considering they are over a thousand years old. Outside the courtyard is the famous spiral minaret, still standing, with the exterior steps curving their way to the top – a masterpiece almost unique in Islamic architecture. Ali insisted I climb to the top while he remained firmly on the ground; in spite of being fearful of heights I managed to get to the top. The view was spectacular, first looking over and beyond the courtyard to the golden domes of Ali El Hadi glistening in the afternoon sunshine whilst in the opposite direction lay the vast brown open desert, and to the left the splendid contrast of the lush green vegetation on either side of the Tigris.

There was yet more to come; first the obvious ruin of a palace about a mile away and then, a further four or five miles across the bare stony desert, the ruins of walls and buildings on either side of the track giving some idea of the huge area that made up original Sumarra in the $8^{th}/9^{th}$ centuries AD. A small minaret was still standing beside a small, well-preserved courtyard as well as the arches and columns of the original mosque. Utterly fascinating.

We made our way back to Baghdad along the Tigris, stopping at two sub-centres and briefly chatting with the staff. Rich vegetation and many date palms grew on both sides of the river, and we saw numerous small villages with mud-brick yards enclosing the primitive living quarters and well-kept vegetable gardens. Everywhere were goats, sheep, geese, ducks and hens pecking away in their inimitable manner, and a few cows and buffalo chained up. Dogs barked, babies cried, women hurried about and children played around; young men played football and the old men sat smoking or doing nothing. Presumably the middle-aged men were still in the fields, harvesting.

As well as Iraqi culture Ali's main interests were current affairs and politics – usually without any direct mention of Sadaam Hussein. At the rural hospital in the Abu-Ghraib district outside Baghdad, whilst drinking coffee after the meeting I got into conversation with a young Polish doctor from Poznan; she was married to an older man, a rich Iraqi lawyer, and they had a son who was then living in Poland at the insistence of the Polish grandmother – obviously to the annoyance of her Iraqi in-laws and their extended family.

"Poland is better for him than Iraq, don't you think?"

Ali was clearly irritated and didn't answer. She continued to talk about Poland.

"Have you heard that Prime Minister Kania has resigned? Do you know?"

"No," was my reply.

"And General Jaruzelski has taken over."

She was really amazed and disappointed that Ali and I, in fact all the other Iraqis present, hadn't heard – as we drove home Ali heard the news both on Voice of America and the BBC World Service. Such conversations were commonplace and I wondered if informers were listening – later events would prove me right.

Fallujah is a town about forty miles west of Baghdad and a visit to the hospital was quickly followed by a longer visit to the local health centre. At both facilities my questions were answered without hesitation and I felt I was beginning to get the hang of things and collecting useful information for my report. By the end of the morning a young Egyptian doctor, three Iraqi colleagues and two dentists had tagged along with us, plus the director of the hospital.

Habbaniya Tourist village was a further fifteen miles to the west on the way to Ramadi. It had been built recently to encourage domestic tourism but was not open for foreigners as the area was the main base for the Iraqi Air Force; there was certainly much military activity to be seen. Anyway, I was able to enjoy an excellent meal and by the time

Ali and I had sat down there were a least a dozen of us round the table – the presence of a foreigner provides a wonderful opportunity to enjoy an outing at the expense of the Ministry of Health. Without any need for alcohol it wasn't long before tongues were loosened and politics were discussed at length, without any direct mention of Saddam. Starting with Palestine, most thought the situation was difficult, complex and virtually impossible to solve. I was asked for my views, and then my companions turned to Northern Ireland. Trying to explain Northern Ireland and the Republic of Ireland, Catholic and Protestant and the IRA, not forgetting the unity brought about by the Ryder Cup and British Lions, was in fact beyond me. We could only agree it was as difficult as Israel and Palestine. Next came a discussion about the Ba-ath party and whether it would hold Iraq together as Saddam had been a long-standing member since its formation. Eventually this led to reflections on Saddam and my views on Iraq and Saddam. I answered with great caution.

Just before we broke up, the young Egyptian, who had said very little, started to talk, hoping, I think, to influence the director of Fallujah hospital. He made it plain he was not sure he wanted to return to his own country following Anwar Sadat's assassination and would much prefer to be allowed to say in Iraq – what should he do? Where else would they suggest? None of the Iraqis had anything helpful to say and it made me realise what mess the Middle East was in.

On the way home Ali insisted on doing a detour over the featureless desert. On both sides of the road army encampments and occasional gun emplacements and a sprinkling of tanks were clearly to be seen, all looking somewhat disorganised and far from threatening. The reason for the detour was eventually explained – Ali wanted to show me the Nuclear Bomb Reactor at Osirak which had been bombed and destroyed by Israel. It was some distance from the road and in truth, without binoculars, it was difficult to see much more than a collection of flattened buildings. Ali told me never to mention to anyone where he had taken me, even his wife; he and his driver clearly trusted each other.

Straight back then to Ali's home where I had already met his charming Russian wife. They lived in a bungalow much the same as you might find in the UK. Inside the home Valentina was in charge – the pictures in the small hallway and in the sitting/dining room were all of Siberia or the architectural wonders of the Russian Orthodox Church. It could have been a Russian home, the only thing missing being the traditional wood burner – instead, an air conditioning unit that sometimes worked and sometimes didn't on account of the increasing number of electricity cuts since the beginning of the war.

A Russian friend and her two children were present as well as Omar and Diana, Ali and Valentina's children, so eight of us sat down to a marvellous spread almost entirely of Russian cookery and recipes. The kids quickly ate what they wanted then disappeared into the small concrete garden leaving the adults to enjoy a friendly couple of hours talking freely about Russia, its literature, politics and life, but I remember no mention of religion. Valentina and her friend chatted away about the infuriating ways of Soviet bureaucracy and Valentina regaled us with the irritations she still experienced at the Soviet Embassy even after living out of the Soviet Union for twelve years.

During my visit all seemed fine with Ali and Valentina with no hint of political worries, so it was a tremendous shock to find out that a few weeks after I departed Ali did the same, but as an emergency, the decision taken in less than a week. It transpired that over the previous six months he on three occasions had been pressured to become an informant for the Ba-ath party and he had refused. A few days before his fateful decision that would mean leaving Valentina, Omar and Diana behind in Baghdad, his colleague, the Director of PHC for the City of Baghdad Governorate, had been arrested and two days later news came through that he had been shot. Ali felt he had no alternative; how he got out of Iraq I don't know and didn't ask.

Valentina and the children eventually managed to get away too with the unexpected assistance of the Soviet Embassy – fortunately they all had dual nationality – but it took nine months and was far from straightforward. Even at the Turkish border disaster nearly struck as the Iraqi border guards told her she would have to leave the children behind. Subsequently she proudly described to me how she had resorted to hysterical behaviour and this, plus the combination of her Soviet passport and her absolute refusal to cross the border without her children, won the day, and forty-eight hours later they all crossed into Turkey.

I have stayed with them in Moscow on numerous occasions and my late wife and I were with them just after Yeltsin had stood on a tank in front of the White House shouting his support for Gorbachev and thus saving him from the attempted coup. It was then about nine years since Ali had left Iraq, but Saddam's people had quickly found him and since then had been keeping an eye on him. One evening Ali told us that a good Iraqi friend was coming to have a cup of tea and a chat; he hoped we didn't mind and asked us to say nothing and just keep quiet. The friend duly arrived, stayed for about half an hour and spoke only to Ali – after he departed Ali explained he was from the Iraqi Embassy and since his escape regular visitors had come, sometimes without warning.

Ali has never returned to Iraq and told me he would never go back until Saddam had either been killed or imprisoned. Unfortunately since his death another obstacle has arisen – secular, religious and extreme violence and chaos. He and his family came from Basra where his three sisters still live; the eldest has become his adviser about when it would be safe to visit Basra. As I write now her advice continues to be 'No'. But as soon as she says 'Yes' Ali will visit his beloved country.

Any free time I had was spent wandering around Baghdad or talking to the young doctors in the military hospital where I was staying free of charge – a magnificent bonus as I had expected I would have to stay in one of the two hotels for foreigners at great expense. All the doctors were doing their compulsory military service on account of the war.

My initial impression of the city was that it was like an enormous building site with excavations and digging everywhere, made and unmade roads and pavements, traffic jams, lunatic driving and horns blowing all the time: an extraordinary mixture of old and new, finished and unfinished mosques and minarets alongside cranes and scaffolding; buildings falling down and others half-completed – difficult to tell the difference; rubble, dust and rubbish along with the unpleasant smell of blocked drains plus the pungent exhaust fumes of cheap fuel shimmering in the heat of the day. All was somehow redeemed by the regular call to prayer. Even the recorded call of most *muezzins* provided a measure of continuity and calm.

Outside all new building sites were large hoardings giving in detail the cost, the planned time of construction and who had procured the contract – architects, surveyors, engineers, builders and so on. Finland, Yugoslavia, Japan, France and West Germany seemed to be the main beneficiaries, no Chinese yet. The United States hardly appeared at all and the UK only featured amongst the architects, which reminded me of a conversation I had had on the flight over with one of the passengers. He had just finished the design plans for a new 450-bed heart and chest hospital for Medical City (the large area occupied by the university medical school). His contract had been for one year and for specification only. I didn't have the nerve to ask how much he had been paid, but he couldn't resist telling me the contract had been very good financially. He was working on behalf of the Department of Trade and Industry and it annoyed me that no one in our government ever seemed to ask what the priorities should be in a country at this stage of development; would the money be best spent on primary, secondary or tertiary care?

On a different tack and with some difficulty I found the rebuilt Armenian church. Architecturally it wasn't worth the trouble but I was interested because of its connection with the Gulbenkian Foundation; the Cathedral School in Wells had recently become one of four specialist music schools in the UK and its development owed a great deal to the Foundation. To my surprise a board on the wall of the church stated that the Gulbenkian had donated half the money for its construction between 1954 and '57, that Gulbenkian was responsible for the formation of the Foundation, and gave the date of his death in 1955. Certainly there was no sign of animosity between Islam and Christianity; Iraq at that time seemed to have a strong secular society.

I was determined to visit a couple of mosques so I caught bus No. 4 to Muadman Square (I was really rather pleased with myself) and the Al-Iman al Adlam Mosque, and then set off on a long walk along the Tigris towards the outskirts of the city to the Kadhimiya or Al Kadhumy mosque with its beautiful golden domes and four gold carved minarets. The walk was fascinating, taking me through crowded narrow streets with the many bazaars full of noise and colour and shouting, and small alleyways with open wooden balconies leaning towards each other, nearly touching, and endless lines of washing strung out between them. All the time there was the constant movement of a seething mass of people and rich interesting smells of herbs and cooked meats.

Quite suddenly I had my first glimpse of the golden domes, and finally Kadhimiya in all its splendour. It was Friday and this being one of the six most holy shrines of Shii Islam it was difficult to pick my way through the bodies. Families were lying on the ground both inside and outside the outer wall of the courtyard and everyone was enjoying an enormous picnic, simply trampling the rubbish underfoot. I didn't attempt to enter the mosque after reading 'NO entrance to anyone who is not a Muslim'.

One of the real pleasures of meandering around was looking at people, especially children and the memorable faces of the elderly with every crease and wrinkle hiding a story and every mouth with a tale to tell – perhaps the end of the Ottomans, the British mandate, the arrival of Faisal I, endless disputes and revolutions, or the Second World War followed by so-called Independence, all quite unimaginable to me who had lived in the security of a democratic nation. I very much wanted to take photographs of these stunning Arab faces but it was not easy with my small instamatic camera. I needed to get very close so I felt it necessary to ask for permission, otherwise I might appear intrusive and rude. This being my first trip to the Arab world I observed another custom – nobody had told me about holding hands, two boys or two young men being far commoner than boys and girls or men and women – just custom, nothing to do with homosexuality.

Had the British left anything behind? I don't mean the influence on medicine or the military, rather I was wondering about everyday things. Yes, we did – the sight of red double-decker buses on every main thoroughfare and our traditional red post boxes and an occasional telephone kiosk. As children we have all played the pavement game immortalised in A A Milne's poem *Lines and Squares* in his book *When We Were Young*. Well, I obviously didn't play like a child but I very nearly became obsessed by the information to be found on the pavements and on manhole covers.

John Taylor & Sons (JTS) was the main company between 1947 and 1955 to build the first sewage system in Baghdad and the first treatment centre and pumping station in Iraq. JTS certainly had the monopoly on sewage manhole covers whilst Haiste & Partners of Leeds took over the street drainage covers much later on. Presumably the red post boxes signified the influence of the Royal Mail and the red double-decker buses must have been supplied by a British firm. I didn't make a note of the smaller companies but I recall that French names were conspicuous by their absence – I imagined Syria would be different and I was right.

And now to return to the young doctors and the conversation in the dining and sitting rooms of the residents' quarters. They had only one topic – could I help them in their careers? Could I help them get further education and training in the UK? Could I contact a pharmaceutical company which might be interested in supporting research in Iraq or the UK? I remember one request being connected with the use of inhaled antibiotics in the treatment of asthma. Would I act as a referee for a recently qualified doctor who was hoping to apply for a junior post in plastic or neurosurgery? The senior doctor in residence aged about thirty was anxious to take the primary exam to become a Fellow of the Royal College of Surgeons of London; at the time he could still take the exam in Baghdad as British external examiners were still coming over – would he then be in a position to become a senior house officer in either liver or renal surgery? And would I act as a referee? Basically all discussions and every request centred on getting experience outside Iraq.

In my report for the Ministry of Health in Baghdad, how did I assess the state of primary care? The illiteracy of adult women had already received special attention as it had been accepted for some years that the education of women was one of the most important factors in improving both maternal and child health; concurrent with this was the great increase in primary school enrolment for girls. However, maternal and child health services frequently took second place to curative work both in the minds of mothers as well as health workers, particularly doctors. The Iraqi authorities had been quite honest in admitting the problem, but as yet their honesty had not translated into much progress.

The development of health centres, sub-centres and rural hospitals had provided a reasonable infrastructure in rural areas, but these government facilities had not produced the hoped-for results. Patients preferred to get help from private physicians in the nearest town, or free at Accident departments. They complained that the buildings were dirty and poorly looked-after and staff hygiene was also poor. In addition the frequent requests for more female doctors had gone unheeded.

Iraq had been one of the first Arab countries to recognise the need to train doctors' assistants and village health workers, and by the time of my visit eighteen Institutes of Paramedical Workers were functioning. In 1965 the Abu-Ghrail Health Centre (which I had visited), in cooperation with the WHO, had set up the first training centre for village workers, and sixteen years later eighteen centres had been opened.

Village midwives/traditional midwives/birth attendants or *dyas* as they were called were being given three months' training and then returned to their villages. This had proved to be a great success and was popular and extensively used. The *dyas* were not employed by the Ministry of Health and payment was a private arrangement with the family. All rather impressive.

Assistant nurses had been retrained for three months as well, after which they were employed by the Ministry of Health to work in health centres. This scheme turned out to be less successful than the *dyas,* first because the girls had not returned to their own village so they had not been as acceptable to patients, who didn't recognise them. But more disturbing had been the speed at which even the simplest hygiene tasks and sterilising procedures had been forgotten. Immunisation routines involving strict adherence to the cold chain, safe injection techniques and reliable documentation seemed beyond them.

A safe water supply had been accomplished in most urban areas but less than 50% of the rural population had clean water to drink. As always, sanitation lagged behind the provision of clean water and was primitive in rural areas with almost no villages having latrines – open pits were often built but seldom used. The situation in the towns was obviously better, but I never managed to get a clear answer as to how many houses had piped sewage disposal.

Medical schools and the medical profession remained dominated by hospital-based, specialist-oriented education and training with the usual entirely predictable results. The UK had to accept some responsibility as they were involved in teaching and examining, but to be fair, the situation was no different from most of the developing world.

Still, all was not doom and gloom by any means. Added to the already-mentioned success of the *dyas* and the introduction of paramedical personnel, the establishment of Popular Clinics must be mentioned. They were an attempt to reduce the reliance of patients in urban areas on private practice. Apart from MCH or health centres, the private sector was all patients could rely on. Although originally staffed mostly by specialists, over the previous couple of years the Popular Clinics had started recruiting more generalists. The doctors were paid a salary, the remuneration smaller of course than in private practice, and patients had to pay only a small consultation fee plus not more than 25% of any investigation. These clinics became popular with patients and soon young doctors were equally enthusiastic. They appreciated a regular salary as the cost of setting up in private practice was becoming almost impossible.

A number of physicians were genuinely self-critical and forward thinking, especially the Director for Health Education and Training, the Chairman of the Institute of Popular Clinics and the Director of the Rural Hospital in Abu-Ghrail; all were agreed about the inability or unwillingness of medical schools to focus on primary care; all were frustrated by the lack of interest or support from the Ministry of Health and were in despair about the profession itself. There was agreement and enthusiasm about developing the training centres for paramedical workers and continuing the training of *dyas*. Ali needless to say supported them and I am certain there were many like him.

None of us could have foreseen the terrible future for Iraq and the total collapse of its health service.

What sticks in my memory about the first Arab country I had visited? It was the first morning and my introduction to meetings proved to be the same wherever I went – a sort of organised chaos. The room was open to anyone who wanted to attend or simply walk through; doors were rarely shut so with two doors left open I felt as though I was in part of a corridor, or that it was just a short-cut to somewhere else. A regular supply of Turkish coffee or a variety of teas with sweet biscuits, chocolate and fruit was provided. Everyone smoked, usually cigarettes, occasionally a pipe. The senior person in the room was always the person I was due to speak to and who had usually organised our meeting – to my surprise he was also available to talk to any colleague, to sign papers and to leave the room without warning or explanation. If five or six were present at the meeting it was the norm for two conversations to be carried on at the same time. Timekeeping or keeping to time was an unknown feature of Arab culture – I hardly remember anyone ever apologising for being late.

On most occasions *as-salaam* or *sabah-akran* (peace be with you) greeted you and *mae'aes saelaema* (peace/goodbye) on departure, whilst every comment, decision, hope, intention – in fact any thought or circumstance always ended with *insha'allah* (God willing).

Changes had had to be made concerning my departure; I could no longer fly Iraq Airways and had been transferred to Royal Jordanian Airlines flying to London via Amman. I never fully understood the reason for this but it was connected with the war and trying to stop all Iraqi flights leaving Baghdad once the sun had set. Ali dropped me at the airport and offered to see me through customs and passports. How I wish I had accepted his offer.

Soon after Ali left I knew something was amiss. Hundreds of people were sitting outside the main building with much shouting and arguing. After a few minutes truncheon-waving police arrived striking out at anyone in their way, including women and children. Their aim was to prevent anyone getting inside the airport and they were soon reinforced by truckloads of armed soldiers. It was becoming rather scary but fortunately I was sitting on the grass with my back to the wall close to one of the entrances. The great majority of the crowd were Arab and the rest were from the Indian sub-continent, the Philippines, and a few from Africa – hardly a white person to be seen.

The aggression of the police and soldiers made me act quickly before I became involved in the violence. By this time it was dark and I managed to squeeze into the terminal building without too much trouble, presumably because I was white. Inside we were packed together like sardines and the dimness of the few light bulbs didn't help. Again luck was with me as I ended up against a wall next to an East German couple who mercifully spoke a little English. The problem was simple – there weren't enough flights to cope with the number of passengers and only a few destinations were available. Fortunately my flight to Amman hadn't been cancelled, only delayed. The largest crowds surrounded the Indian, Pakistani and Indonesian Airlines so it was just a matter of discovering where the Royal Jordanian departure area was. It was a scene of indescribable chaos, but slowly I reached the ticket counter. Many in the queue had no tickets and travelling first-class certainly did the trick as there was no passport or customs control.

Apprehensively I deposited my luggage and around 11pm the flight came up on the departure board, so with no luggage to hinder me I was able to barge my way along a very narrow corridor and finally reach the door of the plane. No one had been asked for tickets and I managed to get on before the last few seats were occupied – many were left behind.

On reaching Amman – relative calm. We were told to wait for our luggage and miraculously mine turned up. Next an announcement; anyone with a first-class ticket was to be immediately transferred to a 5-star hotel for the night . . .

20

SYRIAN ARAB REPUBLIC

In the 1970s and early '80s the image of Syria was grim; a Ba-ath one-party state led by Hafed al-Assad and dependent on the army and the infamous secret police (*mukhabarat*) – a ruthless dictatorship synonymous with corruption, fear, inefficiency, bureaucracy and mass murder.

Like Iraq following the collapse of the Ottoman Empire, Syria was brought into existence by Britain and France as they divided up the Levant, France taking the north and Britain acquiring Jordan/Palestine. Subsequently in 1926 France created Lebanon so that the two countries, Syria and Lebanon, became the home of Arabs, Palestinians, Kurds and Turks. Following the end of the Second World War the situation became more polarised: Sunni and Shii with small groups of Alawi and Druze made up the Muslim population while the Christians were comprised of Greek Orthodox, Catholic and Maronite, a sect of Syrian Christianity. A tiny community of Jews survived in Damascus, and outside the main cities separate tribes ruled the villages.

The military coup of 1963 followed a month after the coup in Baghdad and by this time Hafed al-Assad was Commander of the Air Force. He soon became Minister of Defence and ultimately President in 1971.

It was a lovely spring day in May 1980 and I was in plenty of time for my appointment with the Minister of Plenipotentiary at the Syrian Embassy in London. I was intrigued to meet a Syrian for the first time and to see what sort of man deserved such a grand title.

Nabith Omari introduced himself quietly, without fuss and with a smile. Almost before I had seated myself two cups of Turkish coffee were brought in by his secretary, who clearly was not a Londoner, probably Syrian.

"How can I help? Please explain."

He sat back and listened, no sense of hurry, so I was able to take my time and outline the purpose of my proposed visit to Syria, the information I needed, the people I would hope to meet and the facilities I wanted to see.

> "Yes, that's clear, but I would like you to write to me officially stating what you have told me and then I'll send it to Damascus and tell them I fully support you. I also ask you to write in two parts: first concerning primary care and second that you will need confirmation that the Ministry of Health agrees to your entry so that I'll be able to help with the visa."

I wondered if he really had the authority of a plenipotentiary to act independently; I certainly hoped so. Anyway, so far so good and no sign of corruption, inefficiency or the secret police.

I had expected to be quickly ushered out but tea and cakes arrived and we settled down for a chat. He wanted to know about myself and my family and then told me about his wife and two children who were living in London with him. Yes they were happy in London and the two children went to an International school. We must have talked for at least an hour.

At his suggestion, the next time we met was at his home, a flat in West Kensington:

> "It's more relaxing here than the Embassy."

His wife was present and we all had coffee and chocolates before discussing how things were going. I couldn't believe my good fortune in meeting a diplomat without conceit, genuinely friendly and apparently pleased to help. Without Omari's guidance and his knowledge of how to tackle red tape and Syria's particular brand of bureaucracy, I don't think I could have accomplished what I did. Without a doubt it would have taken much longer.

Nevertheless over the next year I began to wonder if Nabith Omari was the exception. I had written to Dr Araf el Yafi, the Director of International Relations at the Ministry of Health, but it was over two months before I received a reply from Dr Haj-el-Hassen (el Yafi had obviously moved on):

> ". . . with pleasure we acknowledge receipt of your letter dated December 11, 1980, and your further cable asking me for a reply. We truly regret the delay. Concerning your request for visiting Syria and studying primary health care we would like to inform

> you that the Ministry of Health approves of your study subject and has referred the matter of organising a special work programme during your stay to Dr Hairdar Dek-el-Bab, Director of the National Programme for Immunisation . . . He is (sic) gladly answer all your points of information and please don't hesitate in writing him . . ."

Further letters and cables were required, but at last my visa had been safely stamped on my passport through the good offices of Nabith Omari.

On Friday 13 November I boarded a BA flight, less than half full, to Damascus. As we came into land at Beirut for a quick stopover, wonderful views could be seen of the coastline, then the city itself with a backdrop of wooded hills and valleys, small villages, and snow-covered mountains in the distance. As the flight continued the short distance to Damascus the pilot quickly announced it would be a rather circuitous route on account of the local hostilities (who was fighting whom I wasn't sure). Anyway, the detour was redeemed by a spectacular sunset – crimson red, bright orange and yellow, then a plunge into sudden darkness.

On landing about an hour and a half later, I was met by a cheerful doctor from International Relations who knew how to negotiate his way through the hostile-looking passport and customs officials. I was soon outside the airport building where Dek-el-Bab and his ten-year-old daughter were waiting. A long drive into Damascus followed and straight to the hotel. I would be collected at 8.30am.

The Omayyad Hotel was exactly what I had hoped for – old-fashioned, clean, and importantly, not expensive; faded notices and signs from a bygone age were in abundance – *ascenseur, première et deuxième étage, dames et les hommes, cabinets, reception, chaud et froid, postier* and others I have forgotten. Somehow it gave me a feeling almost of being on holiday and I felt quite at home.

I was collected the next day at 8.30am as promised and taken straight to Dek-el-Bab's office; all the main Ministries were actually within walking distance of the Omayyad. Although French was Dek-el-Bab's preferred second language he spoke and understood English pretty well. Two colleagues joined us, one African and the other

Pakistani, and we spent a couple of hours discussing the organisation of the health service. I was then given the work programme he had arranged and at his suggestion I took it away to look it over and ask for any changes the next day.

After the usual chocolates and coffee we went over to the Ministry of Health to meet Dr Ranzi, the Deputy Minister, and some of his officials, to hear his views on primary care and the difficulties in implementing the Declaration of Alma Ata – 'Health for All by the Year 2000'.

Undergraduate and postgraduate education, MCH services, family planning, the EPI (Expanded Programme of Immunisation) which was Haidar's responsibility, and the state of nursing were highlighted as priorities. There followed a rapid conversation in Arabic and it was obvious they had something to say.

> "The biggest difficulty is the military with over 30% of GDP being spent by the Ministry of Defence whilst the Ministry of Health is near the bottom. We have no political clout and no influence."

Later in the day Dr Hag-el-Hussein, the Director of International Relations with whom I had earlier corresponded, was even more forceful about the military and let me know in no uncertain terms that 80% of GDP was a far more realistic figure and as a consequence:

> "At the end of your visit you shouldn't be surprised to find the health service is in a poor state."

He hadn't finished, though, and was utterly scathing about a recent WHO annual report in which Israel, backed by the United States and the UK, insisted the general health of Palestinian refugees was improving:

> "How can this be when they are killing them as well?"

He was unashamedly angry.

Straight after this meeting I made a courtesy visit to his Excellency the Minister Dr Ghasomb-el-Rifa. Here there was a much calmer atmosphere and we mostly engaged in superficial chit-chat about nothing in particular. I was intrigued to see my report on PHC in the WHO's journal *World Health Forum* lying on his desk.

Ranzi and Haidar then suggested it would be a good idea for me to see as many different parts of the country as possible, including sparsely populated desert and refugee zones in the military area near the Golan Heights, not forgetting if possible places of historic interest. I enthusiastically agreed and the day ended happily with more tea and cakes.

The State Health Service provided limited free medical care for certain sections of the population: for a number of specific diseases and medical problems; all emergency and accident cases; the treatment of cancers; infectious and communicable diseases; ante- and post-natal care; children up to five years and primary care for the poor (but no definition of poverty).

A health insurance scheme had been talked about for many years, yet on my second visit to Syria in 1988 no progress had been made and the likelihood of introducing such a scheme seemed as far away as ever. While visiting a women's centre in Midan and two health centres in the districts of Shagour and Zablakani (all within the city of Damascus) I was free to question patients about the cost of care. Clearly it was a major problem, the message being that the majority of families couldn't afford to consult a doctor. No accurate or even inaccurate data was available on this matter but I had no reason to disbelieve what the patients had told me.

The private sector played a significant but limited role for an influential minority – politicians in and out of power, successful businessmen, some religious leaders (mainly Shii although most of the population were Sunni), and aristocratic families. Needleless to say, as Syria was a military dictatorship, the army and the police enjoyed the best medical treatment available.

In 1981 the fifth Five Year Plan was being launched and one of its proposals was the introduction of legislation to compel physicians to work either full-time in private practice or full-time in the State service, but not both. At this time 90% of clinicians were employed part-time by the State although it would be more accurate to say they had been employed mini-time. The profession was to be given two years to make a decision and it was also hoped that newly-qualified doctors would decide to work for the State as the private sector had almost reached saturation point. As with the Health Insurance Scheme, by 1988 nothing had changed.

So much for the financial difficulties for patients, but what about the availability of health facilities and personnel? In the early 1970s, in cooperation with UNICEF who was providing some financial help, it had been decided to upgrade all primary care facilities – dispensaries, MCH centres, health units and health centres. It was stipulated that these new facilities had to be staffed by doctors as well as a varying number of trained nursing personnel.

Furthermore, a new law was passed which pronounced that doctors would be in sole charge of a facility, and unless he or she was working there the other health workers – nurses/midwives/health visitors – were not allowed to perform any task such as immunisation, dressing a wound, taking a blood pressure reading or making any decisions. As a result of this insistence the law of unintended consequences followed.

I visited six rural and two urban health centres one morning and my assumption was that most of them would be busy; in all of them I found the nursing staff twiddling their thumbs, drinking tea, chatting and/or knitting. For various reasons all the doctors were absent – one was ill, one had left early to catch the only public transport back to her home, and three others had simply failed to turn up (according to the nurses this was a very common occurrence). Nobody ever came to check. As for the patients, most of the waiting areas were empty, but a few would-be patients were hanging around in hope. The medical profession remained stubbornly intransigent thus maintaining their stranglehold over the running of the health service.

The poor training of nurses, midwives, health visitors and traditional birth attendants, or *jedas,* was already well recognised throughout the Middle East. In spite of improvements in the number of children attending primary and to a lesser extent secondary schools, girls still lagged behind boys, particularly in biology and chemistry, the consequence being a poor intake into Schools/Colleges of Nursing.

Cultural, social and to some extent religious attitudes seem rather similar to our attitudes to actresses in the UK in the eighteenth and nineteenth centuries when nurses, like actresses, were considered to be little more than prostitutes. There was the added problem that men disliked the physical intimacy with male patients. Neither did men like women working shifts – being away from home during the day or arriving home late in the evening – or worst of all, being absent throughout the night. Also, society at large generally considered girls to be too immature to take on the serious responsibilities that would be required and expected of them.

The vexed question of training medical auxiliaries had quite unintentionally become a political as much as a medical debate. The Ba-ath party, a pan-Arab socialist organisation, had been founded in Syria with the support of Egypt in 1943 and nearly forty years later retained its strong socialist philosophy. Those opposed to the use of medical auxiliaries would argue about why some people should receive medical care from fully-trained physicians and others receive care from the less well-trained auxiliaries and believed everyone should see a physician. In reality of course in many situations it would be an auxiliary or no one at all.

Such arguments were exactly what I was to hear in the People's Democratic Republic of Yemen where the health service had been modelled on Cuba and the philosophy of Castro. The medical profession held the trump card by arguing that auxiliaries didn't have the necessary knowledge or training and would inevitably make mistakes. The irony of the whole situation was that the Ba-ath party, which was strongly opposed to the medical profession, found itself in complete agreement with the medics over the use of auxiliaries.

The day spent in Quanaytra was the perfect mix of medicine and politics. Dr Ahmad Aziz had been Director of Health Services in the governorate of Quanaytra. He was a quiet, dignified, elderly gentleman who was ready to discuss anything. As we drove south out of Damascus towards Jordan with the tops of the hills to our right already sprinkled with snow, he gave me a potted history of the area.

The Golan Heights, overlooking the town of Quanaytra, was Syrian territory until the Arab-Israeli war in 1967 when the Israelis occupied the Heights. Six years later, following the 1973 war, Syria regained a small area of land. However, before their final withdrawal from Quanaytra in 1974 Israel decided that the Arab population would be removed by whatever means and the town was systematically destroyed using explosives and bulldozers. Nothing remained but ruins and rubble.

*

On arrival Dr Aziz wanted me to see his home, his clinic, the medical directorate, his children's school, and the hospital which had been used for artillery and tank practice and by the Israeli air force for bombing practice. All this took place in 1973/74. It was as though there had been a huge earthquake, but as he said:

> "I and my wife and child are still alive. We are lucky."

We wandered around on foot with the Golan Heights dominating the flattened town. The Israeli border ran through the rubble so we had to pass through a couple of checkpoints manned by Israeli, Syrian and UN troops as he wanted to show me un-manned Israeli fortifications and outposts on the summit – they were clearly visible with the aid of his binoculars:

> "We are very nervous about the Golan. These fortifications are just waiting to be occupied again."

I doubt if Dr Aziz is still alive as I write forty years later, but I'm sure his daughter and any grandchildren he might have will echo his anxieties.

From politics to medicine. Quanaytra governorate had a population of roughly 200,000 with 25 health centres. Since the destruction of the town the Medical Directorate had been moved to Damascus. A few of the health centres had incorporated MCH services but the two I visited had not. Khan Arnuabe, about 25 miles from Quanaytra, covered a population of 10,000 and was staffed by one doctor, one trained nurse, two male nurses and an assistant pharmacist; it was planned that a midwife would soon join the staff thus enabling MCH to be provided. In the village itself a doctor had his own private clinic.

Gibbata al-Kachat, with a population of 15,000 had one doctor, a trained nurse and an assistant nurse, but no other staff and no private doctor in the village. Both centres, though small, were of better quality and much cleaner than the others I was to visit. Clean water was available to the majority of both populations but sewage disposal remained primitive. Earth closets, sometimes individual but mostly communal were provided but seldom used.

However, the real interest of the afternoon was the discussion about medical auxiliaries. Dr Aziz encouraged discussion, and widely differing opinions were expressed. How much work could an auxiliary perform? Some said 60% and others nil. Interestingly the 60% came to their conclusion because it was felt that patients were often not really ill, or had self-limiting conditions. Almost everyone thought an auxiliary's work should be focused on screening and connected with relevant health education – 'it's no use talking about the importance of clean water if none is available'. The majority felt limited curative medicine should be provided as a 'carrot', an incentive for patients to come and see an auxiliary. No mother is going to walk miles for ante-natal care if at the same time nobody would be prepared to examine her sick child. About half believed patients would accept medical auxiliaries but believed it would take longer than Dr Aziz thought. There was total agreement that auxiliaries should live in the community – in this way continuity would develop and trust would be established. As if to emphasise the point, the manager/clerk in the Gibatta al-Kachab centre told me that since he had come to live in the village, even though he had no medical training he was often asked for advice and even treatment.

The drive back to Damascus was beautiful as the clouds and rain of the afternoon had disappeared leaving the distant mountains of Lebanon covered by the late-afternoon sun; then there was Damascus laid out at the foot of Mount Kassioun with, sadly, the inevitably expanding outskirts extending beyond Salihiye, a district originally occupied by Ottoman aristocrats, their magnificent homes still standing. Dr Aziz continued our conversation throughout the drive and I noticed he was making notes about the answers I gave to his questions. As we went our separate ways he struck me as being an exceptional person – Haidar agreed.

Homs is one of the four main cities in the country so I was pleased to get the opportunity to visit, but I had no idea how my eyes would be opened and my ignorance exposed.

We set off early on the main road north out of Damascus towards Aleppo, after an hour or so reaching a small village off the main road and nestling in a narrow valley in the foothills of the Anti-Lebanon mountains. I had requested we might visit Ma'aloula and the convent and church at the top of the valley. The main reason for Ma'aloula's fame is because Aramaic, the language spoken by Jesus, is still spoken. The narrow road, not much than a track, was steep, with little cottages painted blue, green, yellow and white miraculously clinging to the hillside in a totally haphazard fashion. The convent at the top is unremarkable, while the church beyond with its simple nave and its dome sitting on a square base reminded me very much of what I had seen in Armenia. It had been built around 500 AD. A rather dirty, seedy-looking priest showed me round (Haidar remained outside) – he was certainly not a good advertisement for the Christian church. In the end, somewhat reluctantly, he put on a tape so I could hear the Lord's prayer spoken in Aramaic. I hoped I hadn't delayed Haidar's plans too much.

Back on the main road we started a steady descent into one of the main grain-growing areas in the country. Aleppo and Homs, as well as Damascus, are surrounded by rich agricultural land. To the east and south lies Syria's endless stony desert.

At the Homs Directorate of Health, Dr al-Ahmed was waiting for us. He was a Palestinian who in 1948 at the age of eleven, along with his family, had left Tiberias on the shore of the Sea of Galilee close to Nazareth. So many of the people I met were refugees, and I was aware how little I really understood about what they've had to go through. He was a dynamic little chap and really clued-up. In the space of half an hour he had galloped through the medical scene in Homs *muhafazat,* (governorate), plans for the hospitals, health centres, MCH facilities, mobile teams for EPI, polyclinics, and lastly Voluntary Health Centres, which I had never heard of. From a public health point of view it was the usual tale – only about 50% of the population had clean drinking water, and the disposal of sewage was a mess, literally and metaphorically.

Haidar, al-Ahmed and I then set off to visit two health centres at Jorataishayah and Talbeesi. In both centres the doctors had already gone home – nothing unusual in that, of course. The nursing staff were sitting around doing nothing and it was not even 11.30am. Between these two centres the villages and settlements looked poor; the most wealthy sometimes boasted a front door or even a window frame.

Our next step was the Voluntary Health Centre – this was how al-Ahmed described it, but the official title was Community Development Centre. It was an undoubted success. The first indication of this was that it was full of patients, particularly mothers and children, and it was well past 1pm. Apart from the strictly medical component there were separate 'departments' for the elderly, and for mothers and young girls who were being taught cooking and sewing and the importance of cleanliness and its connection with diarrhoea and vomiting. The importance of going to school was also under discussion.

The centre was open from 8am to 8pm and during the night it was open but not fully staffed. All the health staff including doctors were full-time and none of the doctors took part in private practice. The ésprit de corps was almost palpable and so different from anywhere else I had visited. The government didn't seem to be involved so I asked who organised and financed the centre – initially al-Ahmed gave a vague rather evasive reply but gradually it became clear it was an Islamic organisation, which had been running it for a decade or so.

"When and where did this organisation begin?"
"In 1928 in Egypt."

My eyes had certainly been opened and my ignorance displayed.

On my return home I discovered that the Muslim Brotherhood and been started in 1928 by Hassan al-Banna. According to Karen Armstrong in her book *Islam 2000* she writes:

> 'When al-Banna, a young school teacher, saw the British living in luxury in the Suez Canal zone, he was moved to tears by the contrast with the miserable hovels of the Egyptian workers. He saw this as a religious problem that needed an Islamic solution.'

The Society of Muslim Brothers became a mass movement throughout the Middle East, bringing their message to the poor. In times of trouble the poor, whether Jew, Christian, Muslim or non-believer, turned to the Brotherhood who produced food kitchens, medical care particularly for mothers and children in rural areas, and clinics and hospitals which they had built. At a really basic level help with clothing and even transport was provided. Whenever and wherever the social fabric of society had been lost, they were there, and as I write we can see on our television screens, amidst the turmoil in the centre of Cairo, the Brotherhood quietly tending the injured. To me it seemed there was a similarity with the support given by the Non-conformists and Quakers to the poor in Britain before the introduction of the welfare state.

A day or so after my visit to Homs, Haidar was keen that I should see the Community Development Centre in Harran Awamid in the Damascus Rural governorate, which had been opened twenty-four years before by the Muslim Brotherhood. In some respects it was similar to what I had seen in Homs; it provided medical and MCH care and its opening hours were the same as those at Homs, but it was divided more rigidly into two other sections – agricultural and veterinary, and entirely separate welfare, education and domestic instruction. It had flourished over the years and was a shining example of what can be accomplished. The participation of the Brotherhood was again not openly spoken about and in fact was kept as quiet as possible, although not actually denied. As I had in Homs, I asked who organised and funded the Centre – the answer was different; it was under the auspices of the Ministry of Welfare and Haidar told me it was actually the same in Homs.

At the time of my visit the extremism of the Brotherhood, as demonstrated in Egypt many years later at the time of the Arab Spring, was not in evidence.

The Expanded Programme of Immunisation (EPI) was Haidar's 'baby' so he was eager to explain and show me what had been achieved. The programme had been proposed and sponsored in 1977 by the World Health Organisation, assisted by UNICEF, and finally became operational in September 1978. It had been decided that EPI should be carried out in primary schools and health centres/MCH, and in rural areas by mobile teams consisting of a public health nurse, two health visitors and a driver. Opposition from the medical profession was strong, teams functioning without a doctor as well as arguments concerning the necessity of having a doctor to decide if a child was unwell or ill and thus not fit enough to receive the vaccine. Doctors slowly lost interest and by 1981 it had been found that rural areas were being better served than in towns and cities – during my visit the introduction of mobile teams into urban areas as well was being considered.

At the First Mouliha Rural Primary School I saw the EPI in action; vans and trucks were going round the villages and hamlets with loud speakers at full blast encouraging mothers to bring their children. The staff from the local health centre were also helping at the school, which was a splendid place – clean and cheerful and full of paintings and embroidery and decorative Arab designs and writings from the Koran. Families definitely found the school environment much more acceptable than an intimidating health centre, especially as teachers were held in higher regard than health workers. Haidar believed that immunisation throughout the country was close to 70%, the target being 80% to 85%. Seventy-six mobile teams were carrying out the programme.

We had one more health centre to visit and as I was settling into the car Haidar turned and quite unexpectedly asked:

"Would you like to see the Garden of Eden?"
"Yes, of course, but where is it?"

The Barada river flows down from the mountains of Lebanon to Damascus where it divides into four streams – I had seen much running water as I wandered around but had thought little of it. Jews and Christians had accepted the words of Genesis following the Creation story.

Chapter ii verse 8:

> 'And the Lord God planted a garden eastward of Eden; and there he put the man he had formed.'

Chapter ii verse 10:

> 'And the river went out of Eden to water the garden and from there it was parted and became into four heads.'

The first was to the land where there was gold, the second to the whole land of Ethiopia, the third east of Assyria and the fourth to the Euphrates. Interestingly, hundreds of years later there are nine separate references in the Koran to the Garden of Eden – always Gardens, in the plural.

Sura (Chapter) ix. 70:

> 'God has promised the believers . . . gardens underneath which rivers flow forever there to dwell and goodly dwelling places in the Gardens of Eden . . .'

Our destination was the vividly green Ghouta oasis about ten miles out of Damascus to the east. We passed through rich farmland extending out to the desert. It was the end of the season; the wheat and barley had been harvested but some fields were still full of maize and vegetables. There were fields of peas, orchards of apples, oranges and plums, many still needing to be picked, and trees lined both sides of the road. Traditional shepherd boys calmly herded flocks of sheep and goats. This could well have been the original Garden of Eden where every tree might hold the fruit which 'woman did eat'.

Beyond Ghouta there was nothing but stony desert and from what I could understand from Haidar, the four streams at different stages had just disappeared into the sand, their final destinations never located. I suggested to Haidar it would be much easier to simply relax and let the Garden of Eden be wherever our imagination took us.

Friday was the Holy Day of Prayer when at noon all men were supposed to attend a mosque for the recital of community prayers, after which a sermon would be preached by a senior cleric, the subject often being religious, or the political issues of the day. Haidar suggested that rather than taking me to Friday prayers we could visit Bosra on the Jordanian border. Bosra was a town of great historical and cultural significance and the centre of the Druze, a small breakaway sect of Shii.

It was to be a family outing; the Volkswagen van was pretty full with his wife and seven of his children before we picked up one of his brothers and a sister-in-law. All in all there were twelve of us plus our faithful driver Yasim Barbari who was already becoming a friend.

We first travelled south to Dera'a, a nondescript town on the Jordanian border where we turned left to drive along the frontier for about twenty-five miles before reaching Bosra. As we approached Dera'a the white headscarves, colourful neckwear and flowing white veils of the women were most striking against their long, dark embroidered dresses. Something else also instantly caught my eye – black basalt rocks, huge boulders and blackened earth had taken over the landscape. As the weather had by this time turned wet and windy the rain highlighted the blackness of the rocks and everywhere looked inhospitable and slightly threatening, a feeling emphasised by the black stone buildings. A strange landscape.

Between Dera'a and Bosra the military were in evidence,

particularly the air force in poorly hidden encampments of jet aircraft amongst the scrubland and boulders. According to Haidar and his brother the planes and all the military equipment were from the Soviet Union.

By the time we reached Bosra we had been in the van for about two and half hours; the children had been as good as gold with not a squeak out of them.

After entering through the main gate we went on to the Central Roman arch and the main street leading to the centre of town. It was an extraordinary place with black basalt buildings and rocks stretching out in every direction, and stone and brick from the time of the Romans providing the foundations of the present town. The only remains of Christian architecture were the ruins of the cathedral which had collapsed and been rebuilt over hundreds of years – now nothing more than crumbling walls, doorways and windows and a number of apses clearly visible.

The jewel in the crown was reached through Doric and Corinthian columns, often part of a colonnade. Here was one of the best-preserved Roman amphitheatres in the Middle East. It was vast, with seating for 15,000, quite incredible, as were the acoustics – I was able to hear Haidar and his brother as they were standing on the stage whilst I was walking along the top row of seats. The Citadel surrounding the amphitheatre had been built in the 12th-13th centuries as a massive fortress to resist invaders, but also to act as a *caravanserai* on the busy trade route running north and south.

As we came to the end of our visit the rain had stopped and the cold wind was dropping. Yasim Barbari, bless him, had stayed behind and by the time we got back to the van the primus stove was alight, ready for tea with masses of sugar and iced cakes, chocolate, sweets and fruit. Soon everyone felt better. What a star Yasim was!

Once we were back in Damascus the sister-in-law invited me back to her home in the heart of the old city - down a narrow cobbled street with blank walls on both sides, and just an occasional heavy wooden door and small window strategically placed so that you and your family could look out but passers-by weren't able to see you. The home is very much a private affair, especially for women. Once through the front door it was another world – a square courtyard with a small central fountain surrounded by a tiled floor. On three sides of the ground floor there were doors and glass windows. Above on the second floor were beautiful wrought-iron balconies.

I was invited to see some of the rooms – heavy dark antique furniture, much china on display, brass fittings hanging from the walls, and Persian carpets and rugs on the floors. Flowers and plants even as winter was beginning completed the scene. As in Japan, shoes were left at the door and everyone wore thick socks or slippers. Arab music played gently in the background and I was quite unable to hear the noise of Damascus street life. Enchanting.

The sister-in-law explained that she and her husband had only her father and mother and sister living with them. In most similar situations, certainly amongst the poor, as many as forty to fifty people would be living in such a house. It became self-evident that Haidar and his brother had a different status in society, quite apart from his brother having no children. I never found out what business he was involved in or how he made his money, but he certainly didn't work for the government.

Damascus, according to serious historians, has existed for 3-4,000 years. How much of this city would I be able to see? Maps were difficult to find and were in any case next to useless as the jumbles of alleyways and small streets were represented by straight lines so that much time was spent turning the map this way and that – people were very ready to help, but to no avail. Nevertheless, as a tourist, luck was on my side as the Old Town, lying within the city wall which remains largely intact, holds most of the history, culture and tradition and virtually all of its sublime architecture. I decided I needed to walk and whenever possible on my own. Progress was inevitably slow with the criss-crossing labyrinth of small winding streets and tiny alleyways canopied with trellises of vines, blocked by goats and donkeys with their carts, while motorbikes twisted through the crowds and even cars tried to force their way through the covered *souks*.

The Umayyad Mosque is argued by many to be the peak of early Islamic architecture. It is reached through the extensive Al Hamidya Souk which is covered by a metal roof and contains hundreds of shops and stalls selling everything you can possibly imagine. I reminded myself never to make eye contact with a vendor unless I was prepared to spend half the day arguing and bartering. The aroma of coffee and spices, cooked meats and blocked drains was a constant accompaniment: plus the occasional rat.

On reaching the end of the *souk* I had my first glimpse of the Umayyad Mosque between a row of Roman columns. The mosque was built at the beginning of the 8th century AD on the site of a Christian church named after John the Baptist; this in turn had been constructed on the site of the Roman temple of Zeus. For over a thousand years the Umayyad had been damaged and/or half destroyed by earthquake and fire, the most recent catastrophe being a great fire in 1893, but the most careful restoration has managed to preserve its breathtaking beauty.

The courtyard is an immense area containing the famous blue dome of the Prayer Hall and three minarets, the most impressive being the minaret of Jesus Christ. The walls are decorated with Islamic mosaics and the floor is smooth marble. A curious octagonal structure built on top of eight Corinthian columns stands on the east side of the courtyard – I forget its purpose.

The Prayer Hall takes up one side of the courtyard and is colonnaded on both sides of three long aisles – it's just staggering. The tomb and shrine of John the Baptist, along with his decapitated head, is placed behind the prayer area and close to the main pulpit. I felt really pleased with myself; it was a Friday and contrary to what Haidar had said the previous Friday I had managed to get into the Prayer Hall to watch and listen – no one had queried whether I was a Muslim or not. Even though the hall was less than half full it was crowded, the men at prayer in front and the mothers and grandmothers sitting or lying on rugs and matting, their children quietly running about. Picnics were laid out and they seemed to be having a good day.

The wars between Christendom and Islam have always been referred to as the Crusades – in fact there were eight separate Crusades over a period of about two hundred years. Salah ad-Din's name (Saladin) entered Western history after the Second Crusade when he was portrayed as a great leader of the Arab/Islam cause. His reputation for military skill and chivalry was well founded and even more the mercy and compassion he showed to his enemies.

I had been told that his mausoleum lay just outside the Umayyad courtyard; it was difficult to find as there were no signs anywhere – it was all wonderfully un-commercial, almost as though it was a secret for Damascenes to share with each other and hide from strangers. Actually his tomb is close to the northern gate of the Umayyad, lying in a small square mausoleum surrounded by a ribbed cupola quietly hidden in a garden of lemon and orange trees close to a small *medrasa.* The mausoleum is decorated with beautiful Arabic and floral designs; running around the top is an inscription from the Koran with, interestingly, a further inscription on one of the walls written in Turkish and giving thanks to Salah ad-Din for 'having saved Jerusalem from being defiled by the infidels'.

The Azem Palace, originally the residence of Ottoman governors, was taken over by rich Damascene families, and by the 1950s was occupied by the government. In 1981 it had become the Museum of National Folklore. On entering the Palace precinct the quietness and sense of peace was immediately noticeable in contrast to the shouting and bustle and noise of traffic outside. The marble courtyard with a central tree and mosaic paving stones was surrounded by simple small arcades and further trees half hiding a number of perfectly proportioned buildings. The main palace was built of black basalt, presumably from Bosra, and local limestone, which together produced a striking effect with alternate black and white stones positioned both horizontally and vertically. I sat under the tree and breathed in the wonderful atmosphere and sense of tranquillity and when I closed my eyes all I could hear were the wood-pigeons and starlings.

Time was marching on and I was thinking about the 'Street Called Straight', the Roman street that runs from east to west in the old city and was visited by St Paul (Acts of the Apostles, chapter 9), when by chance I came across a nondescript house in a narrow street, its large wooden double door wide open. Inside on both sides were metal beds and long stone benches lining the walls, while at the back two small rooms displayed medical instruments and old-fashioned bottles filled with plants and herbs; sheets, blankets, bandages and a variety of slings were lying about. Leaflets were available but only in Arabic. However, the elderly man in charge spoke a little English and told me it had been a hospice for weary travellers. It had been built hundreds of years ago and represented an important aspect of the Arab way of life. People could stay for a few days and if they were ill they would be looked after until they died. The old chap didn't understand English well enough for me to discover whether it had originally been set up by Christians and then taken over by Islam, or vice versa.

By now it was nearly dark, so the Street Called Straight would have to wait for another day.

Bab al-Jabriya has a large Ottoman facade with a central entrance and two small pedestrian archways leading to Suq el Kumeileh which lies at the western end of the 'Street Called Straight'. It was desperately busy with struggling shoppers and their children; it had little to recommend it and was a disappointing start to what I was hoping for. I left the *souk* and entered the equally disappointingly busy 'Street Called Straight' – cars and motor scooters everywhere, donkey carts ignoring the traffic, everyone shouting and the police endlessly blowing their whistles. But the two minarets on my right, the dramatic domes of the Khan (a place for displaying merchandise) of As-ad Pash on my left, and ahead a Roman arch across the road, made me feel I was about to enter a part of history.

The story is of Saul's experience on the road to Damascus; how he fell to the ground following a flash of light and heard a voice saying to him: 'Why do you persecute me?'. The voice told him he was Jesus. On opening his eyes Saul found that he could not see, and he was led back into the city. He was blind for three days. A disciple of Jesus, Ananias, had a dream in which he was instructed to go to the street called Straight, ask for a man called Saul of Tarsus and restore his sight. This he did, whereupon Saul was baptised and became a follower of Jesus. (Acts of the Apostles, chapter 9)

Nobody I asked had heard of Ananias. As for the Gate of Paul where Paul was said to have been lowered over the wall in a basket, it couldn't have been more unlikely. Nowhere was there any sense of history, far less of holiness or prayer. It was just another tourist trail and a rather poor one at that. It was so disappointing.

As I wandered back rather disconsolately for a meeting with the Director of the British Council I was feeling decidedly downcast. I wasn't looking at a map and suddenly I had the good fortune to come across something that quite made up for the 'Street called Straight'. The railway station was part of the original Hijaz Company and was a real gem, built at the top of a long incline in the centre of the city in the traditional Ottoman style of the nineteenth century. Inside was a large rectangular wooden hall enclosing balconies of dark wood on three sides and a fine wooden ceiling that would have graced any banqueting hall. I managed to persuade the elderly railway official, dressed in the uniform of a by-gone age and wearing a fez, to allow me onto the two platforms. The four single tracks were rusty, as were the manually-operated points for diverting coaches and trucks onto sidings. The platforms were covered with dying weeds and the whole area was swathed in ragwort, meadowsweet, bindweed, nettles and brambles; willow herb was being blown everywhere. It was great to see the old traditional lever signals operated from an aged wooden signal box with a signalman inside. There was even a steam engine shunting trucks and coaches about. It might have been the turn of the century – I felt really cheered up.

On the day before departure, following a final meeting at the Ministry of Health with the Deputy Minister, for some unaccountable reason we visited three hospitals – a university hospital, a paediatric hospital within the confines of the city, and a rural hospital about fifteen miles away. I could only assume Haidar had been instructed by the Deputy Minister. I didn't want to embarrass him as he had organised such a good programme for me, so I didn't ask. I learned nothing new and it merely confirmed my view that physicians working in urban hospitals had no interest in or knowledge of primary care and never gave it a second thought, whilst those working in a rural setting were really pessimistic about attitudes to primary care ever changing.

The Pakistani Airways flight was due to leave at 8.30am. Haidar and Yasim promised to be at the hotel around 6am, and they were. I was sad to say goodbye to both of them and was taken aback when Yasim gave me his string of prayer beads, a sort of Islamic rosary. It had been his constant companion for prayer and contemplation throughout my visit and I was deeply touched.

Flight PK 701 from Damascus to London was delayed – nothing

strange in that. After about an hour and half I was getting impatient and was looking aimlessly at the tarmac when a Pakistani Airline plane arrived from Karachi. At least sixty young men, all Pakistani, got off and were soon in the departure lounge. Curious. Within half an hour flight 701 was called and all the young men rushed back to the plane. The rest of us, about fifteen Europeans, followed. I was the last to board and in front of me I heard Moscow being repeated several times. Grabbing the attendant at the top of the steps I asked:

"This is the plane to London, isn't it?"
"No. Moscow."
"But my ticket is for London."
"It's been changed to Moscow."

He slammed the door.

The arrival at Sheremetyevo was in the late afternoon. It was late November so there was a great deal of snow piled up at the sides of the runways. All the young men disembarked shouting and laughing while the rest of us remained on board. I was quickly reminded I was back in the Soviet Union when, as soon as the last person was at the bottom of the steps, armed soldiers came to guard the two doors at the front and back of the plane. The doors remained open and the freezing wind blew through the plane, covering the soldiers' boots with swirling snow. No entreaties to shut the doors could persuade our Soviet comrades, or the Pakistani attendants.

The flight attendants were also unwilling/unable to explain why flight 701 to London had ended up in Moscow, nor could they tell us how long it would be before we were on our way again. The reason for the continuing delay was eventually explained – the plane was waiting for food and drink to be brought on board by the Aeroflot caterers. Quickly a couple of us went round our fellow passengers asking how many wanted to wait for food – the answer was a resounding NO. Next we demanded this message was passed through to the pilot, and after several false starts with soldiers clumping up and down the steps, the doors were closed and we taxied onto the runway for takeoff. Heathrow was reached soon after midnight.

Pakistani Airlines refused to give any explanation about the young men being deposited in the USSR, nor would they comment on the International Civil Aviation Organisation's regulations which stipulate that a change in destination could only be sanctioned for reasons of weather or an emergency in flight. Curious to say the least.

In October 1986 I had arranged to attend a meeting of the Regional Committee of the East Mediterranean Region of the WHO in Kuwait, and afterwards with the Chairman of the Council of Arab Health Ministers. At the time I had not decided whether I would attempt to write *PHC in the Arab World* or whether I would content myself with the individual reports on the countries already visited, which had been my original intention. Cambridge University Press were still interested and I was keen to find out what support I might get from the Arab Health Ministers regarding publicity and maybe some financial help. And would I need to visit other countries?

The overall response was supportive and there was general agreement that the book would be a good idea. However, it was made clear that I would be required to visit other countries if I was expecting full support from the Council. The two Yemens, Bahrain, Qatar and the Gulf states comprised the minimum. This was going to be a massive task: first, arranging visits to a further five countries; second, the difficulty in getting up to date statistics and further information from the countries already visited; third, direct financial support was not mentioned although I felt some help might be given with accommodation and travel arrangements.

I had to make up my mind quickly before the final meeting with the Chairman. Rightly or wrongly I decided I would go ahead with the book. The additional travel/time/cost was daunting, and whether I was capable of getting everything organised filled me with anxiety, not enthusiasm. Looking back I'm ashamed to say my decision was little more than personal vanity to have another book published.

In 1987 I wrote to His Excellency Minister of Health Dr Lenghi in Libya requesting up to date data and information about any changes in their health service. We had first met in his bedroom at Selfridges Hotel in London along with Professor Awad Abudjaja of the Department of Community and Family Medicine at the University of Garyounis, Benghazi. My letter was passed on to Awad who contacted me later on in the year. He had left Libya and taken up a new position as Secretary General of the Arab Board of

Medical Specialisation with its headquarters in Damascus.

If I was to meet Awad in Damascus, I thought why not try to meet some of my Syrian colleagues at the same time in order to get up to date on their situation? However, everything had been made a hundred times more complicated and difficult as the UK and Syria had broken off diplomatic relations. This meant visas were hard to get and could only be organised by the Syrian Embassy in Paris or the Syrian section of the Lebanese Embassy in London. It was a complete nightmare requesting the Ministry of Health and Ministry of Foreign Affairs in Damascus to send telex messages with covering letters of invitation sometimes to London, sometimes to Paris, and to get it all repeated when the telexes had been lost or mislaid. The final straw came when the embassy in Paris, having finally agreed to issue the visa, suddenly called to say it would take at least six weeks to organise. How I wished Nabith Omari, the influential Minister of Plenipotentiary at the Syrian Embassy, was still around.

Awad had a request to make; his son Nael was to have an operation for hypospadias at Guys hospital later in 1987 and his wife would of course be accompanying him. Could I therefore arrange for Nael and his mother to see an ophthalmologist privately with a view to having his squint corrected at the same time? This I was able to arrange with a specialist in Wimpole Street. How Awad could afford this I couldn't work out.

We finally arranged to meet in Damascus in February 1988 directly after I'd visited Bahrain, Qatar, and the United Arab Emirates.

Damascus was cold and windy, but mercifully no rain. As I was queuing at passport control I heard my name on the tannoy. I couldn't make out where I was meant to go, but almost immediately someone took my arm and asked if I was Mister Stefan. On saying yes, within a minute Dr Hag-el-Hussain, the Director of International Relations, appeared. In spite of it being seven years since I had last seen him he was much the same. What a pleasant surprise, it was like coming home. El-Hussain knew how to manage the grim-faced passport officers and joked away with customs – little did I know how different things would be in a couple of days.

*

My first meeting at the Ministry of Health with the Deputy Minister was worthwhile; it turned out he was also Director of Primary Health Care, which was a great step forward. Haidar soon joined us and it was really instructive listening to their discussion about the continuing difficulties between primary and secondary care and their agreement that medical education was the main problem. I interrupted at one point to say there must have been some improvement with the Director of PHC now being the Deputy Minister, and they agreed. The following day the Department of Medical Statistics provided as much up-to-date information as they could. It had proved to be a valuable couple of days – once again Haigar had turned up trumps.

Haigar and Awad had arranged that the three of us should meet at the Arab Board of Medical Specialisation. First, however, Haigar and I went to the MCH Training Centre I had visited eight years before and found that Dr Mardini was still the Director – again something really positive as he was able to tell me about the considerable increase in the number of both urban and rural health centres and the improvement in MCH services since my previous visit. Finally he outlined the changes in statutory training for traditional birth attendants and the new training programme for assistant public health nurses and midwives who were now only working in MCH clinics. It was all most impressive and Mardini was justifiably proud of what had been achieved. Irritatingly I have forgotten whether nurses and midwives were now able to work without a doctor being present.

Everything had been organised so well that as we made our way to the Arab Board of Medical Specialisation I feared something might go wrong. I had no need to worry. Awad was there to greet us and treated me like a long lost friend. I hadn't realised that he and Haigar had never met and it felt extraordinary for me to be introducing a Syrian and a Libyan to each other. A few colleagues had joined Haigar and it was obvious that none of them, including Haigar, knew much about the Board. They listened carefully to its history and the explanation of its raison d'être and the progress made over the previous five years. After Turkish coffee and chocolates Haigar and I returned to his office at the Ministry of Health for an update on the EPI programme – like Mardini he was proud of it and justifiably so.

Again we said goodbye and the authorised driver, sadly not Yasim, took me back to the Board of Specialisation.

Awad then told me about the successful operation for hypospadias at Guys and the appointment with the ophthalmologist which also had led to a successful operation. He was genuinely grateful, but further help was needed – he was in the middle of writing a book, *Epidemiology & Community Medicine,* and wanted to know if there was any way I could help in finding a publisher in the UK as he wanted the book to be published in English. I talked to him about how difficult it might be and explained that a draft of three or four chapters would be required before any consideration might be given. I never received the draft.

The headquarters of the Board was halfway up the slopes of Mount Kassion, beyond the fashionable district of Salihye and with a commanding view of Damascus. Awad and I sat there musing about medicine, politics, Qaddafi and our families – I didn't think he would be returning to Libya. I was beginning to feel cold and we parted with an Arab embrace.

As I got into bed that night I found it difficult to believe this was likely to be the end of my time in the Arab world. In some ways I would be sorry, but I was running out of steam. The KLM flight to Amsterdam (no direct flights to London) was due to leave at 10.30am so I set the alarm. Around 4am I awoke with an acute attack of benign labyrinthitis with vertigo, vomiting and nausea. How the hell was I going to get to the airport and onto the plane?

The taxi was late which gave me enough time to get to the top of the front steps of the hotel with all my luggage; provided I kept my head vertical and didn't turn from side to side and walked at the speed of a snail I thought I would be able to cope. The drive to the airport brought back my nausea and my apprehension.

Inside the airport there were few people about, which was encouraging, but then I realised I couldn't look up at the departure board without feeling I would topple over. I made my way very slowly to the customs leaning on my trolley like a zimmer frame. It took me an eternity to lift my luggage onto the tables. Whether it was my slowness when asked to open my cases for the customs officer to see what I had bought with the hundred US dollars (which was compulsory for foreigners to spend), or because I couldn't find what I had purchased, nor the receipts, the customs officer was furious. He moved my cases to a separate area where he rummaged around and pulled out half the contents. Somehow I think it was entirely political as the UK had broken off relations with Syria and this was an easy way to humiliate someone.[8] Anyway I was next forced into an open cubicle and told to undress; in full view of anyone who wanted to look I started to undress very slowly and with difficulty, which only served to increase the officer's fury. Eventually I was standing in my pants. By this time I was beyond caring even if I had been asked to walk around stark naked. How I wished I spoke Arabic and could explain I was ill. Nothing was found on my person, in my clothes or in my luggage, and I was allowed to get dressed and re-pack my cases.

Thankfully the KLM flight had been delayed for an hour, so I found my seat, said nothing to the flight attendant and managed not to be sick before take-off. Once airborne the vomiting started and the unfortunate passenger next to me was quickly moved; the attendants kept me supplied with vomit bags for the rest of the journey. At one stage the senior steward arrived to say it was felt I needed a doctor and the pilot had decided to turn back or make an emergency landing. At this point I explained I was a physician, that there was nothing to be alarmed about and thanked them for their attention and supply of bags. KLM impressed me.

On reaching Amsterdam it had been arranged for me to be first off and put on a motorised trolley to be taken to the medical centre. A couple of hours' wait for the connecting flight to Heathrow gave the treatment time to stop the vomiting and improve the unsteadiness and nausea. To my relief BA agreed to take me.

Heathrow and a three-hour bus ride to Bristol meant I was nearly home.

In 1993 I visited Syria once again but on a quite different journey – to celebrate Rachel's 60th birthday. However, while we were there a

---

[8] In 1986 at a trial in London the Syrian ambassador was found to have been implicated in a plot to blow up an Israeli airliner on its way from London to Tel-Aviv, in mid-air. The Syrians rigorously denied the charges.

number of things occurred that emphasised the closeness of medicine and politics as well as the influence of religion on everyday life.

As we drove north from Damascus we spent a day and a night in Hama, an attractive town on the Orontes with its famous *norias* – wooden waterwheels up to eighty feet in diameter, built to keep the water flowing freely along the stone channels running through the old part of the town. Abdul our driver said little except to mention the trouble here some years ago, and as we wandered around we started to question him about the badly damaged buildings and the bullet holes everywhere. We sat down for a cup of tea and he launched into a full account of the uprising in 1982 against Hafiz al-Asad's regime; basically it comprised the poor, plus supporters of the by-then outlawed Muslim Brotherhood, against the army and the police. The massacre of 20,000 civilians had taken place only a few months after my visit to nearby Homs when I had encountered the medical and social support given to the poor by the Muslim Brotherhood, its existence half hidden from me. I certainly had no idea the Brotherhood had been an outlawed organisation. I told Abdul of my experience around Homs and Damascus:

"Yes, I believe they help the poor."

Abdul Khadev Najjar, before becoming a taxi driver, had been a Professor of English at the State university in Aleppo, but after a long struggle had decided he could no longer look after his family on an increasingly meagre salary. By the time we reached Aleppo he had told us the sad story of one of his daughters (he had four children). Sehan was ten, and about fifteen months previously she had become ill and was quickly diagnosed with acute renal failure requiring renal dialysis twice a week for two months. Unfortunately it was not reliable, due either to electricity cuts or the equipment needing repair. With the aid of an Italian doctor who had been a passenger in his taxi, Sehan had been transferred to the University of Padua's teaching hospital for six weeks. Here she was dialysed regularly three times a week and her condition saw enormous improvement. She returned to Aleppo in the hope of continuing this regime – this proved to be impossible and she was taken back to Padua where it was decided she needed a kidney transplant.

Abdul realised that Rachel and I were doctors and asked if we would come to his home to have a meal and see Sehan for ourselves. Of course we agreed. A simple meal and a long discussion ended with Abdul asking if we could make enquiries in the UK about the possibility of a transplant. I remember clearly two questions we asked; why not get Sehan seen in Saudi Arabia or one of the Gulf States – after all, they were over-run with high-tech medicine. He and his wife just looked at us in disbelief and smiled sadly:

"Do you not understand that as a Syrian it would be almost impossible to even get a visa? And even if she went it would be too expensive."

They had heard that the UK was like Italy and they wouldn't be charged. We changed tack. Our second question:

"Would any member of the family be prepared to donate a kidney?"

Again they looked at us in disbelief as well as horror. How could we have asked such a question? Abdul gave the reasons and explanations while his wife sat silently by him. First it would be impossible for any man to do this as at some stage he would be head of his family and such an action would reduce the respect society would give the family. Second, women need to have two kidneys to have a child and a safe delivery, and in any case such a woman would never be able to marry – to remain unmarried would be her fate and no increase in her dowry would make any difference. In the end it became clear to Rachel and myself that it would be either the family or childbirth or the inability to get married that highlighted the attitude of Arab culture.

We spent the next day travelling to the early Byzantine church at Qala'al Sama'an which had been dedicated to St Simeon, famous for establishing himself on top of a 60-foot-high pillar for nearly forty years, and preaching to anyone who would listen. It would be a long journey but Abdul had insisted Sehan came with us – an exhausting day and she slept on Rachel's lap all the way home. As we climbed out of the car Rachel whispered to me:

"She's a very sick little girl."

On our return to the UK I wrote to Dr Paulo Tedesco in Padua about our mutual friend in Syria and by return of post he updated me on the situation. Sehan was on a waiting list but it would be about eight months before she reached the top, so at least another eight months' dialysis in Syria would be necessary. Her stay in hospital in Italy would be free and the operation would cost nothing.

The news from the UK was not good at all; kidney transplants were not available to foreigners, but a live donor transplant from a member of the Najjar family could probably be arranged at the cost of around £18,000. The NHS turned out to be more like Saudi Arabia than Italy.

Abdul and I kept in contact for about ten years, writing once or twice a year in peace and friendship. I always asked after Sehan but strangely I never received a clear answer and never knew when she must have died.

Our journey by train from Aleppo to Damascus provided some interesting conversation; the journey normally took about three hours but ours took over seven. The train was fairly clapped out and once the sun had started to go down it became very cold. We had settled down in a carriage which was virtually empty – it took us a mere quarter of an hour to discover why; we hadn't noticed the broken windows. We quickly moved to another carriage which was much warmer and nearly full and managed to get seats facing each other. People started looking at us, the whispering began, and finally an extremely large fat man stood up and asked our nationality. He then spoke slowly:

> "Do you like Syria? What do you think of Assad? Why do the British hate the Syrians?"

All the questions were directed at me. It was as though Rachel didn't exist. I was surprised by the questions, particularly as we had been warned the secret police were everywhere. I answered carefully and discretely and as honestly as I thought prudent.

> "Do you like the Queen? What do you think of America? Do you like Americans? What is your job?"

Immediately things began to change as by now the sweating fat man had been superseded by other passengers, women as well as men.

> "What do you think of the Syrian health service?"

After answering this I saw my opportunity and suggested questions could also be directed to Rachel as she was a doctor too. The carriage really woke up then and the nature of the questions changed.

> "When should women have children? What is the best number of children? How can you stop having children? What is the best operation for bleeding? How many children do you have and how old are they? Are children better looked-after in England?"

Rachel coped really well and everyone seemed satisfied to the extent that men now joined in:

> "What is the best contraceptive? How often should we make love?"

At this point I was beginning to wonder how much more detail might be asked, so I interrupted and said we were tired and wanted something to eat. Smiles all round and no more questions. I had been questioned about politics whilst Rachel had been asked about the family and personal matters, which interested people much more. Both of us were astounded by the number who spoke English, often haltingly but at least they could make themselves understood. So much for poorly educated Arabs, particularly when French would have been their natural second tongue.

Damascus was reached about 12.30am, sadly not at the old station in the middle of the city, which apparently had been closed, at least for passengers. The new station was a fair distance out, but finally a taxi arrived and took us to the Iwan hotel – only to find that our room had been re-let for the night as reception thought we weren't coming. Disaster. What to do and how to find another hotel? To our complete surprise the driver immediately suggested we spend the night with him at his family's home in a village outside the city. Everyone was in bed and asleep but he organised two settees and we slept like logs.

Rachel washed and I shaved in a basin the taxi driver had shown us in the corridor – it was nerve-wracking as we didn't know what to do or expect. A most pleasant younger brother was the first to appear. He spoke French fluently and was followed by a sister, very shy and quiet, but by the time we left we had managed to get her to talk a little and even express an opinion – she spoke English. Gradually all the family appeared and introduced themselves, mostly in English, sometimes in French, the mother and other members staying in the background in the kitchen.

Finally the taxi driver asked us to sit in the sunny courtyard surrounded by flowers and shrubs and here we were introduced to his father who was already sitting there reading his paper. The mother brought in the breakfast and wonderful coffee; nothing would persuade her to join us and she returned to the kitchen. We talked easily, mostly with the father but also with two of his sons – his daughter of course knew her place. We were asked about Palestine and what we thought of Syria. The father's views on Palestine were pretty standard and I asked both his sons for their opinions and whether they agreed with their father. The answer was Yes. Interestingly, the father spoke directly to Rachel, even when talking about politics; it was all quite relaxed and without any sort of tension.

After saying goodbye to everyone we were shown where to catch the bus. Mercifully it wasn't too crowded. On reaching the Iwan Hotel the reception staff couldn't apologise enough for the previous night and on going to our room we found a bouquet of flowers and a token for a free evening meal that night.

Around Christmas a letter arrived from Syria:

'My family and I were so happy to receive your letter. And I hope we could express all our welcome to you during your visit which was too short. Perhaps in your next visit we might have more time together.
Anyway, you left good and happy memories in our minds and hearts.
We are all waiting for the time when peace and wells (sic) prevail all over the world generally and in our area especially
Until you next visit we wish you all the happiness and Merry Christmas and Happy New Year.
Your sincerely
Ma'an Al-Sabbagh

21

HASHEMITE KINGDOM of JORDAN

Jordan, of all the countries included in *Primary Care in the Arab World,* has had stronger ties with the UK than the rest, in part due to the close relationship between the Jordanian royal family and the British military, but also on account of two Englishmen – 'Lawrence of Arabia' T E Lawrence, and Glabb Pasha, Lt General Sir John Bagot Chubb.

In his book *A Soldier With The Arabs,* Glubb Pasha wrote:

> 'I strenuously opposed an idea that East was East and West was West and that the two should never agree. I had expressed in myself, as I thought, the feasibility of living simultaneously as an Arab amongst Arabs and as an Englishman amongst Europeans. Why should the two not work hand in hand . . .'

He spent thirty-six years living amongst Arabs. During the first nineteen years he lived almost entirely in their company, rarely meeting Europeans and sometimes not speaking a word of English for weeks on end. He had resigned his commission in the British army and in the early 1920s came to live in Trans-Jordan, subsequently becoming the Commander of the Arab Legion, the tiny army of a little State. Finally, in 1956, following a disagreement between the government of the United Kingdom and the King of Jordan, he left Jordan.

Lawrence of Arabia in *Seven Pillars of Wisdom* and *Revolt in the Desert,* described his dramatic, romantic involvement with the Arabs in their opposition to the Turks in the First World War, thus contributing to the final collapse of the Ottoman Empire. Lawrence never recovered from the deception of the British government that affected both him and the Sherif of Mecca, and brought lasting shame on Britain.

Nobody, either in Azrak (which had been his HQ), or in the rest of Jordan had heard of Lawrence or his exploits as the British Liaison Officer in the Arab Revolt, or his involvement with the Arabs, whom he loved and respected, especially the Bedouin. Probably even more surprising was the equal ignorance of Glabb Pasha who after all had lived in Jordan for nearly forty years. Rather disheartening, really.

Britain was given the Mandate of Palestine in 1921 and a year later the artificial state of Trans-Jordan was created. In 1946 Trans-Jordan became the Kingdom of Jordan in the land east of the river Jordan; west of the river the rest of Palestine remained a British Mandate until the State of Israel was created in 1948, totally against the wishes of the great majority of Palestinians. At the end of the Arab/Israeli war in 1949, a small area of the West Bank, now in the State of Israel, was returned to the Arab Palestinians, and finally, in 1950, this small area and the Kingdom of Jordan became the Hashemite Kingdom of Jordan.

The result of most of the West Bank being occupied by Jews was that thousands of Palestinian refugees fled to Jordan, amongst them the Palestine Liberation Organisation (PLO) and its leader Yasser Arafat. At the time of my visit the total population of the Hashemite Kingdom was 3.15 million, of which 7-800,000 were Palestinian refugees. Since that time the number of refugees has dramatically increased with more and more refugee camps having to be set up.

It is no surprise that Jordan was and remains a poor country: no oil, uncertain tourism, anxiety about water and the socio-economic problems resulting from 15% of its population being refugees. The country is divided into eight governorates (*muhafazat*) with corresponding health directorates – Amman, Balga, Irbid, Kerak and Ma'an in Jordan, and the remaining three – Hebron, Jerusalem and Nablus – being still under Israel's control. What a ghastly muddle.

The separation of health care between the private and public sector was absolute. In both urban and rural areas, care was provided by a variety of private specialists as well as so-called general practitioners. In rural areas private physicians had their office in the nearest strategically placed small town in order to cover the neighbouring villages. However, almost always they lived in the nearest large town. In both urban and rural areas it was of course more profitable to practice as a specialist even if you held no additional qualifications – the fees were higher and the status greater. Work carried out in the private sector was almost exclusively curative and this affected both the care of children and pregnant mothers – immunisation, ante- and post-natal care, developmental paediatrics and health education were ignored. By law the private sector had to ensure that out-of-hours cover was provided and this was organised by the Jordanian Medical Association in association with the Ministry of Health. This law worked only in theory. In Amman, for instance, with a population of over one million, only two private physicians would be 'on call', whilst in the countryside virtually all private physicians had closed their offices by late afternoon and were at home in the nearest large town.

The Ministry of Health had made no provision for primary care until the early 1970s. However, by 1982, 66 basic, 22 comprehensive, 76 MCH and 283 village centres were in existence. I was able to visit five comprehensive, three basic and four MCH centres, giving me an excellent opportunity to talk with the staff and speak to the patients.

At the time of my visit the long-term strategy had been to increase the number of comprehensive and upgrade the basic centres. In theory this seemed a good idea but it was completely unrealistic when only eight percent of the health budget was spent on primary care – my impression was that nobody really believed this plan was feasible, including those who were proposing it. In addition a number of simple facts made people doubt the wisdom of the policy and it didn't take me long to see why.

First, all the primary health care facilities were seriously underused – they were meant to be open for nine hours per day but in fact were only used for between thirty minutes and at the most four hours, so were unavailable most of the time. The second issue concerned the dirty, badly repaired and ill-maintained premises with poor furnishings and inadequate medical equipment along with poorly-motivated staff. Finally, perhaps the most serious reason for dissatisfaction concerned the lack of women doctors. Between 80 and 100% of women patients wanted a female doctor and the majority of women would simply leave the premises as soon as they were told that only a male doctor was available. It was commonly said that to increase the number of MCH centres without increasing the number of female doctors would mean they would never be used. Or more briefly, the policy was described as 'silly and stupid'. Very few patients thought that the Jordanian Medical Association or the Ministry of Health were listening or were in any way concerned.

Restrictions placed on those working in primary care by the Ministry of Health was a further reason for the service not working effectively. Doctors were not permitted to order x-rays or even, very often, laboratory tests. Every physician I spoke to in primary care was adamant it was like working with their hands tied behind their backs. They were angry and frustrated and it reminded me of the early days of the NHS when GPs couldn't arrange physiotherapy without referral to either an orthopaedic surgeon or a rheumatologist – and even sixty years later GPs have only recently been allowed to refer patients directly for CAT and MRI scans.

The general consensus amongst those involved in primary care was well summed up at the Department of Community Medicine, University Medical School, in Amman:

> 'What's the use of putting forward plans for the next 5 years if the plans for the last 5 years haven't been carried out?'
>
> Or:
>
> 'What's the use of putting forward plans for the next 5 years if the mistakes of the last 10 years haven't been corrected?'

My first meeting with the new Director of PHC went well. Dr Suleiman Qubain had spent nine months in Bristol in 1968 attached to the Department of Community Medicine whilst preparing for his Diploma of Public Health. During this time he had come to understand the importance of primary care, and since returning to Jordan he had attempted to point out the appropriate relationships between primary, secondary and tertiary care. As far as he was concerned, sanitation or rather the lack of it, available safe drinking water, refuse collection, the care of mothers during pregnancy, the immunisation of children and the need to change the education of doctors and nurses, were his main priorities. His wider interest was to reduce the domination of private practice vis-à-vis the state-run health service. A slight change in emphasis:

> "Do you know the privileges of the Army?"
> "No."

"They and their families get everything free, particularly the officers. Do you know about hi-tech medicine in Jordan?"
"Well, yes, I know a bit – but tell me about Jordan."
"Right. Jordan was one of three very poor countries to introduce ultrasonic foetal examination, fibre optic endoscopy, cardiac catheterisation, CAT scanning, renal dialysis, cobalt isotopes, open heart surgery and laser beam therapy, all by 1978. What do you think of that?"

I told him we were all on the same wavelength.

At the next meeting Qubain started to describe the plight of the Palestinian refugees, who had been virtually imprisoned in camps under the supervision of UNRWA (United Nations Relief and Works Agency) in the Near East since the early 1950s. I never had a formal meeting specifically about the refugees, but in any discussion with anyone an identical scenario was given: their plight was grim and included a lack of medical care. I requested a visit to such a camp – the nearest was at Barqa'a on the road out of Amman towards Jerash. I was only able to view it from the outside – endless tents, muddy tracks and thousands simply standing around staring towards the road from behind the barbed-wire encampment. There were queues for food and many were struggling with buckets of water – some of it collected from outside the barbed wire, it seemed.

As we left Barqu'a Qubain's thoughts again turned to the military and he asked me once more if I knew about them. Again I answered 'No'. He explained that although he had already told me about their separate and privileged arrangements, he wanted me to understand that all high-tech medicine had been concentrated in military hospitals and not in the university teaching hospitals – the smarter and bigger the hospital appeared, often looking like a five-star hotel, the more likely it would belong to the military. I never found out how many of these military hospitals there were or how many beds they had.

About twenty miles south of Amman lies the small town of Madobar, famous for its unique mosaic maps of Palestine and one of Jerusalem. Not surprisingly this was not the purpose of my visit. The comprehensive health centre covered a population of 40,000 and was staffed by five doctors, a dentist, two midwives, three nurses, a laboratory technician and an assistant pharmacist. Eight village clinics were also its responsibility. It was in a different league to anything I had seen before. The MCH centre was separate and staffed by a trained midwife and two assistant nurses – a small unit with only a few deliveries. Madobar hospital gave me an opportunity to meet some doctors and try to find out their attitude to primary care; unknown to me there were no private or military hospitals in the vicinity so it was responsible for all referrals and emergency care.

I decided to visit three departments – paediatrics, obstetrics and accident & emergency. The paediatricians were very clued up about the wider issues of their speciality. They considered the main problems were related to poverty, poor housing and ignorance. They were unanimous in believing that improving female education would benefit children's health more than many medical interventions. The obstetricians also mentioned education but they were focused on the fact that over fifty percent of confinements presented as emergencies – ante- and post-partum haemorrhage (APH/PPH), toxaemia, eclampsia, retained placenta, obstructed labours and ruptured uterus. It was agreed that ante-natal care (ANC) was totally inadequate and frequently non-existent, yet when questioned none would accept that the presence of male and the lack of female doctors was likely to be a significant reason for this lack of attendance at clinics. The midwives and nurses strongly disagreed with them and were not afraid to say so. Traditional birth attendants (TBAs) or *dyas* were mentioned and the majority of staff felt they were a good idea, but more training was needed and they must be officially licensed. Regarding accident & emergency I could have had exactly the same conversation in many parts of the world – too many patients turning up with simple problems not requiring hospital treatment or even advice. It was noticeable, however, that the nursing staff were far more sympathetic to patients, particularly to mothers with their children, and were able to understand the reasons they turned up.

Estimates of the number of Bedouins living in Jordan were uncertain as, due to their tradition and culture, they were always on the move in search of grazing, wandering north into Syria, east into Iraq and south into Saudi Arabia. The estimate was between thirty-five and forty thousand, but who knows? They were nearly always to be found in small groups of strikingly handsome men and women wearing colourful clothes, surrounded by many children, chickens, goats, sheep and camels.

A day had been set aside for a visit to the Dead Sea and to look at medicine in rural areas. Rafiq Abdel, a Jordanian colleague, was to be my companion. A pleasant drive from Amman to the town of Salt took us from a fertile plateau to a twisting rapid descent through a verdant wooded *wadi.* The town was a charming, attractive place with many buildings and ochre-painted dwellings reminding a traveller of the influence of the Ottomans and the French. It had been built on a steep slope and the *wadi* continued its way down to the river Jordan.

With a population of around 30,000, Salt had a comprehensive health centre close to the Health Directorate. The centre proved to be a delightful stop for the first Turkish coffee of the day. A valuable discussion regarding immunisation took place; the triple vaccine of diphtheria, pertussis and tetanus was offered, plus cholera and typhoid, but no polio, measles or rubella. Even though the manufacture of these vaccines had commenced in 1968 they were used mainly for export. I never received a satisfactory answer to this extraordinary decision.

The National Immunisation Programme initiated in the Eastern Mediterranean Region in 1975 didn't start in Jordan until 1979. It involved the triple vaccine, cholera and typhoid as well as oral polio and measles, but still no rubella. However, by the time of my visit, according to reports written by the WHO in 1982, immunisation was becoming a real success and was recognised as the most important factor in the recent improvement in children's health. I decided I would test these claims and when possible use the Bedouins as my subject matter.

Beyond Salt the road was bleakly spectacular with bare limestone hills and peaks intersected by numerous dry *wadis.* The road twisted and turned its way down to the Dead Sea passing a surprising number of trees growing out of the arid stony ground, whilst on the other side the brown barren hills of an occupied land could be seen – the West Bank of the State of Israel. It is incredible how such a small piece of land could have been, and continues to be, the source of so much fighting and bloodshed. It is equally difficult to forget the extent to which my own country has been responsible for much of the misery and anger in this part of the world.

Health centres in the villages of South Shuneh and Rawda were visited before reaching the shoreline. Strangely neither place could be found on any map or bus timetable. Both centres were in a good state of repair, both were clean and the staff seemed professional. In fact South Shuneh had recently been upgraded to a comprehensive facility with eight doctors, a dentist, a midwife, three trained nurses and some auxiliary nurses plus an assistant pharmacist and laboratory technician. Interestingly two of the doctors lived locally, but none were female. Six outlying village clinics along the Dead Sea were the responsibility of South Shuneh. Rawda was much smaller but had also been upgraded eighteen months before to include some maternity services and the appointment of a trained midwife.

As we were coming down from the hills I could see an encampment of Bedouins and I asked Rafiq if we could stop and ask them about their children's immunisation. He was somewhat taken aback as it was not included on the programme and I hadn't told him what was in my mind. He agreed, rather reluctantly.

There were six main tents, and as we got out of the car the women stopped what they were doing and eyed us warily. Only the sheep, goats and a couple of camels took no notice. The children kept close to their mothers; there were no men to be seen. Eventually two old men came out of a tent and walked over to us past lines of washing moving slightly in the gentle breeze. Their faces were a deep mahogany with wrinkles and furrows like dried-up *wadis*. Their eyes gave nothing away and the reputation of Bedouin hospitality remained hidden. Rafiq went over to them to explain – what he said I don't know but the atmosphere immediately changed, the women relaxed with broad smiles all round and finally the old men talked to the women again to make sure they gave their approval.

It took a little time for the documentation about the children's immunisation to be found and then eight or nine mothers gathered around so I could ask some questions:

"Are you happy to have your children immunised?"
"Yes."
"Where do you have to go to get them immunised? Was it at the health centre or the MCH centre or school?"

"No, the mobile team comes."
"Do you like that?"
"Yes, very much."

There were too many children for me to check all the documents so I took a sample from each tent. All had been filled in with the date of immunisation and the date the mobile team were next coming. It was very impressive. My visit had been without warning, so clearly no preparation had been involved, and anyway they couldn't write. It was a great success for the immunisation programme.

After everything had been tidied up we sadly had to refuse their hospitality – already food was being brought out and in spite of the time of year it was getting hot and nothing could have been pleasanter than lying on their carpets sipping tea and eating fruit and cakes.

The shore of the Dead Sea was initially a disappointment. Rafiq had taken me to a government entertainment park where the restaurants and cafés were now closed and the empty chairs and tables with protective umbrellas were surrounded by rubbish and plastic bottles. It looked like most holiday resorts do the world over when out of season. Rafiq managed to find a water pump so that he and the driver could wash themselves before going off to pray. They found a quiet corner and returned to get their prayer mats.

While they were praying I was thinking about this extraordinary place 1,000 feet below sea level. I was surprised how clean the water looked and how even a single drop of water or moisture tasted like raw salt. After the prayers had been completed we had the lunch we had bought in South Shuneh – fruit and cakes and a couple of bottles of orange juice. We made our way slowly along the shore and came across a number of bathers, mostly families, and I was intrigued by how Rafiq instantly recognised their nationality – Iraqi, Saudi, Egyptian, Yemeni, Iranian and so on. He tried his best to explain the differences but with no success.

Neither Rafiq or our driver wanted to bathe and neither did I, but I felt duty-bound to at least paddle, and so I did – Victorian style with rolled-up trousers. As I wandered around in the water a curious prickly feeling started to irritate my feet and legs below the knees and it became much more noticeable when I got out. We were about halfway back to Amman before I realised my trousers were becoming noticeably stiff. By next morning they could almost stand up by themselves in the corner of the room and of course were quite unwearable. Once back home, even after being soaked for twenty-four hours and then washed, they had to be thrown away.

My programme had been organised carefully, so being told without warning that the next day was to be taken as a public holiday – it was King Hussein's birthday – and everything had to be cancelled, was like having two Fridays in one week! I had realised already that it was going to be impossible to find the time to visit Petra, Jordan's most famous tourist site, so here was my chance and (unknown to me) I was going to have the opportunity to see how the health service really functioned.

I set off by public transport from the central bus station at 7am. Most of the passengers were Jordanian with a sprinkling of obvious foreigners – a couple of Germans and Italians, three blue-rinse Americans and a charming Frenchman who was sitting next to me. We took the main Aquaba road, the Desert Highway, which is the quickest way to reach Petra. The Hejaz Railway runs parallel with the road and they criss-cross each other until Ma'an is reached. Every thirty or forty miles, small stopping places on the line would coincide with a cluster of sheds and mud houses along the road, and usually there would be a few stalls selling coffee, tea, drinks, cakes and chocolates, with kebabs spitting on their skewers. Ma'an was such a place – like a minor oasis – with date palms providing protection from the sun. A monotonous rocky desert had been our companion with an endless line of electricity pylons disappearing into the distance.

Quantrana was our next stop, about a hundred yards of mud-brick and concrete houses and an open shed with the carcasses of four decapitated sheep hanging from hooks, flies swarming all around them. The driver invited us to 'make use of the facilities' – a wall at the back of the shed. There was enough time for a cup of very sweet tea but not enough to enjoy the wonderful-smelling *shashlick* and fried eggs – the swarming flies hadn't put me off, surprisingly .

At Quantrana we turned off to join the King's Highway lying to the west. Mercifully this road was much less busy, but it seemed to encourage our driver to drive faster and the Frenchman and I were beginning to feel nervous at the speed we were going, especially as on a couple of occasions the bus had slipped off the edge of the banked-up road, and ahead we could see a curve in the road – almost the first bend we had encountered. The inevitable happened as we veered from one edge to the other and back again before leaving the road and overturning, eventually ending up on our side. The ground was a combination of sand and stones; miraculously we had avoided the large rocks and boulders. There was no fire and no other traffic involved. The windows were broken on one side and the front of the bus was smashed, the driver escaping with only superficial cuts, although two passengers were lying on the ground, one with a broken leg and the other a broken arm, but no one was trapped.

Some panic and much anxiety quickly surfaced so I realised it was necessary to admit I was a physician. I insisted the woman with the broken leg wasn't moved and just made as comfortable as possible, while the broken forearm was fixed up with a sling. All we could give them was paracetamol from the first aid box in the bus. Otherwise it was a matter of making sure everyone remained calm and in the end telling the blue-rinse ladies to stop complaining.

Initially the road and the surrounding desert appeared to be empty yet within fifteen minutes a car could be seen approaching from the direction of the King's Highway – it was an Englishman, who promised he would raise the alarm. Within a further ten minutes a Bedouin appeared from nowhere and was quickly followed by others – how we didn't spot the lumbering camels sooner remains a mystery.

Within three-quarters of an hour of the Englishman leaving us, a police van turned up; we managed to immobilise the injured woman's leg and get her into the van. Despite having only had only a couple of paracetamol the woman, a Jordanian, never complained, and it was just the same with the woman whose arm was broken. The police van then set off with the women for the nearest orthopaedic department in Amman.

Finally, and barely an hour and a half since the bus had overturned, another bus arrived driven by army personnel and accompanied by a couple of army trucks with an officer who seemed keen to take control of everything. To complete the picture we were by this time surrounded by Bedouin and anyone else who happened to be passing.

The Frenchman and I were very impressed that within two hours we were on our way. We reached the King's Highway at Kerak, renowned for its ruined Crusader castle of which we saw nothing as we were driven straight to the local health centre. It was a large building in obvious need of repair, scruffy and dirty inside with little equipment and few facilities, but at least it had a resident doctor. I introduced myself and together we did the necessary, which was mostly reassuring people they didn't need anything more than simple dressings, although a couple needed sutures. A young Jordanian teenager who up to then had kept quiet, was found to have severe bruising and swelling around her ankle and lower tibia. The doctor quickly arranged for her to be taken to Amman for x-ray, using the ambulance car attached to the health centre.

The three American women were really tiresome, at least to me. They cornered me and asked me to examine them and fill in their medical insurance forms which they pulled out of their handbags. I examined them but refused to sign any forms as I had no desire to be badgered by three different American insurance companies regarding the inadequate treatment and inappropriate reassurance I had given their clients. They were highly incensed and indignant that I could be so uncooperative – it was fascinating, if dreadful, listening to the discussion about how much money they could hope to get from their respective insurers.

On reflection I was impressed by the Jordanian response to the accident – the police, the army, the health centre, and the doctor with the ambulance car being immediately available, and perhaps as much as anything by the remarkable stoicism of the Jordanian people.

We were about three hours late in reaching Petra but felt lucky to be alive and uninjured and with enough time for at least a glimpse of the magnificence and beauty of some of the stunning monuments hidden away in this valley at the southern end of the Dead Sea Rift, dwarfed by the spectacular rocky mountains surrounding Petra.

I was full of anticipation and excitement as I entered the narrow *siq* (path) which would take me to the dramatic architectural treasure, the Khazheh, but the atmosphere was spoilt by the majority of tourists, American and German, who, rather than walk, were awkwardly sitting on horses which were as stubborn as mules and blocking up the *siq*. It was their clothing, though, that struck the note of contrast between the two cultures – Hawaiian shorts, Bermuda tops or other garish tops, or blouses and skirts that revealed more than Bedouin Arabs wished to see. Grossly obese in addition and singularly unattractive, none of them appeared to be in the least aware they might be offending the locals. Or if they were, they didn't care.

We left the *siq* and passed close to where Bedouin Arabs were living in the nearby caves. We watched young men, some just boys, riding bareback at great speed and with unbelievable skill on their splendid Arab steeds. The women could be seen busying around at the entrance to the caves, hanging up washing or cooking on a fire. The girls in their brightly coloured garments whispered together and played while the older men chatted and smoked and gazed at us in a most dignified way. I would love to have known what they thought about us tourists – I imagine they must have been mystified by the apparent vulgarity of western culture.

A good friend, a knowledgeable ornithologist, who had done his national service in Iraq in the 1950s, told me it was a must to visit Azrak because it was a great area for birds, particularly migrating ones. When, therefore, it was suggested I should visit Azrak as part of the rural health service I was delighted, not only for the birds but also because it was Lawrence of Arabia's main encampment in his support of the Arabs in their fight against the collapsing Ottoman Empire during the First World War. Rafiq didn't understand my enthusiasm as he had no interest in birds and had never heard of Lawrence. However, he was keenly interested in the early history of Jordan, about which I knew nothing.

We took the northern route to Azrak that would take us past Qasr (castle) al-Hallabat. The road to Kuwait and Iraq was badly pot-holed with large lorries towing unstable trailers thundering along in both directions – thankfully Rafiq had told our driver to go carefully. Qasr al-Hallabat, built on a small hill, could be seen from miles away. Originally it was the main fort of a Roman encampment and was later occupied by Muslim invaders. Obviously water was a necessity for any encampment, and grass and weeds were still flourishing among the ruins; Bedouins continued to cultivate the surrounding countryside –

strangely there appeared to be no problem with the surface water in this region. We stopped to look around and while we were wandering about the ruins Rafiq suddenly shouted "Stop!" I had no idea what was going on until he pointed out a black snake wriggling out of the foundations of a collapsed wall. He assured me it was highly poisonous.

Around al-Hallabat clusters of bright green grass, shrubs and the most beautiful purple flowers took me by surprise. There were even occasional trees. The distance between the ruins and Azrak was seventy miles and very quickly we returned to a grey featureless rocky desert with nothing green or even growing to be seen. Surely the ground water level must be dropping.

Unashamedly I asked first to see the lakes and the marshes. All that remained was a large dirty shallow pond with two motionless cranes standing on the edge and no evidence of any marshland at all. This was a shock for which I was quite unprepared, although the seventy miles from Qasr al Hallabat should have forewarned me. When in 1922 the village of Amman was chosen to become the capital of Trans-Jordan, its population was barely 3,000; by 1982 the estimated population of Jordan was 2,500,000 of which 140,000 lived in Amman. At the time of my friend's visit in the mid '50s, the lakes and marshland covered an area of ten square miles and now all that remained was a polluted pond. I never had the opportunity to speak to a water engineer about ground water levels and when the pumping of water from Azrak to Amman started.

The health centre was a new two-storey building and was responsible for a population of roughly 5,000 including two village clinics, one of which was three to four miles away and the other thirty. The staff consisted of a doctor, a midwife, two assistant nurses and an assistant pharmacist. The doctor and his family lived in a second-floor flat which was rent free, as was the accommodation for the midwife and her family. Patients requiring x-ray or a laboratory referral were sent to the nearest hospital – Zarka, sixty miles away. Almost next to the centre an ambulance and fire engine were garaged. The nearest village was visited every day by either the doctor or one of the nurses, and the more distant one was visited by the doctor once a week.

The MCH department had a separate entrance. Eighty percent of confinements were carried out by the midwife in the department. It was clear that a level of trust had developed between patients and midwife which was undoubtedly related to her having worked in Azrak for over six years, thus providing continuity of care. Breast feeding was the norm as in all rural areas, while in towns and Amman it was 50:50 breast to bottle. The midwife attributed the difference to powerful advertising by western companies, and both she and the nurses were constantly irritated that the packaging of milk powder always showed a white European baby, never an Arab one. I suggested tentatively that perhaps this was just as well as otherwise bottle feeding might be even more popular. My comment was ignored.

The opinion of the midwife and nurses merely confirmed what I had already heard – the need to have more female doctors and the refusal of most women to be examined by a male, although it was conceded that some were prepared to talk to a man about their children and perhaps some of their own problems.

All the staff seemed content with their work and reasonably content with the pay, particularly the doctor and midwife who enjoyed free accommodation. The responsibility of visiting the two outlying villages appeared to be taken seriously although I had no way of verifying this. The five members of staff spoke freely when I asked them questions but only the doctor spoke spontaneously.

Although nobody either in Azrak or the rest of Jordan showed any interest in or knowledge of Lawrence of Arabia, I found the entrance to the old fort he used without difficulty. It had been part of his headquarters for most of the time he had spent supporting the Arabs against the Turks. He wrote:

> 'Azrak's unfathomable silence . . . a famous place, queen of these oases, beautiful as ever . . . I had promised everyone a bath . . . and a little later its shining pool was brilliant with the white bodies of our men swimming . . .'

When it was time to leave, Rafiq explained that we weren't going to be able to visit either of the village clinics, in part due to my interest in and curiosity about the lack of birds, the disappearance of the lakes and marshland, and finally in Lawrence. A little hard, we thought.

We stopped on the edge of Azrak at a small petrol pumping station as otherwise the nearest would have been more than fifty miles away. It allowed Rafiq and our driver to take their prayer mats and wander off to a quiet spot to say their prayers. I sat on some stone steps with an old Arab man who, on Rafiq and the driver's return, insisted on giving us a cup of tea in the shade of a few date palms. I had vaguely noticed him fiddling around with an old primus stove and sure enough he brought cups of boiling hot tea and a collection of biscuits and small cakes – all arranged on a silver tray. He would accept nothing from us, only our thanks. I was sad to leave and suggested we might stay the night, but was firmly told there was nowhere to stay. This I didn't believe and felt sure that Rafiq was thinking there would be nowhere good enough for a foreigner, who would be expecting a swanky five-star hotel.

The return to Amman was on the southern much smaller road so Rafiq was able to show me something of the early history of the region. Qasr Amra, Qasr al Kharranah and Qasr Mawaqqar all had elements of Crusades and Muslim architecture, but mostly it was Ottoman, largely in ruins but still recognisable as the remains of castles. Rafiq came into his own and explained that Amra, built around 710 AD, had originally been a hunting lodge for nobility. The official notice board for tourists stated it was a castle.

Before leaving Jordan, quite out of the blue I had been summoned to a meeting at the Ministry of Health as the Deputy Minister of Health wanted to meet me. Fine by me.

On arriving at the Ministry Rafiq and I were shown into the deputy Minister's office where we waited mostly in silence. After a while I asked Rafiq what I was meant to do and what were we waiting for. Slightly irritated he answered 'His Excellency the Minister, of course'. Shortly afterwards His Excellency the Minister of Health and Deputy Prime Minister arrived and I was introduced. I could see why I was confused as one man held both titles! He wanted to fully understand why I was in Jordan, and asked what other Arab countries I had visited, what work I had done in the non-Arab world and whether I could send him a copy of *An Analysis of Primary Medical Care*. On further questioning he was clearly surprised and interested that I wasn't connected with any university or medical school or any institute or official organisation such as the WHO or UNICEF and received no government support – that I was literally on my own. This seemed particularly to please him and he hinted he was most supportive of my endeavours.

Some months later after sending my report to the authorities in Amman I received a letter from Dr Zuheir Malhas His Excellency the Deputy Prime Minister. He wrote:

> '. . . it was quite fair and objective . . . some of us did disagree with a few of your assessments but on the whole all feel that you have completed an admirable work. We should like to inform you that our appreciation of your work has been enhanced by the knowledge that you are your own sponsor.'

This letter encouraged me to believe that my original decision to work on my own had some merit.

My second visit to Jordan in 1993 was at the same time as my late wife and I were visiting Syria. I had arranged that during our holiday I would have a meeting at the Ministry of Health concerning *Primary Care in the Arab World.* The meeting was with the Minister of Health and I went armed with Dr Malhas' letter in the hope I could persuade the Ministry to purchase some copies and gain the book some publicity. Unfortunately Dr Malhas had retired from both his posts, but nonetheless the meeting went quite well and it just remained for negotiations Arab-style to decide on the number.

Rachel and Fares, our driver, had dropped me at the Ministry and were left to wander round the shops until the meeting was over. In the evening Rachel told me that it had been slightly awkward with Fares until he realised she was a doctor. He then started talking about everything – the Koran, Mohammad's teaching on morality, various other topics and then on to AIDS and what her thoughts on the disease were – he was really disappointed when my meeting ended! Unknown to either of us she was going to have an even more outspoken Q & A session on the train from Aleppo to Damascus.

22

The Mediterranean Coast

DEMOCRATIC & POPULAR REPUBLIC of ALGERIA

Five Arab countries, Morocco, Algeria, Tunisia, Libya and Egypt stretch along the southern coastline of the Mediterranean Sea from the Atlantic to the shores of Turkey, Syria, Lebanon and Israel. This area of north Africa is known as the Maghreb, whose southern border lies along the northern frontiers of central Mauritania, Mali, Niger, Chad and Sudan. The harsh and inhospitable Sahara desert covers most of central Magreb and the frontiers of all these countries are basically nothing more than imaginary lines drawn in the sand.

Algeria is roughly divided into three regions running from north to south and east to west. The Tell zone or coastal strip is 60 to 120 miles wide; south of the Tell is a high plateau, nearly 90% of which is uninhabitable stony desert and bare rocky mountains including the Atlas range extending from Morocco to Tunisia. The southern region is sand and stony desert.

The indigenous people of Algeria are often referred to as Berbers and comprise many tribes and nomads, differing dialects and languages. Their land has been occupied for two thousand years by Romans, Muslim Arabs and the Ottoman Turks. France began her occupation with the capture of Algiers in 1830, and over the following 130 years the official policy was to extend the power and influence of the French settlers rather than cooperate and integrate and educate the locals. Algeria was assimilated into France and in reality became another Département of the Second Republic. The government in Algeria was administered by the military.

By the end of the Second World War over a million Europeans, almost exclusively French, lived in the country and three-quarters had been born there. The Berbers referred to these local indigenous Algerian-born French by the insulting term *pied-noir*. One of my oldest friends was born in Algeria during the First World War, where she lived with her mother and elder sister. Her father had been an officer in the French army and had been killed on the Western Front in 1916. Odile remembers at the end of the Second World war that she and her friends were often referred to as *pied-noir*: the origin of the expression is shrouded in mystery and there is much debate about its meaning – perhaps it refers to the black boots worn by French soldiers as they figuratively trampled on the local people. Much later in her life Odile became a close friend of Albert Camus' third wife; he had been one of the main targets of the Berber people. Odile and Camus were the same age; she had remained in Algeria during the war while Camus had returned to Paris to become involved with the Résistance and the communist party. He was born in a village close to the Tunisian border, the son of a poor farm labourer, but his parents were Breton and Spanish so in fact he qualified as a *pied-noir*. After his death in 1960, three years after winning the Nobel Prize in Literature, I had the great good fortune to meet his wife on several occasions and due to these brief contacts I quite absurdly felt I knew a little about Algeria.

Odile, who adored the country, admitted that as she was growing up she was totally unaware of the terrible and pervasive poverty surrounding her. Her own mother and her friends and relatives were typical of their generation and it was interesting to hear from Odile their views on the occupation by Allied forces before the invasion of Sicily and Italy, and how complicated politics became.

The Algerian War of Independence(1954 -1962) was ferocious and barbaric with terrorism and counter-terrorism being conducted on both sides. The Front de Libération Nationale (FLN) was the political party striving for independence against the French, and the Armée de Libération Nationale (ALN) represented the military resistance to the settlers. In the late 1950s the Organisation de l'Armée Secrète (OAS)was set up consisting mainly of extreme right-wing French Algerians who seemed prepared to torture, rape, kill and maim anyone who opposed them - in particular they turned on the Muslims. In 1959 General de Gaulle became President of France and almost miraculously, through his realism and political *nous*, he eventually managed to persuade the French people that the independence of Algeria was inevitable and should be organised as quickly as possible.

In July 1962 independence was proclaimed and hundreds of thousands of *pieds-noirs* left Algeria.

Three years after I first wrote to the Ambassador in London I arrived in Algeria – it was January 1985. Since independence over twenty years before I hadn't realised that the influence of France had remained virtually unchanged – culturally, commercially and linguistically – far more so than I had found in Syria. French seemed to be the first language and Arabic the second, certainly as far as journalism, broadcasting and politics was concerned, but for the vast majority of the poor, Arabic was their first choice.

The atmosphere in the centre of Algiers immediately struck me; cafés and small restaurants could have been transplanted direct from France, the cars were almost all French, though a few were Italian, and virtually all the number plates were in Roman numerals, not Arabic. In fact Algeria was the only Arab country I visited in which this was the case.

The kasbah had a distinctive, picturesque charm with its muddle of houses clinging to the hillside, and narrow streets, blind alleyways and steep steps leading to terraces and minute squares. Everywhere balconies almost met overhead, creating a sort of canopy. Parts of the kasbah were very poor, many houses in urgent need of repair and streets full of uncollected rubbish with rats scurrying around and the all-pervasive smell of poverty in the air. Outside the kasbah I could see minarets poking out of this densely populated area. The elderly tended to dress traditionally whilst the younger generations favoured western dress.

I had been warned it was an expensive country and so it proved to be. The hotels I stayed in were down-market, built in the twenties and thirties, and as in Syria the French language lingered on faded notices – *étage, assenseur, la réception* and so on, but other countries were now in evidence, particularly those from Eastern Europe. In my diary I wrote:

> '. . . also kicked myself for forgetting a plug, my room compared well with the Soviet Union – no plug in bath or basin, lukewarm water not filling the bath even half full, which emptied into a bidet which had a blocked exit pipe; after numerous attempts with bits of wire and coat hangers the bidet remained full and leaked onto

> the floor through a wide crack. Still more delights – the central ceiling light had a clasp for four bulbs with only two working, while the lamp next to the bed would only stay alight if frequently tapped.'

I went down to reception to see if I could change my room, only to find the receptionists were busy with three large buckets collecting the rain steadily dropping through the ceiling.

Changing the room provided me with a lavatory, a plug in the bath, three dim bulbs in the ceiling and a lamp without a bulb next to the bed. The bath would sometimes have warm water but only sometimes; the final solution was a bucket of hot water left outside my door each morning and evening. A large old-fashioned radiator added to the charm but leaked continuously with a steadily increasing wet area spreading over the carpet until finally the entire floor was wet to walk on. A final irritation was when the receptionist informed me it was obligatory to eat one meal a day in the hotel restaurant, which needless to say was twice the price of a café or bistro. The so-called socialist and democratic countries certainly know the all the tricks of the trade.

The first day started badly with the reception staff unable or unwilling to explain how to get to the Ministry of Health, or even what bus I should take. This was followed by the taxi driver charging me 100 dinars, which I refused to pay and gave him 20, only to discover the Ministry of Health had recently moved. The first pedestrian I came across was really helpful, spoke a little English and pointed me in the right direction.

Professor Koudri with whom I had been in correspondence for the best part of a year and who had agreed to organise a programme and provide transport and interpreters, had left the Ministry – whether he had retired or been moved or sacked I never discovered. His successor, Dr Bellamma, had no idea who I was or why I was in Algeria and definitely wasn't expecting me. She spoke as much English as I spoke French so we definitely needed an interpreter. My luck began to change when Dr Ouchfoun turned up – he spoke English and had read *An Analysis of Primary Medical Care*. Perhaps all was not lost. After much discussion it was decided that I would come to the Ministry the next day at 2pm and hopefully there would be news. In the meantime they gave me *Le Developpement d'un Systeme National de Saute: L'Expérience Algerienne* which had been presented at an international conference in Algeria in 1983 and was crammed full of information and data.

Mr Whitell, the Representative of the British Council was my next port of call, first to report my arrival and also to thank him for the help he had given me by putting me in touch with Professor Koudri. He was a likeable man who explained the ways of Algeria to me. No, he was not surprised about Koudri as it was routine for people to be moved quite frequently and without warning, and he thought it inevitable that his successor knew nothing about me; all of which rather reassured me. He was surprisingly well-informed about PHC as the previous year his sister had been involved in setting up the organisation *Medicine Unlimited* which was chiefly concerned with the difficulties of PHC in the developing world. He warned me that most Algerian physicians didn't want to hear any criticism regarding the introduction of high-tech medicine and the miniscule effect that such a policy would have on the main health problems in their own country.

We must have spent a couple of hours talking, during which I was struck by how small his office was, and indeed the initial impression was unimposing. The Council's attempts to interest Algerians and persuade them that it would be worthwhile to visit the UK and study there seemed to be limited to leaflets about Chaucer, Shakespeare, and various poets of the eighteenth and nineteenth centuries. Universities appeared to be recommended mainly on their history and tradition – I could find no reference to the particular strengths of individual universities. There was no mention in any leaflet that few of us in the UK speak French well and almost no one speaks Arabic. I visited Mr Whitell on three occasions and only a few people dropped in. I found this very dispiriting and sadly it seemed to be an accurate reflection of the UK's influence in these parts. What a waste of Whitell's undoubted talents and intelligence.

The evening was taken up with *L'Expérience Algerienne* – translating was going to take a lot of time when I got home. At the end of my first day a feeling of foreboding prevailed. What on earth was I going to do tomorrow if the Ministry were unable or unwilling to organise a programme. So ended January 13.

January 14 was better in every way, even though the unexpected heavy snowfall of the previous day remained in the streets. I reached the Ministry promptly at 2pm to find Drs Ouchfoun and Naceur from the Ministry and Dr Belhamma representing the Council of Ministers, there to greet me. Much work had been carried out on my behalf. No records or letters belonging to Professor Koudri or letters from the Embassy in London could be found, but I was assured that once the Minister of Health had been contacted there would be no problem in getting a programme organised. There was just one snag – the Minister was out of town. However, Dr Ouchfoun had quickly contacted the Council of Ministers about me and clearly had made some complimentary remarks about *An Analysis of Primary Medical Care*. As the discussion continued it seemed that permission had been given by Dr Belhamma, although I wasn't sure I had fully understood the conversation. Anyway, a telephone call from the Council confirmed that my visit had been given official approval.

Without Ouchfoun and Naceur, especially the former, nothing could have been achieved. In addition Ouchfoun had decided to be my interpreter and guide in and around Algiers. I was to be responsible for getting myself to Biskra on the edge of the Sahara about 270 miles south-east of Algiers. Once in Biskra transport would be provided and then it only remained for me to find an interpreter.

Several long meetings with both Ouchfoun and Naceur gave me basic information about the organisation of the health service since independence. Naceur pointed out the difficulties there were in educating and training sufficient numbers of doctors and nurses – prior to independence it had been the deliberate policy of the French not to educate the local Algerian Arabs. Ouchfoun concentrated on the complexity of financing the service and the totally unresolved policies concerning priorities. All in all I got the impression that having first been embarrassed by my arrival, they then took pity on me and quickly decided I could help them lay bare the poor state of PHC to the English-speaking world. The French, and de Gaulle and his followers in particular, were anti the United States and the UK as well as countries such as Canada, Australia and New Zealand. In fact French doctors attending international conferences wouldn't receive any travel or hotel expenses or any support paid by the government unless they spoke in French and never in English.

In 1984 the final administrative reorganisation took place. The country was divided into 48 *wilyas* (areas), 160 *dairas* (districts) and 1,540 *baladaias* (communes), this being the smallest French territorial division for administrative purposes. Pari passu the health service followed suit. The Directeur de la Santé was in charge of a *wilya* and his headquarters and office was always in the *wilya* hospital – this had the obvious disadvantage to PHC in that specialists working in the hospital had immediate access to the Directeur with regard to equipment and resources.

Arranging the journey down to Biskra was more difficult than I had anticipated. I was advised to take an Air Algeria flight in a small plane carrying a dozen passengers, but all the seats were booked. My next stop was the central railway station, only to find the line between Algeria and Constantine had been cleared, but between Constantine and Biskra it was blocked by snow. Finally I made my way to the chaotic bus station with one of the Ministry secretaries offering to help me. She was told it was impossible to book a seat for the next day as the bus was not running today because the roads were still blocked. Anyway, I at least found out the bus departure times.

The following morning there was still plenty of snow lying around as I walked to the bus station. I found the right queue and after about twenty minutes we were told to buy the tickets on the bus although the officials were still unable to tell us whether the bus would come or not. From where it came I don't know, but come it did and we departed almost on time.

Packed with baggage and people, the bus first travelled along the coast with views of undulating hills dotted with grazing sheep in the charge of shepherd boys. Soon we turned south and climbed steadily, snow lining the winding road and filling the deep wooded gorges of the Tellian Atlas mountains. The summit, around 3,300 feet, gave panoramic views of rugged snow-covered ridges radiating in all directions. As we began a gradual descent to the High Plateau the snow disappeared to reveal curious angular rock formations that covered the bare plain. It was a featureless desolate landscape with steppe as far as the eye could see, which often was not very far as a gale-force wind often reduced visibility to a few yards within minutes, sand and earth blowing everywhere, causing vehicles to drive with their headlights on. Brief stops in the middle of nowhere were a feature of the journey letting people on and off, although where they lived was impossible to see. On two occasions we all got off to have a pee and eat our food which I had managed to get at the bus station. On both occasions there was a coffee stall and a few houses – white-washed mud-brick dwellings with flat corrugated iron roofs straggling both sides of the road; sparsely populated is an inadequate description.

We had been travelling for about six hours when suddenly and spectacularly the first Ziban oases appeared – famous for their dates, reputedly the finest in the country. Their flavour and juiciness and the vivid green of the oases was due to successful irrigation from artesian wells. It was really quite dramatic and for another half an hour we were able to enjoy this ever-changing landscape before we reached Biskra, the chief town of the Aurès range of mountains stretching east and west.

The 270 miles from Algiers had taken over seven hours; it had been a terrifying experience and almost a miracle there hadn't been an accident. The driver attacked bends and corners with almost suicidal intent and at one stage as we came off the High Plateau it took him nearly ten minutes to put on his Arab headdress, all the time driving at high speed and turning round to chat with the ticket collector. Needless to say he smoked continuously. I resolved to try and book Air Algeria for my return journey.

The person Ouchfoun had arranged for me to meet wasn't at the bus station but I managed to get someone to phone the Directeur de la Santé. To my surprise an ambulance car turned up quite quickly and drove me to the most expensive hotel in town. I decided to walk around to see if I could find somewhere cheaper. I was successful and found somewhere old, much more my style. Even here, however, the evening meal was expensive, so off again into town where I soon found a workman's eating place. It was little more than a square room that had been dug out of the side of a hill with enough space for cooking and a few tables for customers; bits of chicken in a soup with a lump of bread for fifteen dinars was much better than eighty dinars at the hotel.

The ambulance driver had explained to me I would be picked up at 8am the following day; luckily it wasn't far from the original hotel so I was able to walk back to where the authorities would presume I was staying. Soon after 8am I was duly picked up and taken to meet an electrical engineer from Algiers who happened to have come home for a few days. Mr Zahn spoke good English and had visited the UK – Newcastle-on-Tyne and Bournemouth – and he was to be my interpreter. My luck was changing as he was to be paid by the Ministry.

The first stop at the Secteur Sanitaire enabled the Directeur to fill in many gaps in my understanding and slowly the framework of the service took shape. Zahn had no medical knowledge, but Dr Sadek Lebal who came with us provided the necessary background. By the end of the meeting it was obvious that both of them had a real understanding of the battle between PHC and hospitals. The Directeur outlined the PHC facilities which he had contacted and arranged for me to see. Unfortunately I was never able to adequately thank him for the preparation he had given to my visit and at such short notice.

M'Chounèche was our first stop, a village at the head of a barren valley which suddenly became an oasis with spectacular views up the radiating gorges of the Aurès mountains rising all around. The Salle de Soins et de Consultation covered a population which included many small settlements. It was a facility only found in rural areas and was staffed by aides *adjoints medicaux de la santé* (medical auxiliaries) who like the rest of Algeria were middle-aged men. The building was new and impressively clean as was all the equipment – dressings, syringes, needles, bandages, and a refrigerator containing all the vaccines used in their immunisation programme – the triple, the oral polio and BCG. After the introduction of the measles vaccine in 1984 only two deaths were recorded in 1986 as against sixty deaths in 1984. The water supply was tested every three months when porous clay bricks soaked in chloride of lime were laid out at the bottom of community and private wells; the adequacy of the chlorine concentration was then tested by means of a hand-held device lowered into the wells.

On returning to the main road we continued east towards the Tunisian border, again a featureless landscape of flat stony tundra, stunted shrubs, occasional clusters of bright blue and yellow flowers and oases filled with Bedouin tents and grazing flocks of sheep and goats. Sidi Oqba our next stop was really just a huge oasis of palm grove estimated to be about 100,000 individual trees. We made straight for the maternity hospital, where we had lunch.

At last some women were involved; a female doctor, two *sage-femme* (midwives) and four *assistant rurale* (assistant midwives). The delivery room had two beds, eight ante-natal beds and ten for post-natal care. An excellent atmosphere was evident and probably accounted for the increasing numbers of young women who were prepared to come for their confinement – a number that had steadily increased over the last few years. Nonetheless no father had ever attended a birth and they were compelled to enter the hospital through a separate entrance.

All the babies were in tight swaddling clothes from head to toe as mothers were convinced that babies slept better if swaddled. The midwives were less certain about this but felt it was traditional and ingrained in society so that it would create uproar amongst the mothers, grandmothers and great-grandmothers if efforts were made to change. In addition, in areas such as this about half of the deliveries were carried out by *matrones* (traditional birth attendants) under poor hygiene conditions in the home with an inevitable increase in maternal and peri-natal deaths, and if swaddling was disputed the number of mothers willing to come into the hospital would drop.

The Centre de Santé was staffed by two male doctors, a male dentist and a number of male *aide-soignants* (assistant nurses) and again their work was greatly restricted on account of their sex. I found this out later in Ain Naga at their Centre de Santé where again there was only a male doctor and mostly male *adjoints medicaux*. A brief visit to a Salle de Soins et de Consultation (a place for treatment and consultation), a facility found only in rural areas, was staffed by three *aide-soignants,* all male.

Our final destination was Zeribet el Ouel about seventy miles from Biskra, a small nondescript town but situated at an important junction of roads close to the Tunisian border. The Centre de Santé's chief doctor was an Egyptian whom I found really cooperative. In answer to one of my questions he let rip on the difficulties and frustrations he was experiencing in trying to run the centre. For instance, a reasonably stocked pharmacy, a simple laboratory and a radiological unit were in theory part of the centre, but in reality the x-ray machine had broken down five months previously and no one knew when or if it would be repaired; the laboratory had run out of simple dip-sticks for blood and urine testing, while the supply of drugs was uncertain and anyway completely random. In addition he also had responsibility for five other Salle de Soins, each of which had to be visited on a weekly basis, which he said was simply impossible. Likewise the responsibility for the medical examination of children in primary and secondary schools could only be carried out in a most cursory manner. The Egyptian doctor acknowledged that these were his own personal views, but throughout our discussion Dr Lebal never interrupted or disagreed, just listened and often nodded in agreement.

An absolutely fascinating and useful day ended back in Biskra looking for somewhere to eat. Eventually I ended up with an omelette supper in an even smaller place than the previous evening – just room enough for an array of black pots and pans hanging from the blackened wall, an open fire, a primus stove and a great variety of skewers to grill the meat. Bread brought in from a nearby bakery was stacked on the floor. And so the day ended with the glorious smell of cooking filling my nostrils.

I needed to book the flight back to Algiers, so the next morning in the company of my interpreter and Dr Lebal I made my way to the local aerodrome. Unknown to me and seemingly to them, Air Algeria shared the runway with the military; two MIG fighters and a number of army trucks could be seen. It was surrounded by a barbed-wire fence and two armed soldiers guarded its only entrance. Bizarrely they refused to allow either the engineer or Dr Lebal through the gate, but on looking at my passport they somewhat paradoxically let me in. It was a fairly long walk with my baggage to what looked like the local bus station, reminding me of Samarkand, or Bristol in the late '50s. Mercifully a couple of seats were still available.

Returning to my companions, we drove in a south-westerly

direction towards Tolga, finally reaching the edge of the desert with dunes stretching out as far as the eye could see. Aïn-Benaoni was a small village with a collective-farm type of regime (à la USSR), described by Lebal as socialist farming. The Centre de Santé was small, supervising only 120 families with the aid of a male assistant nurse and a female assistant midwife plus a doctor from the polyclinic in Tolga visiting for half a day twice a week. Lichana, another flourishing palm grove, had a bigger Centre de Santé as it also supervised the population of a neighbouring village.

The polyclinic in Tolga had been open for only two years; it was staffed with two male doctors, a dentist, and a mix of trained and assistant nurses. The doctors were trying to get a variety of specialists, initially in dermatology, ophthalmology and ENT to carry out regular out-patient clinics. I asked Lebal when this was going to happen but he was unable to give a definite answer. The day ended with meeting the mobile team which was based at the polyclinic – they were positive about their work, and the immunisation programme in particular gave them a lot of satisfaction.

What I had been able to see in these two days was more than I had dared to hope as everything had had to be arranged at such short notice. The response to my questions had been informative and if they didn't know the answer they said so. There is no doubt that the absence of officials and bureaucrats enables people to talk more freely – a great bonus from my point of view.

I returned to Algiers in a small, twin-engine plane that flew low over dry arid steppe, just clipping the mountains before the green fertile coastline suddenly appeared. As we turned, the most glorious view of Algiers in the fading evening sun and the widely curving coastline of the long bay was visible, reminding me this had been a safe haven for shipping for hundreds of years and brought to mind the romantic schoolboy tales of adventure and pirates. I could see as well the unique line of reefs and inlets that gave added protection against strong winds.

In spite of the country's socialist orientation, with the visible evidence of the Boulevards of Che Guevara and other revolutionaries, along with the influence of Eastern Europe and Cuba, medical education remained utterly traditional, and, likewise, the expectations of physicians for whom hospital and high-tech medicine represented the pinnacle of ambition and achievement. Since independence, the effects of social deprivation and female illiteracy on both maternal and child mortality had been highlighted, yet the government had done nothing to try and rectify these deficiencies. Neither had the medical profession been even remotely concerned.

Primary care was officially accepted in Algeria as the way forward following the Alma Ata Declaration 1978, but the reality was different. PHC had been incorporated into the Départment de la Prevention Génerale, Ministère de la Santé Publique – a Départment with little power or influence; the least that might have been expected would have been the creation of a new, separate Départment – and of course this hadn't happened.

The shortage of nurses was no different from the situation in every other Arab country and this couldn't be blamed on France. Until the cultural, social and religious framework of Arab society changes its position towards women, there can be little prospect of improvement.

However, in 1976 a remarkable advance did take place when contraception, or birth spacing as it was referred to rather than birth control, was introduced. Interestingly birth spacing was discussed under three headings: improving the socio-economic condition of families; improving the education of girls and married women; and setting up birth-spacing centres. By 1984 over 600 centres had been opened. The oral contraceptive pill and the intra-uterine device were the most commonly used methods; condoms were conspicuous by their absence. What was not known was the percentage of women who practised birth spacing. But it was a step in the right direction.

The financing of the health service was difficult to understand. Between 1963 and 1973, except for the really poor, patients had to pay for all services both in primary care and in hospital. In 1974 a new epoch began with the creation of a national health service which was intended to be free at the point of use. At the time of my visit both hospitals and primary care remained free, in theory, but the exchange of money between patient and doctor was routine – in other words the poor and less well-off remained without care. As people's expectations started to increase, so the popularity and use of the health service began to decline amongst the middle classes and they resorted to private practice. This occurred even though by law doctors who were employed in the state health service were forbidden to carry out private practice. The reasons given by patients were ease of access and doctors who were more sympathetic and responsive and spent more time with them. Doctors truly have it in their power to make or break a health service, particularly in the developing world.

After returning home I remained surprised by the Algerian attitude towards France which had so recently been an occupying colonial power and against whom such a bitter and bloody war for independence had been fought. French tradition and culture has remained part of everyday life, and amongst the middle and ruling class the French language remains more commonly spoken than Arabic. In the same way the traditions of French medicine continue to dominate in a country with a socialist background which had been advised on health matters by Cuba and Eastern Europe.

As I write this now, thirty years later, I realise how fortunate I was to visit Algeria when I did. At the time there didn't seem to be any indication of what was to come. The Front de Libération Nationale (FLN) had ruled Algeria since the end of the war of independence in 1962, a military dictatorship masquerading as a democracy. An election was to be held in late '91, early '92, and for the first time since independence, support for the FLN was declining in parallel with the rise in popularity of the Front Islamique de Salut (FIS). The appearance of the Islamists was the inevitable consequence of decades of corruption, and the neglect and indifference of the FLN to the majority of the population – the poor.

The first round of the election had been monitored by independent international observers; they judged it to have been fair and well-run. It was won by the FIS, but within twenty-four hours the FLN, in fact the military, announced the election null and void. The government in Paris, and most of the West, supported this action. The civilians of both sides then experienced unimaginable cruelty and horror with death squads roaming the country, killing and butchering women and children and the elderly. Neighbouring villages that had been co-existing happily together were simply slaughtered. This senseless bloodshed continued right into the 21st century until both sides became exhausted by their own insanity.

23

LIBYAN ARAB *JAMAHIRIYA*

Libya, like Algeria, is a large country, most of which is part of the Sahara Desert where major oil deposits were discovered in 1959, the rest being a narrow coastal plain bordering the Mediterranean Sea where 95% of the population live. Niger, Chad and Sudan extend along its southern border. Tunisia and Algeria lie to the west, and Egypt to the east.

The original inhabitants of this sparsely populated coastal strip were the Berbers from the Magreb and Bedouins in a number of extensive oases throughout the desert region. From the eighth century BC when the Phoenicians settled in Libya, a succession of foreign powers have followed – Greeks, Romans, Islamised Arabs from Egypt, Ottoman Turks, Italians and finally the French and British towards the end of the Second World War.

Certainly by the end of the First World War the antagonism between the local population and the Italian colonialists who had annexed Libya in 1912 was obvious for all to see, so the action of Benito Mussolini in 1922 to send in troops was no surprise and within a few years the population had been subjugated.

The Second World War was the scene of heavy fighting between the Germans and Italians on the one hand and the Allies on the other; Libya suffered greatly – Benghazi and the main cities and towns along the coast were virtually destroyed with many thousands of civilians being killed. Tripoli the capital was least damaged as the Germans and Italians had surrendered by the time the Allies reached the city. It was a matter of intense resentment, particularly amongst the young, that a conflict in which the Libyan people had no interest and in which they had taken no part, had been fought by the nations of Europe on their soil. I wondered how these nations would have felt if the roles had been reversed and, say, the tribal disputes between Tripolitania and Cyrenaica had been fought on the mainland of Europe or even the Isle of Wight.

A French/British military establishment was set up after the German surrender in North Africa and it was not until 1951 that Libya was granted independence by the United Nations with Idris, the leader of the Senussi sect, as king. Prolonged unrest against this weak, corrupt, incompetent monarch followed, ending with a military coup in 1969 when a radical revolutionary leader came to power.

In 1962 the exporting of oil had started to change Libya from being one of the poorest countries in the world to one of great wealth, but by the time of my visit in 1983 the behaviour of the western oil companies was understandably giving rise to increasing anger as oil revenue was quite openly being siphoned out of the Libyan economy. Initially, though, at the time of the coup, Libya's economy was beginning to flourish, much to the benefit of the new leader. A Republic was declared under the rule of a twenty-nine-year-old army officer, Muammar Qaddafi, and a twelve-man Revolutionary Council. In 1973 the country became the Libyan Socialist People's Arab *Jamahiriya* (State of the Masses) and was finally renamed in 1986 the Libyan Arab *Jamahiriya*.

Qaddafi loathed the West in his early years, especially Britain, and gradually transferred his loathing to the United States as well. This dislike of Britain was in part related to a four-month military training course on which he was sent in 1966, initially in Beaconsfield for a month to learn English, and then at the Royal Armoured Corps HQ in Bovington, Dorset, for three months. During this time his opinion that the British were arrogant and treated the Arabs with contempt, was confirmed. A further resentment was that British troops were still stationed in Libya twenty-five years after the end of the Second World War and fifteen years since independence.

His reputation for being a supporter of terrorism was largely due to his readiness to offer help and training to anti-western 'liberation movements' and in particular his support for the IRA, both with arms and training. As a member of the non-aligned group of nations under the leadership of Marshall Tito, he was considered to be a maverick, unpredictable and often unreliable, whilst the Arab League and many fellow Arabs were never certain of his reactions, intentions or support; quite simply, he was not trusted.

My first contact with the Libyan People's Bureau, never referred to as an embassy, was in 1980. Relations between the two countries were poor – from the UK point of view his support for the IRA was our main point of contention, whilst from the Libyan point of view Qaddafi had always insisted that Britain was the main haven for members of the National Front for the Salvation of Libya (NFSL). In 1980 two members of the NFSL had been killed in Britain, which gave rise to much celebration in Libya that these 'stray dogs' (as any opponent of the regime was always called) had been tracked down. As far as I can remember, the Foreign and Commonwealth Office maintained that the two murders were committed by one of Qaddafi's death squads which had crept into the country.

Dr Omar Sodani came to the UK in 1979/80 to continue his postgraduate medical training which had been organised by the Royal College of Surgeons in cooperation with the medical school at the University of Garyounis in Benghazi. It turned out subsequently that he was representing the Revolutionary Council in Tripoli and had been dispatched at the personal insistence of Qaddafi. The aim was to ensure that the People's Bureau was not losing its revolutionary enthusiasm and to keep a check on the hundreds of Libyan students at universities, colleges and language schools, and also to guard against any infiltration by the NFSL. According to David Blundy and Andrew Lycelt's book *Qaddafi and the Libyan Revolution* published in 1987, Sodani had become head of the People's Committee in the Bureau in London, and in 1983 there had been debate as to whether he or the ambassador was in charge. Whatever the truth of the situation, he managed to set up about twelve revolutionary cells in different parts of the UK.

I of course had no inkling of such activity and he was the only person I met or spoke to in the Bureau. He seemed genuinely supportive of my intended visit and eventually organised a meeting on 13 June, 1980, in London with Dr Murad Lenghi, the Minister of Public Health, who was also a practising surgeon at the Medical School at Tripoli, and Dr Awad Abudejaja, Vice-Dean and Professor of Community and Family Medicine at the Medical School at Benghazi.

It was all rather cloak and dagger stuff with a touch of Le Carré. First I met Sodani at the Bureau and we proceeded to Selfridges Hotel where Lenghi and Abudejaja were staying. We were not permitted to meet at the Bureau in St James' Square or even at the consular section at Princes Gate; he took me into the foyer at Selfridges, introduced me quickly and departed immediately.

We didn't talk in the foyer but went straight up to one of their bedrooms – Abudejaja and I sat on the bed and Lenghi sat in a comfortable chair. The meeting went without a hitch – Lenghi gave permission for me to visit Libya and Abudejaja agreed to arrange my programme of study. Both seemed enthusiastic and keen to keep in touch with the medical scene in Britain. This surprised me as I had expected Italy or maybe France might have had a greater pull, but by this time English had become their second language and virtually all international meetings, medical reports, journals and articles were carried out, or spoken or written in English.

My last face to face meeting with Sodani had been in February 1981 when he had been particularly helpful in answering questions and reassuring me that I would receive my visa in good time. So three years later on 17 April 1984, following the shooting of WPC Yvonne Fletcher outside the Libyan Bureau, it was a great shock to see Sodani's face endlessly on television, and over the next few days to hear about his position and activities in the Bureau. For a time he was the prime suspect in the shooting, although in the end it turned out not to be the case. Rather he had organised the secret arrival of firearms, ammunition and explosives which were later found in the Bureau. At this point the UK government broke of diplomatic relations with Libya.

Monday 21 February 1983 was the date of departure and I woke to the news that a Libyan airliner had been hijacked overnight on a flight from Tripoli to Malta. I phoned Heathrow and was reassured there would be no difficulties with my flight. I checked in with Air France as Libyan Airlines had withdrawn their staff. There were no problems although there was massive security on boarding the plane, which was half empty. During the flight I got some idea of Qaddafi's strange behaviour since the implementation of the *Jamahiriya.* Immigration and customs declaration documents were written only in Arabic thus making it impossible for the majority of passengers to fill them in.

Curiously he hadn't ordered that the air stewardesses should only be Arabic – some in fact were British and those that were Libyan spoke English. How would they have coped if the plane had been full? Perhaps the documents would have been issued before takeoff.

At Tripoli all notices including arrival and departure information was in Arabic, and within a day or so it was obvious that this regulation applied to everything – road signs, street names and all public signs written in English had been removed; the same applied in cafés and hotels. It reminded me of Japan in 1972, but there it was not to make a political statement, simply that Japan had for centuries been an extremely isolated nation. In Japan there was one exception – Coca Cola was in English. In Libya there was one exception to the Arabic-only rule – political slogans and propaganda in public places had accompanying English translations as did Qaddafi's infamous *Green Book* which had been translated into English in toto. Like all totalitarian dictatorships pictures of the leader were everywhere.

After a delay at Tripoli for two hours I was met at Benghazi by Dr Ratan Singh and his twelve-year-old son – they had been waiting for over three hours and no information about the delay had been announced. I was surprised that he was of Indian nationality and even more surprised to find that in the Department of Community Medicine, excluding Professor Abudejaja, there was only one other Libyan, the rest being Indian, Pakistani and Egyptian. I was dropped off at the Kasr Al Jazeira, the only hotel available to foreigners. It was pleasantly situated on the seafront and from the small balcony of my room I could see a large civilian harbour, and to the left a small (naval) military dock. In retrospect rather foolishly, I took a number of photos of a destroyer and two submarines at anchorage – a later incident confirmed that if I had been seen I would have been in serious trouble.

The Secretariat (Ministry) of Health in Tripoli was my official host along with the Department of Community and Family Medicine at the University of Garyounis. Professor Abudejaja and his small staff enabled me to visit all the various primary care facilities, and as they all spoke reasonable English it was relatively easy to communicate with both patients and staff.

At my second meeting with Abudejaja he explained there were a number of things he needed to tell me. Unknown to me, permission to visit Libya and obtain a visa depended on a number of things. It was required that I be given the position of Visiting Professor of Family Medicine, and a number of things followed from this. The new Al-Keesh polyclinic was to become a training facility for family medicine and it was to be supervised by Abudejaja and his department; I was to visit the polyclinic and within two months produce an official report. Next I was to amend two articles in the *Garyounis Medical Journal* both as regards factual correctness and the use of English. In reality this meant re-writing them in the hope it would be published either in the *Lancet*, the *BMJ*, the *Journal of the American Medical Association* or the *New England Journal of Medicine.* Finally, my report on primary health care in Libya had to be in the hands of the Minister of Health (Dr Lenghi) within three months – this of course would be quite separate from the chapter in the book I was intending to write.

None of this had been mentioned in London, nor the generous payments I was to be given – the cost of the return flight from London to Tripoli and the cost of the hotel in Benghazi. Immediately an obvious caveat stood out – was this just a simple bribe to make sure I followed the party line of the Colonel? Inevitably I would find things to criticise and problems to be discussed openly – was I expected to keep my mouth shut?

Administratively the country had always been divided into municipalities (*balidiyas*), but following the military coup everything changed when the country became a *Jamahiriya* (State of the Masses) in 1973. Each *balidiya* was represented by the basic unit of government, the Popular Committee. This was enacted by law and covered every aspect of daily living – agriculture, housing, education, industry, transport and health. In 1977 Popular Committees became responsible at the regional level to Basic Popular Congresses which in turn elected representatives to the next level of government, the General People's Congress from which members were chosen to become the General Popular Secretariat or Cabinet.

Health policy and planning was carried out by the health

committees in the Basic Popular Congresses in conjunction with the Health Secretariat. Their combined decisions were then passed up to the General People's Congress for approval, at which point laws were passed and budgets approved. Wait for it – the implementation of any plan was then decentralised back to the health committee of the local Popular Committee. PHEW!

In 1978 private practice was forbidden by law and the first article of the Public Health Law No. 16 stated that medical and health care was to be the lawful right of all citizens and to be guaranteed by the state. Health care was to be free for the entire population both in hospital and in primary care, and was to include foreigners as well.

Community participation and involvement was intended to be one of the cornerstones of primary care. Such a concept is obviously easy to talk about but much more difficult to implement. By the time of my visit it had been realised that the position of hospitals vis-a-vis primary care was largely unchanged. The reasons were largely straightforward – the ordinary citizens on the Popular Committees were unaware of the importance of primary care and had been easily seduced by the glamour of high-tech medicine, but without understanding the costs involved. Undoubtedly the blame could not be directed just at hospital doctors: rather the Secretariat of Health had failed to accept that ordinary people needed educating and the pros and cons of debate required sophisticated understanding. Sadly the Libyan endeavour was no worse, but certainly no better than no involvement at all.

Medical services were organised at three levels: locally, with basic health care units (originally referred to as dispensaries) and MCH centres; at the intermediate level, polyclinics (combined units) in urban areas and rural hospitals in the countryside (a more accurate definition of urban and rural would be coastal and desert); finally, at what was called the central level, were regional and specialist hospitals.

The polyclinic had been a new concept and the first had been built in 1969, mainly on the advice of Czechoslovakia. Progress had been slow so that by 1983 only 28 were operational – again the reasons were self-evident with the hospitals continuing to dominate the medical scene and continuing to receive about 80% of the budget. My visit to Al-Keesh polyclinic convinced me that the idea of trying to combine primary and secondary care was sound and the decision to introduce a training centre for family doctors was a big step forward – and absolutely essential. During my stay I was to learn that a polyclinic similar to Al-Keesh had been set up by the Faculty of Medicine at the University of El-Fatah in Tripoli and the two polyclinics were starting to cooperate closely.

My request to visit the rural area, basically the coastal strip, was finally organised and Dr Appa, a kindly Indian doctor in Abudejaja's department, accompanied me as we set off on a beautiful warm sunny day. We drove south west from Benghazi along a straight flat road through scrubland, stony desert and occasional oases with flocks of sheep and goats wandering over the road. Our destination was a rural hospital in the small town of Ghemenis, some thirty miles away. Clearly Appa had no idea how to get there and after a time he stopped to wave down a lorry to ask the way. It was getting hot by now and the old car over-heated and wouldn't start. Appa removed the radiator cap amidst a fountain of steam and near-boiling water and scalded his hands – how he didn't more seriously burn himself I don't know. We had stopped close to a well – these were periodically to be found at the side of the road – so fortunately we were able to refill the radiator. We set off with Appa gingerly holding the wheel with his sore hands; we had to stop on three further occasions before reaching the hospital.

Ghemenis is a small coastal town with a population of about 8,000. The hospital was responsible for a total population of 35,000 and was opened in 1981with a surgeon, anaesthetist, gynaecologist, internal medical specialist and a paediatrician, plus trained nurses. By the time of my visit all the original medical staff and most of the Filipino nurses had left, and the current staff of two GPs, three dentists and an ophthalmologist could provide only a limited basic service. The MCH department had a gynaecologist and a paediatrician – both male, and one trained midwife and other trained nurses (possibly from Bulgaria if I remember correctly) who couldn't speak Arabic. The hospital obviously demonstrated many of the problems of the health service.

Mohammad Badri, a Libyan and director of the hospital invited us in for lunch after I had had a good look round and an instructive chat with the two GPs. After an embarrassingly lavish lunch Appa announced he didn't want to stay so Badri offered to drive me back to Benghazi when we were done. Although Badri was totally unaware of my programme for the rest of the day we managed to have a good discussion about polyclinics even though by then there wasn't time to visit one. A Red Crescent dispensary and home visits remained – I was particularly interested in the latter.

Badri however had an additional agenda and was intending to visit as many government supermarkets, unofficial private markets and even *souks* if they could be found – he was in search of a jacket and trousers for one of his sons and anything else he could find for the rest of his family. He also had friends to visit en-route back to Benghazi. However, almost before we were seated in his car he explained he wanted to take me to see the new Omar Muktar grave and memorial. He assumed I knew who he was talking about but eventually I had to ask him to explain. Apparently at the time of Mussolini's original occupation of the country in the late 1920s, an elderly school teacher became a guerrilla leader of perhaps 5,000 men, who constantly attacked the Italian forces and their supply lines. In 1931 he was captured and executed and became one of Libya's heroes and a martyr. And so we made our way inland to the small town of Soluk, about ten miles from Ghemenis – yes, it was an impressive memorial.

We progressed to Magroom, a small town under the responsibility of the hospital, to visit a Red Crescent dispensary. Although private practice had been abolished in 1979, these dispensaries had been permitted to continue as a sort of outlet for patients who were prepared to pay a small fee in the hope they would get more time and a more personal service with the doctors, as well as some drugs and investigations. Between 4pm and 7pm a simple free consultation service was provided – the doctors were not paid by the patient but received a salary from the Red Crescent. At that time only twenty-six dispensaries were operational and patients were impatiently demanding that their number should be increased.

*

The local supermarket had proved to be unsuccessful but Badri asked if I would like to see something else. Reluctantly agreeing, we walked across the town square to a large shed – dirty, rusting and in need of paint, and inside offering only half-full shelves. As I dutifully wandered around this dismal warehouse I was taken aback by the small shoe section – it had been completely taken over by Clark's Shoes, High Street, Street, Somerset, UK!

Gerdina was our next port of call, another government supermarket where again Badri had no luck with the jacket and trousers, but on the way he had stopped and managed to bargain for an assortment of bits and pieces at various roadside stalls. His friend was the head teacher of the primary school and we dropped in for a cup of tea. He was a friendly talkative chap who spoke English and we quickly got on to politics and *The Green Book* by the Great Leader.

"Have you read it?"
"No"
"Why not?"
"Because I don't have a copy and I haven't seen it in any shop."

Obviously disappointed in me he said he would try and get me a copy and true to his word, two days later, the three slim volumes had been left at the reception desk of the hotel.

By this time the sun was beginning to set and still I hadn't made a home visit. Badri was bemused by my insistence and quite unable to understand why it was important to me. However, the head teacher immediately suggested a family with many children, two of whom were ill and had been away from school. He explained they were Bedouins and proudly told me they had recently been re-housed in a new three-storey block of flats – one of the great achievements of the government to help the poorest members of society.

He led us to a collection of concrete buildings, the grey already dirty and stained and most depressing to look at. I was assured this was much better than a tent and there was electricity and piped water to a tap outside each block of flats. My first impression was the sheep and goats had surrounded the flats with excrement, including all the steps leading up to the third floor. The head knew where to go and we found the door of the flat ajar, with sheep and goats on the stairs and along the corridors. We knocked, and introductions and explanations to the mother were made whilst her six children stared at us. The two sick ones were quickly separated and presented to me.

I had a stethoscope with me (just in case it might be required sometime) which gave me a certain authenticity, and the mother was very happy and eager to talk to me and finally asked if I would examine the two children who were clinging to her like limpets. Both had upper respiratory tract infections but were not ill. I advised steam, should they develop a croupy cough, and the mother seemed reassured – at least, she was smiling as we left.

As we were leaving the husband arrived and I decided to ask the question I had been wanting to ask – what did he and his wife think of their new home? It was like an explosion as they both let rip and were quite uninhibited and fearless about what they were saying. After about ten minutes a rough translation was that the flat was no compensation for their tent and the way they had been used to living surrounded by their animals. They intensely disliked urban life and the inability to move around as they wished; they had no freedom. Grudgingly they accepted that the water tap attached to the flat was an improvement but they were less enthusiastic about the electricity. Badri and his friend were genuinely surprised to hear these criticisms – one of Qaddafi's proudest projects being so dismissed and undervalued.

We didn't reach Benghazi until 9pm and drove straight to Badri's home for coffee and cakes. His wife kept out of sight but the children came in and out while he gave them the small gifts – sadly no jacket and trousers for one of the boys, but he didn't grumble. It was quite late when a neighbour, an ophthalmologist, dropped in. There was no hesitation in talking about politics, and conversation swiftly turned to Qaddafi and his regime. Neither Badri nor his friend were happy with his domestic policies and not being able to criticise the government at the local Popular Committee. Both however were satisfied with his foreign policy and the manner in which he opposed the United States and other western countries including the UK. Furthermore both were pleased that Libya was involved with the non-aligned group of nations. The domestic situation could be tolerated provided he maintained his present policy towards the West.

Another invitation is worth mentioning – different from Badri's but equally enjoyable. Unlike Badri's home where only Arabic was spoken, this was a home where no Arabic was spoken. Dr Ratan Singh, who with his son had picked me up at the airport, invited me round and quietly introduced me to his Indian wife and their four children.

> "Please come into the sitting room, leave your coat where you like and my children will talk with you. I must go now."

No explanation. The smallest boy was in fighting mood, much to the annoyance and irritation of his brother and sisters. Mercifully everything soon calmed down after two electricity cuts and the candles had been found. After some whispering both girls said they would recite three English poems they had learned at school, while the younger boy redeemed himself by speaking three English nursery rhymes. They all attended the local International school. Finally Ratan's disappearance was explained when he returned with friends of his – an Indian ENT surgeon and his wife who was a paediatrician, and their two boys, and soon afterwards a knock on the door produced a close neighbour, a Pakistani statistician with his wife and baby. The meal was spicy and Indian but the ambience of the evening had a strong British feel. Neither the Indians nor the Pakistanis could hide the fact they had all attended private schools influenced and run à la British public schools. Their colonial past was obvious. The Libyan health service and Qaddafi were discussed freely and when I questioned them they assured me they had no problems whatever living amongst Arabs.

It was fascinating that in spite of living under a strict military dictatorship a foreigner could be invited without fear into both an Arab and an expatriate home, and everyone was able to talk about politics and even criticise the dictator.

The three volumes of *The Green Book* that had been left for me at the hotel were subtitled a) *The Solution of the Problem of Democracy, the Authority of the People* b) *The Solution of the Economic Problem, Socialism,* and c) *The Social Basis of the Third Universal Theory.*

The first volume heralded the beginning of the era of the *Jamahiriya*, the State of the Masses, and to Libyans he portrayed himself as a thinker, almost a philosopher, who understood the oppressed, the deprived and the grief-stricken. One of his aims was to do away with the economic theories of the past and bring down the exploiters of such economics. In the final volume he announced that he would be able to provide a genuine solution to man's struggle in life as well as the unresolved problems between men and women. Quite a handful of promises.

To an outsider these three volumes are little more than the thoughts of an idealistic young man, perhaps in his last years at school or first year of university, impractical but full of compassionate, even noble thoughts, however mostly just childish rubbish and meaningless rhetoric. Interestingly there is no mention of Islam.

With Qaddafi and similarly-minded young men in charge, the General Popular Secretariat or Revolutionary Council, made an appeal in 1978 to the medical profession that was utterly naive and absurdly Utopian. The leadership of the *Jamahiriya* was keen that medics should discontinue their traditional attitudes of being entrepreneurs, of being a social and professional elite, and undertake a revolutionary change of heart and behaviour by listening to the needs and hopes of the society in which they were living. Implied in this ideal was the certainty that in many countries physicians were more interested in their own professional and personal ambitions than in the aspirations of society. To quote from *The Lancet* in 1982:

> 'The Revolutionary Council's hopes were that the medical profession remains accountable to the needs of the Libyan people and does not become a wealthy, professional elite replacing one type of privilege with another.'

How far the profession would respond to that call would be watched with genuine hope by a few, but with cynical scepticism by the majority, both within and without the *Jamahiriya* – to them such a call merely reinforced the childlike naivety of the Great Leader.

The university of Garyounis had a very pleasant campus with laid-out gardens, and as I was leaving one day I stopped to take a photograph of a large circular tiled sculpture with water flowing gently over its surface. Apparently the water symbolised knowledge and the sculpture itself represented knowledge as yet undiscovered. It was elegant and made me stop and ponder. It was close to the main entrance and almost immediately a young student approached, followed by others, to ask if I realised it was illegal to take photographs. I answered 'No' and he replied, with the obvious approval of his fellow students, it would be permitted this time but I must not repeat the offence. Perfectly polite but deadly serious.

One evening, in a rather grim café attached to the hotel, I was drinking coffee with a quiet, earnest young chap in his early thirties who was working for the Libyan State Bank, and like another student several days later, was totally committed to the Revolution. He insisted I read *The Green Book* and was convinced that within five to ten years Libya would be transformed into a perfect society for the masses, although during our discussion he had to agree with my feeling that by and large the elderly didn't understand or agree with the Revolution. The response from both students had been similar: it didn't really matter as soon they will have died. So much for the perfect society. Subsequent meetings and discussions with other young students confirmed that they believed Qaddafi and his government was the only way forward for the young, even if their parents and grandparents thought differently.

Women were rarely seen in the streets unless they were shopping; this was a young country dominated by men. The majority of the women I saw or spoke to were in MCH centres or on a few home visits. Otherwise it was old women I saw, sitting chatting, carrying mountains of shopping, truly beasts of burden. The old men just sat and smoked.

Within a day I had noticed the streets were strangely empty with all the shops boarded up – I was informed this was part of Qaddafi and the Council of the Revolution's recent decision to try and eliminate private business. Not only the shops had been shut up but the traditional *souks* and markets had suffered the same fate; everything had been replaced by the new government-run supermarkets that were stocked with very little other than the basic requirements for life.

To an outsider such as myself this action seemed crazy, completely contrary to Arab culture and custom where bartering and arguing over the cost of everything in a *souk* or roadside stall was part of everyday life. As I wandered around I couldn't be sure, but it seemed that the *adham*, or call to prayer, when the faithful are summoned by the *muezzin* five times a day, was less noticeable. In my limited experience of the Arab world, the *adham* was the most frequent sound to be heard, other than the traffic.

Strangely there were few cars and almost no cyclists, but trucks and lorries thundered along full of workers being taken to and from construction sites for road building, bridges, overpasses and government buildings. Most of the workers were Korean, Pakistani and some Africans. What a mix of cultures and what an awful life for the young men in their camps at the end of the day – lonely, alienated and trapped, as their passports had been taken from them. I suppose they had employment and a little money to send home, but it must have seemed like a prison. It was the same story in the health service in that most of the workers were foreigners – the physicians were mainly Indian, Egyptian, Pakistani and East European, while the majority of nurses were from the Philippines. These nurses and any other expatriate nurses had to surrender their passports, but in the case of doctors this only applied to the East Europeans.

On Fridays I was a free agent and on one occasion I was wandering aimlessly along looking for somewhere to eat when I was confronted by a crowd of excited young men waving flags, shouting and singing and moving towards a large circular concrete stadium. I joined the throng, who were evidently going to a football match. Queuing for tickets was surprisingly orderly, the cost only a few dinars – I didn't notice the police to any great extent and the military not at all.

The stadium was a circular bowl with concrete benches and no protection from the by-now baking sun. Toilets were either non-existent or hidden. Who was playing I wasn't sure but I think it was Benghazi against possibly Tobruk. The standard of play was pretty poor and performed at half pace, but by this time it was pretty hot and there was no swigging of bottles of water by the players. The crowd screamed and shouted but there was no violence between the rival supporters as we filed out. In fact there was a good deal of bonhomie on both sides as we queued for ice-cream and fruit drinks. It was quite an experience and there is no doubt in my mind that being alcohol-free made all the difference to behaviour.

As I wandered back from the match I was beginning to find this rather unattractive city becoming more interesting. Old parts were still standing and the colonnaded streets usually led down to a *souk*, now bizarrely empty on account of Qaddafi's new plan. However, people were defying the government and briefly behaving like traditional Arabs selling toothpaste, matches, combs, picture frames, sandals, children's clothes, pots and pans, in fact anything they could lay their hands on. To my further surprise the whole *souk* area was full of women, only rarely veiled, wearing long, brightly-coloured cloaks and long dresses. Boys played football and the girls chatted and giggled.

It was sometimes difficult to decide whether damaged buildings were falling down as a result of the Second World War or from general neglect, or a combination of the two. My freedom to wander around on a Friday gave me the opportunity to see how the large open dusty squares and crescents displayed the influence and beauty of Italian architecture, which I had previously failed to notice. The sight and sound of hens and sheep and goats brought about a feeling of normality. There was only one thing I found really scary and that was the packs of wild dogs roaming the streets. They certainly made me anxious.

Someone, I forget who, told me an intriguing story about an Italian Renaissance church built in the early twentieth century which had recently been converted into a mosque. I knew vaguely where it was and whilst searching without a map I came across a British War Graves cemetery for the dead of the Second World War. It covered quite a large area with around 2,000 graves neatly divided by sandy/gravel pathways. It was surprisingly well looked-after and I was just about to leave when I spotted an elderly man slowly coming towards me carrying a broom and fork. He stopped and spoke. He knew no English so we nodded and smiled at each other for about ten minutes. We then shook hands between the railings and I tried to convey my gratitude for the way he was looking after the graves. More smiles and then we went our separate ways.

Oh for a map – but eventually I found the church. It proved to be difficult to photograph so I walked down a road away from it in the hope I would at least be able to get a picture of the spire. As I was walking I failed to notice high walls on both sides. Loads of bricks and mounds of sand were heaped up against the walls and I clambered up to get a good view. I was pleased with the photo and just as I finished I felt I was being watched. Turning round I saw an armed soldier walking towards me. After much gesticulating and mimicking I was handcuffed and marched off towards the nearest entrance. As soon as I was through an inner gateway I realised I was in a large military barracks. I was made to stand against a wall and my passport and camera were taken. By this time half a dozen young soldiers had turned up and couldn't decide what to do. After about half an hour a sergeant arrived who managed to explain that an officer was coming. Thankfully the sergeant spoke a little English and told me it was absolutely forbidden to photograph anywhere near a military establishment. I tried to explain I was taking photographs of the church/mosque but he told me to shut up and wait for the senior officer. He asked if I would like a cup of tea to which I said 'Yes', so we went inside and I sat down to await my fate.

The senior officer returned my passport and camera and then asked me to give him the film, all requests and conversation being carried out very politely. I was sent on my way, but not before insisting on shaking hands with the senior officer and even getting smiles from the other soldiers. Unwittingly I had been foolish and it could have been awkward for Abudejaja.

A further surprise awaited me when I got back to the hotel. The reception staff had been anxiously looking for me because I must vacate my room immediately; every other room on the same floor had been emptied so I must act at once. When I asked why, I was told an important guest was expected.

I had just finished emptying the room when a car horn could be heard blaring, and from the balcony of my new room I could see a small cavalcade of black limousines with a police escort. It stopped directly beneath my balcony thus giving me a perfect view of the important guest who was eventually helped out of the biggest car. He was a small slim extremely black African, his age difficult to judge, but probably mid-thirties, elegantly dressed in a dark, pin-striped, double-breasted Saville Row-style suit, the whitest of white shirts, a sombre tie and large gold cufflinks ostentatiously visible. His black shoes were polished so they almost twinkled in the fading sun. Who was this man displaying such flamboyant wealth? Where did he come from? It transpired he was the Prime Minister of Upper Volta which, according to the World Bank and the WHO, was one of the ten poorest countries in the world: depressingly true that wealth, poverty and corruption are inseparable.

By the final day in Benghazi I had managed to complete the report on the Al-Keesh polyclinic and was rather pleased with my efforts. It only needed to be typed when I got home. I had a slight worry over the post, which was slow and unreliable, but I hoped I might be able to persuade the Bureau in London to send it back to Benghazi via the diplomatic bag.

The flight to Tripoli went without a hitch and by chance an Indian doctor and his wife were on the plane – he was returning after holding the post of Professor of Surgery for the past five years; we were able to talk about the health service ad nauseam. As we took off he pointed out about thirty to forty Soviet MIG aircraft on a neighbouring airstrip – the Soviet Union was here in strength.

The outskirts of Tripoli were as poor and dreary as Benghazi but it was a much more bustling and exciting place. In the centre much of the old town was still standing and there were a number of old mosques and minarets, small beautifully-proportioned arcaded streets and enchanting brightly-coloured courtyards filled with flowering shrubs. Several *souks* were intact although closed, as were the boarded up stalls and shops. The impressive fortress castle was in an excellent state of repair and had been converted into a natural history museum with a collection of mammals and birds. From the walls surrounding the castle a splendid view of the attractive seafront, esplanade and harbour was laid out. I think the difference between Tripoli and Benghazi was almost entirely due to the fact that most of the fighting between the Allied and Axis forces had taken place in the eastern part of the country and by the time the Germans surrendered barely a shot had been fired in Tripoli.

It is now thirty years since I was in Libya. At the time it seemed that Qaddafi's domestic policies would be accepted, particularly by the young, even if they didn't agree with all his ideas. Provided he pursued his foreign policy of strong opposition to the West, society would probably remain fairly stable. I don't think anyone could have predicted the capture and gruesome killing of the Great Leader in the culvert in his home town of Sirte in 2011 – and by his own people.

24

ARAB REPUBLIC of EGYPT

Egypt was a daunting prospect – its size, its history and culture and its rapidly increasing population. At the end of the Second World War, the continuing presence of British troops following the previous seventy-four years of occupation, became increasingly unpopular as did the degenerate lifestyle and corrupt rule of the British-backed King Farouk. Colonel Gamul Abdul Nasser and the coterie of Free Officers all had angry memories of the military incompetence of Egypt, Syria, Iraq and Transjordan following the partition of Palestine in 1947 and the creation of the State of Israel in 1948. In 1952 he finally led the popular revolution to get rid of Farouk and his family, which led to the creation of a republic.

In 1954 Nasser became president and immediately became involved in the Arab Ba-ath Party which had been created in Syria with the aim of uniting Arab countries under the umbrella of nationalism. Egypt quickly became a powerful voice. By 1956 the last British soldiers had peacefully left Egypt and yet within four months the British, alongside the French and Israelis, had invaded Egypt.

Nasser, in an attempt to overcome some of his country's economic difficulties, had decided to build the High Aswan Dam in order to increase agricultural production, particularly in the delta region between Alexandria and Cairo. The Americans and the British had agreed (without much enthusiasm) to help finance the project, mainly in an endeavour to keep out the influence of the Soviet Union. However, Nasser's almost constant anti-western propaganda finally made Eisenhower pull out. Nasser's response to Eisenhower, and Eden in the UK, was to nationalise the Anglo-French Suez Canal Company, declaring he would take the revenue it provided to help his country's ailing economy and to finance his dam. (Ultimately the Soviet Union assisted with the project.)

The response of Britain and France, along with the duplicitous involvement of Israel, is now a shameful part of history, which left

Nasser the hero of the Arab world along with the final certainty that Britain and France could never again be trusted.

Unfortunately the presidencies of Nasser and Sadat did nothing to reduce the corruption and nepotism that had been part and parcel of everyday life in Egypt for as long as anyone could remember. On my arrival in 1984 I was informed that corruption was getting even worse and was endemic in every branch of society as well as in government, the military, the police, the law and business. Medicine was no exception. Over the last thirty years since then, Mubarak and his cronies have maintained the tradition of corruption whilst the United States and other western countries have considered Egypt to be one of the strongest allies in the region.

During the early 1970s the *Times* newspaper produced a series of special articles concerned with Third World countries explaining the progress they had made since de-colonisation, or independence. In May '72 it was the turn of Egypt and one full page (before becoming tabloid in size) highlighted *The Health Service in Egypt* and its plans for the next ten years. The plans were well set out and most impressive – Preventive Health Service, Health Education, Rural Health Service, Industrial service, Family Planning, Maternity and Child Health, Nursing and Cost/Insurance. What was immediately obvious was that it had been written as though everything was already fait accompli – a perfect example of believing one's own propaganda.

Two years later in 1974 Geoff Watts, a highly-respected independent science writer and correspondent, wrote in *World Medicine* an outline of the Egypt's health service entitled *Patience and the Sphinx*. Ten years later, on my visit in '84, one thing had not changed and rang true – it was not connected with the health service but was about the Egyptian's attitude to life. Watts had written:

> 'Scene: the Ministry of Information's press office in Cairo. An office. A desk with two telephones. A man sitting at the desk making two calls at the same time. Extreme pressure of work obviously. Also in the room a group of armchairs: people sitting smoking, drinking coffee, doing nothing in particular. Other visitors waiting their turn – or so I assume. Minutes pass, nothing happens. I chat idly to a man next to me explaining why I am here, what I want. Slowly it dawns on me he is not a visitor, they all

work here. A dreamy pool of stillness disturbed by a lone ripple of activity.'

'Every country has its bureaucracy and every bureaucracy has its singular characteristics. The desk-bound multitudes of the British Civil Service may or may not be doing something useful but they are certainly doing something. Paper, files, forms, letters or whatever; the keynote – in accordance with Parkinson's Law – is activity. Egyptian bureaucracy on the other hand defies Parkinson; its work does not expand to fill the time or occupy the energies of those available for its completion. And so much unutilised manpower hangs like a dead weight on the administration of every activity, on the organisation of every detail no matter how trivial. To confront a bureaucracy that lacks the time to help you is maddening: to confront one that flounders out of surfeit of time is not only maddening but incomprehensible to boot. During ten days in Egypt I learned many things about the health system and how it works. But I could never quite understand how it avoided asphyxiation in the soft and bottomless bureaucracy which presumably sustains it.'

Ten years later Watts' description remains unchanged – or more realistically, I suppose, unchangeable. I have been able to add my own glimpses into Egyptian ways, although perhaps it would be more accurate to say into the ways of the Arabs.

Early in September 1980 Dr Badran, Medical Attaché at the Egyptian Embassy in London, became my first contact with Egypt. He agreed to contact Dr Mobarak, First Under-Secretary at the Ministry of Health in Cairo, about my intended visit and thought it would be a good plan for me to write at once to Dr Mobarak explaining the purpose of my trip.

I took his advice but received no acknowledgement or reply. Over the next eighteen months I wrote two further letters, and two new medical attachés in London contacted him on my behalf. It was all to no avail and I had virtually given up when two and half years later, out of the blue, a letter dated 14 April 1983 arrived from Dr Mostefa Hammamy, Director General of Rural Health Services, to say that following discussions with Dr Mobarak it had been decided my visit could not be organised. Yes, I was disappointed, but at least I knew where I was.

*

Six weeks later another letter from Egypt arrived, again from Dr Hammamy, dated 28 May, this time to say how delighted he was to confirm I could visit Egypt and how he was looking forward to meeting me. No mention of his previous letter. He asked for my passport number and a photograph so that my security papers could be issued before my arrival, otherwise it would take ten days or more to get security approval after I arrived. It all seemed quite serious although I do remember wondering if another letter might arrive . . .

Clearly I was pleased, but totally confused by the delays as well as the fact that I had already had a meeting with Dr Hammamy in 1982 after my visit to Jordan. I had briefly stopped off in Cairo on my way to a number of meetings at the WHO Regional Office for the Eastern Mediterranean in Alexandria. At the stop-over I had arranged to meet Dr Hammamy with the express purpose of finding out the likelihood of getting agreement and permission to visit his country – he had seemed genuinely optimistic at the time. Not surprisingly Geoff Watts' *Patience and the Sphinx* sprang to mind!

Three and a half years after my original contact with the Embassy in London, on 20 January 1984 I was finally on a plane to Cairo. The plane was less than half full, which was fairly standard on flights to the Middle East at that time. Although only half an hour late it wasn't until 2am I found a taxi and set off for the Windsor Hotel with mercifully only minor haggling over the fare.

The Windsor proved to be a delightful small family-run business hidden away in a narrow street in the centre of the city. It had been recommended to me by two medical students recently returned from Egypt and had the added attraction that it was reasonably inexpensive. It had an old-fashioned air with dark heavy furniture and dark wood panelling in the bar, the sitting room and the restaurant. The doorman and the bartender wore traditional dress and fez hats.

What I hadn't bargained for was how cold it would be at night – washing in a dribble of cold water at 3.30am on that first night was rather grim.

The Ministry of Health was within easy walking distance and I arrived spot on time for my meeting with Dr Hammamy – he wasn't there and I was ushered into his room and rather unconvincingly told by his secretary he would be arriving shortly. Two cups of Turkish coffee and an hour later he still hadn't arrived and I was just beginning to wonder what to do next when he appeared. In excellent form, looking much as I remembered him, we chatted briefly with no mention of our past correspondence and then got down to my programme. Much to my relief he was well prepared for my visit and had appointed one of his staff to be my interpreter, guide and general adviser; Dr Mohammad Samir Saad El-Din proved to be a great help – Egyptian style of course.

The first few days were spent mainly at the Ministry of Health where I was given a lot of information about urban and rural primary care, plus the broad framework of the service and basic health matters such as mortality, morbidity rates, life expectancy, availability of clean water, the effectiveness of sewage disposal, malnutrition and illiteracy, as well as more specific data concerning health manpower, the training of doctors and nurses, the school health service, family planning, the complex financing, the muddle over health insurance and the extent of private practice. Most of the discussions took place in the Ministry, but I also made visits to the Nutritional Institute in which, inexplicably, the Department for the Strengthening of Rural Services and the Second Population Special Project resided – the Special Project had been set up in 1979 because family planning had failed.

Over my first four days in Cairo I got a very clear picture of the virtually continuous traffic jams, the endless honking of horns, the manic driving, the smell of cheap petrol and the ineffectiveness of both the traffic lights and the traffic police – on reflection it is amazing that Cairo with its huge population isn't in a permanent state of unrest. In 1983 the population was estimated to be 48 million and it was forecast to reach more than 70 million by the year 2000. In fact the 2006 census revealed 'an Egyptian is born every twenty-three seconds pushing the total to 76 million'. Despite being such a large country 95% of the population are living in only 4% of the land. The population pyramid merely outlines the complexity of the problem with 40% under 15 years, 56% between 16 and 64 years, and only 4% over 65 years.

*

Meetings at the Diarrhoea Disease Control Project, the Second Population Special Project, a Nurse Training School and the Strengthening of the Rural Services Project all provided perfect examples of the inefficient and completely disorganised Egyptian way of doing things that was accepted as normal and nothing unusual. The clash with the culture of the western industrialised world was glaringly obvious – never any embarrassment about the inability or indifference in keeping to what had been arranged or promised, no shame about incompetence and no awareness about keeping to time. Never once did I hear 'I'm really sorry about this cock-up'.

However, it is important to point out that my criticism is largely related to organisation, and good work had been carried out by public health doctors. The most crucial problems had been identified as infant, child and maternal morbidity and mortality, with respiratory infections and diarrhoea in children under five years being the commonest causes of death. In fact Egypt was one of the first countries to introduce oral rehydration therapy (ORT) as the main treatment for diarrhoea, and in order to focus on the problem the Diarrhoea Disease Control Project had been set up in two governorates, Alexandria and Sohag, and by 1984 plans had been made to expand the project to the entire country.

Heavy smoking was common both in adults and children, and specific diseases such as tuberculosis, hepatitis, typhoid, bilharzia and hookworm were prevalent, although an extraordinary omission concerned syphilis and gonorrhoea. HIV was still in its infancy and as yet on the horizon. The rapidly increasing number of road traffic accidents in young men had also been included.

Whatever health problems were being considered, there was unanimity about the need to improve health education, particularly amongst mothers, whilst female education in general was seen as an urgent requirement. All this tied in with the relentless increase in the population due to failed contraception.

The difference in organising a professional meeting or a private discussion stood out. It was as though we were in a café with people coming in to join us whenever they liked, and often half a dozen extras would tag along with Samir and myself – who they were and what they were doing remained a mystery and they rarely contributed anything. Open doors gave the impression we were sitting in a corridor with people wandering past us in both directions. Fellow professionals would talk in an ad hoc way to the person in charge of the meeting, but more often it was just people clutching bits of paper to be signed. Obviously this took up a significant amount of time and inevitably curtailed my meeting. As a foreigner it was fascinating to watch, but I hadn't come to study anthropology.

A definite meeting had been arranged at a Nurse Training School for 10am so it was necessary to be at the Ministry no later than 9am in order to find a driver. Samir and I sat for a while as our driver couldn't be found and quite by chance a colleague from the Rural Health Department could be heard talking, so Samir collared him, introduced me, and we had a good discussion about the unpopular but obligatory legislation which compelled newly qualified doctors to work in rural areas for a minimum of two years. By this time it was way past 10am so instead of trying to get to the Nurse Training School Samir decided to try and set up another meeting. The first door he found open turned out to be the Department of Finance and Health Insurance and although this was not a pre-arranged meeting it proved to be most useful. Samir eventually found a driver to take us to the original meeting and by this time we were two hours late. Again we waited until it was obvious the meeting wasn't going to take place, which was not surprising under the circumstances. The situation was really quite absurd as we weren't in the Nurse Training School but at a Technical Training School.

By this time I was beyond being angry and frustrated and just accepted Samir's suggestion we should return to the Ministry of Health to talk with the woman who was supposedly in charge of nurse training. Who was I to argue? After the usual problem of finding a driver we set off, but lo and behold in less than a mile we stopped at the Diarrhoea Disease Control Project where we wasted another half hour for an un-arranged meeting with the Director – he of course was not expecting me and was in another meeting. Samir insisted on barging in and dragging the unfortunate Director out; far from being irritated or annoyed he was quite charming and the ensuing discussion proved to be really useful. All these experiences taught me one thing – the Egyptians were very much more flexible than I was. Needless to say we never made it back to the Ministry and I imagine that the woman we were going to talk to was probably by then collecting her children from school or doing a bit of shopping, blissfully unaware of a meeting she had not been told about.

The following day the Strengthening of Rural Health Services Project was our destination and so as to get there on time I needed to be at the Ministry no later than 8.30am. I arrived promptly but, now realising that drivers never turn up before 9am, I persuaded Samir we could go by public transport. The bus was crowded beyond words but it was a simple journey. The meeting was attended by an American adviser from the American International Development Agency (AID), a Panamanian adviser on rural health services and two Egyptians from the new university/medical school in Ismailia. An interesting discussion about Ismailia ensued, but as far as I was concerned the purpose of the meeting had been forgotten. I spoke to Samir and told him I wanted to start talking about the Rural Health Service Project, after all why else had he arranged the meeting. To my astonishment he replied that there wasn't any time as we had to get back to the Ministry for a visit to an MCH centre. By this time six other Egyptian colleagues had joined us so two vehicles were now needed plus two drivers. Eventually we arrived at the MCH centre which, no surprise, was a mere ten minute walk from the Rural Health Service Project. I couldn't believe what I was experiencing and words failed me.

It took me several days to understand how Samir functioned; when he said he had made an appointment or arranged a meeting, what he meant was that they were vaguely in the plans for the day – *insha' Allah* (God willing). He also believed that meetings should be organised in a totally flexible way and again *insha' Allah.* In my limited experience this disorganised way of doing things was more common in Egypt than in any other Arab country. On the day we were to visit the Nurse Training School, Samir and I had planned to meet in a small public garden near my hotel to save me walking to the Ministry, the School being close to the hotel. I clearly remember we walked back to the Ministry and set off in the opposite direction. Quite baffling.

There were exceptions to this muddle, one being a meeting with the Director of a hospital on the outskirts of Cairo. First, the meeting took place in the Director's office and both doors were kept closed. Second, the meeting started with him explaining he was sick to death of the bureaucracy, inefficiency and incompetence to be found throughout the health service. He asked what my experience had been and I replied that I thought his description exactly fitted what I had found. It was so refreshing to talk directly to him and without any interruptions, just like a meeting in the UK. He asked if I would like a brief look round – I felt I should say Yes but I think he was hoping I would say No.

The hospital was in need of paint and was dirty with an unpleasant smell of drains. The majority of doctors and nurses were just sitting around smoking and chatting. The corridors were full of old iron beds, bits of furniture, cardboard boxes and old packing cases. Even the new out-patient department wasn't much better. With great expectation I entered the Dental Research Unit – three empty rooms, no patients or staff. The Director was very embarrassed and ashamed:

"I have no excuses."

I was sorry to say goodbye as we functioned on the same wavelength and he had been so honest.

The next port of call with Samir was a school polyclinic and we were joined by the Director of the School Health Service. We couldn't find the polyclinic and eventually picked up a young lad at a bus stop who showed us the way. I couldn't believe that neither the Director nor Samir knew the way or hadn't even bothered to find out before we set off. The polyclinic was a scene of complete inactivity.

Health care in the urban setting was a mix of government and private in an estimated ratio of 1:7. In fact accurate information about private practice was non-existent, but the main provision in both primary and secondary care was obviously private in spite of 75% of physicians being employed in the state sector. Fees were negotiated between doctor and patient. Rightly or wrongly I decided to concentrate on what the government were providing. During the 1950s and '60s hospitals were virtually the only facility being built and it wasn't until the early '70s, just over ten years before my visit, that any thought had been given to primary care. A decision was then taken to set up health centres in which MCH and adult curative care was to be provided in one facility – in addition a health bureau was integrated into the centre, which was to be responsible for the registration of births and deaths, the inoculation of the adult population, the supervision of food hygiene and the notification and follow-up of parasitic and infectious diseases. No clinical work was undertaken by the bureau. From my limited observation the supervision of food hygiene was poorly carried out, largely due to inadequate numbers of well-trained staff resulting from the squabbling between local and central government about whose responsibility it was to provide the funding. It was impossible to discover whether the statistics regarding the registration of births and deaths was accurate or not.

MCH units had a surprising number of female doctors, supported by assistant midwives and nurses. The majority had one or two beds available for confinements, but around 80% of births still took place at home under the care of the traditional birth attendants. The adult unit provided simple curative medicine and was staffed by GPs and male nurses and it goes without saying the stipulated staffing levels were rarely met.

In 1980 the concept of the polyclinic was accepted with the result that the out-patient departments of new hospitals were transferred to the health centre at the centre of each community. It was hoped this would be more convenient for patients and, as importantly, would improve the cooperation and ease of referral between primary and secondary care.

All 'out-of-hours' work remained rooted in the nearest A & E department, leading to the usual problems of overcrowding, and irritability and frustration on the part of medical and nursing staff on account of the numbers of patients who should have been dealt with in a primary care setting.

The planners' intentions couldn't be challenged, but in the facilities I visited in and around Cairo the quality of work being carried out was on the whole embarrassingly poor. I wondered what the situation would be like in rural areas.

When the British started their domination of Egypt towards the end of the nineteenth century, no doctors or nurses worked in rural areas. One health inspector, untrained in clinical medicine, was deputed to the capital town of each governorate and became responsible for the health of between 100,000 and 250,000 people. Two additional groups were recruited at the same time to help the inspector. The 'health barbers' became responsible for vaccination against smallpox and for supplying simple first aid. They were further trained to distinguish between natural and criminal death and to notify the police if necessary. The second group consisted of the traditional birth attendants or *dyas* who in theory had been trained to attend normal births and to recognise the abnormal.

In the early part of the twentieth century the British introduced a variety of public health measures – the maintenance of primitive toilets and washing arrangements in mosques, the installation of electric pumps for underground water, and as many wells as possible. They also undertook the filling or drying out of swamps to reduce the presence of bilharzia.

In 1930 the construction of the first rural hospital commenced and in 1936 the Ministry of Health was established. In the middle of the Second World War while the Axis and Allied armies were fighting each other, quite amazingly the Rural Health Reform Decree was announced. Its principal objective was to build 860 rural health centres with up to ten beds, each covering populations of up to 15,000. Progress was very slow, partly because of the war and its aftermath, partly through lack of money, and partly from lack of enthusiasm from most of the Egyptian medical profession. However, in 1954 rural health centres were combined with local primary schools and local agricultural development centres to create what came to be known as Combined Units. Regretfully this broad-based approach to primary care didn't take root as it was never properly funded or supported by the medical profession.

Doctors involved in public health recognised, however, that the use of these centres was directly related to their accessibility for patients and in 1962 smaller centres that covered a number of villages not more than a mile apart were created to provide for no more than 5,000 people. Progress again was slow, but in 1970, following the Nasser Project, 400 rural centres were built; a very important element of Nasser's philosophy was the involvement of the community whereby they had to find the necessary land and were responsible for 50% of the money for construction. Between 1962 and 1976 the number of centres increased from 200 to 1,661 and further improvements came about in 1975 when the more remote centres were upgraded into rural hospitals by increasing the number of beds to forty and providing simple laboratory services and a simple x-ray machine. Admittedly it was slow, but by the time of my arrival in '84 eight rural health centres had been upgraded – only one per year, but in a country where money was directed mainly towards the military or the police, or was siphoned off through widespread corruption, it was some progress.

The trip to the Nile Delta to assess the state of rural health care was a real success. We all met at the Ministry at 7am – Samir, Dr Negaty who was in charge of the Strengthening of Rural Health Services Project, a fully-trained male nurse with experience of the rural scene, a Panamanian adviser to the Rural Health Project and Dr Allwardt, a West German adviser to the Programme on Family Planning.

I remembered the train journey I had taken two years previously from Cairo to Alexandria and back, the train packed inside and passengers sitting and standing between carriages and surviving precariously on the carriage roofs. By car I was able to see more and I was surprised how lush and fertile the countryside looked, and more wooded than I recalled, not only from date palms.

The two-hour drive north through al Zagaziq, capital of Sharqiyyah governorate, to al Sinbillawayn in Daqahliyah roughly followed the railway but we passed through many small villages, all much the same with small mud-brick single-storey dwellings with children everywhere, hens and ducks and geese behaving as they do, goats and sheep shepherded by young boys or old men, women carrying water or cleaning clothes, camels and buffalo lying down or just wandering, and the men mainly sitting and smoking. The roads weren't too bad, although in most of the villages they were just rutted tracks. Everywhere were irrigation channels which, fed by the Aswan Dam, enabled the land to be cultivated for most of the year. This allowed a form of subsistence agriculture to flourish, but these channels and irrigation waterways also encouraged fresh water snails to thrive which acted as the intermediary host for the flatworm Schistosoma, the cause of the disease biliharzia (now known as schistosomiasis). The sluggish filthy grey water where children were swimming or playing at the edge and women were vigorously washing clothes, provided perfect conditions for contracting schistosomiasis. There were even young men swimming under the water along the bank, getting as close as possible to clumps of reeds that apparently were the best place to catch fish by hand. I was surprised in fact to see feeding fish rising to the surface and wondered how they could possibly flourish in such foul water.

In most of the fields the traditional wheel for grinding corn could be seen, driven by an ox going round and round in circles. At the village wells, buckets lowered with chains were operated by donkeys that then brought the water to the surface – immensely picturesque for a tourist but very hard work for the villagers. What happened to the electric pumps provided by the British in the early years of the twentieth century?

At al Sinbillawayn, Dr Ahmed Gomoa, Director of Rural Services in al Mansurah governorate, was waiting for us. A well-prepared talk on the problems being experienced at the time led to worthwhile discussions and a question and answer session. As the meeting was drawing to a close the mood changed. Samir and Negaty seemed determined to find out what Dr Allwardt thought about the Nazis, the concentration camps and the Jews. Both were dismayed by his reply – he explained that in spite of the folly of the Versailles Treaty and the economic straitjacket the Allies had imposed on Germany, he saw no excuse for the behaviour of Hitler and the philosophy of the Nazi party. Both the Panamanian and I strongly supported him but Samir and Negaty vehemently disagreed – to them Hitler was a brilliant leader in spite of Stalingrad, el Alamein, the D-Day landings and losing the war! I had had previous chats with Samir and felt his opinions were closely related to his views on Zionism and Zionists rather than the Jews, plus of course the manner in which the State of Israel had been created by the United Nations.

The next day Samir couldn't resist returning to the subject and explaining his beliefs. The Palestinians had been part of this region for thousands of years, just like the Jews, and both had the same rights. He then started on modern history – the Sykes-Picot Agreement, the Balfour Declaration, and the perfidious behaviour of Great Britain and France. Gerald Butt, the correspondent reporting on the Middle East for the BBC wrote in 1987:

> 'I don't think it is fully appreciated in Britain how much the Palestinians blame the British (and French) for creating the Palestinian problem.'

As we came to the end of our discussion Samir looked me straight in the eye and spoke with absolute conviction:

> "We are a patient people, this is our home and we will outstay all of you."

Interestingly two subsequent publications in English have somewhat supported Samir and at least made his views more understandable and acceptable. *Cairo in the War 1939-1945* by Artemis Cooper published in 1989, and *Monty and Rommel: parallel lives* by Peter Caddick-Adam published in 2012, have both graphically pointed out how unpopular the British were compared with the Germans (and Italians) and have described the almost decadent way in which a number of politicians, the majority of journalists, many high-ranking military men and most of the officer class flourished in the luxurious living in Cairo. Nobody gave a second thought to the poverty that surrounded them.

After this political interlude let's return to the Egyptian Delta. The plan was for Samir, Ahmed Gomoa and I to visit a district hospital in Sinbillawayn, followed by rural health units in two small villages, al Zahaila and al Zoreqi and finally a rural health centre in Gharita, a larger village of 10-12,000 inhabitants. We passed by the district hospital which I was told we were too late to visit, so proceeded to the two villages, then finally to Gharita, only to find no doctors had bothered to turn up. My companions took this in their stride without any hint of embarrassment.

The last destination was in al Mansurah to see a newly-built polyclinic. We were met by the Director, who showed us round – it was well-designed but all the departments had been closed since midday and only a couple of cleaners remained. We quickly gravitated to the Director's office where he spoke candidly about poor productivity and performance, poor training, poor pay and a laissez-faire attitude about almost everything. He was not allowed to dismiss anyone however much they deserved it, and he became extremely angry and complained bitterly to Ahmad Gomoa who after all was the Director of Rural Health for the governorate. It was utterly depressing and I couldn't believe I had been able to see so little of the polyclinic. Any health service of course only reflects the society in which it operates and this was particularly true of Egypt.

Even in my superficial appraisal there were obvious differences in the rural and urban way of life – it was easier to get food for the family in the countryside whilst it was easier to find schools and some form of medical care in the towns. Nevertheless poverty united peasant farmers (*fellahin*) and their families with the poorly paid workers and their families in the grim urban sprawl on the edges of Cairo and Alexandria. A definite hopelessness and weary acceptance was evident. Little was likely to change and the one certainty was that both the urban and the rural poor would always remain at the bottom of the pile. And nothing has changed over the last thirty years.

On our return to Cairo, Samir and I were joined again by the Panamanian, who kindly invited us back to his house for the evening. First we had to collect his car, a brand-new Volvo estate covered in a dust-sheet. He was obviously not without money – or perhaps advisers are well-paid. Anyway, off we went to pick up an American friend living in the fashionable Hilton Hotel – he was an adviser to Westinghouse, a company involved in the building of health facilities in Cairo; living permanently at the Hilton was considered to be quite natural. The Panamanian's home was in an upmarket suburb in a delightfully quiet, tree-lined avenue – the scents in spring and summer must be unimaginable. We had a most pleasant evening with his wife and three children; they all enjoyed living in Cairo and had settled well into the lifestyle of the ex-patriot international community.

Family-planning had not been started until the early 1950s and then in a somewhat limited and almost hidden back-street way, nobody quite daring to speak about it. In reality, most women continued to resort in desperation to 'tradition women' who would do their best, often in the most brutal and unhygienic circumstances.

Those with more money turned to the private sector where abortions were widely carried out in rather more desirable surroundings, often government hospitals, even though abortion was against the law.

The National Assembly took until the middle '60s to recognise that the country needed an official family-planning programme, and by the time of my arrival the educated urban middle class used the oral contraceptive pill (OC) and intra-uterine device (IUD).

The Second Population Special Project, which had been started in 1980, was a recognition that family-planning for the majority continued to fail. Dr Allwardt had been working with the Project for about eighteen months and felt progress was being made – at least contraception and abortion were now officially discussed and a number of women's organisations that were standing up for women's rights were now being heard, if not immediately acted on.

By the end of the meeting there were ten of us and the conversation turned to the inappropriateness of western advice and advisers. My Egyptian colleagues were adamant that the great majority of foreigners failed to understand their different social, cultural and historic traditions. Allwardt and I had no difficulty in accepting and agreeing with many of their criticisms.

After this Allwardt said he would like to talk about some of the difficulties he had experienced whilst in Egypt and suggested all of us would be surprised by what he had to tell us. I remember a couple of examples. Part of his work had been to recruit suitable people from West Germany for Fellowships to work on the Project; he astounded us when he explained that few of the applicants understood that the Project would be closely connected with primary care, and quite a few of them knew very little about primary care. He recalled one candidate who, on being asked what serious health issues were facing Egypt, responded that he imagined discoloured teeth would be near the top. Quite beyond belief! Allwardt assured me that similar responses were far from being unusual when primary care or the social aspects of health care were under scrutiny. He added he would have no problem on the other hand finding a suitable Fellow for the hospital service. Sandwiches and tea followed and by now everyone seemed to be sufficiently relaxed for me to ask about the present government.

I started with Samir:

"I've been told that in 1980 a huge celebration took place to mark the anniversary of some major historical event. I'm ashamed to say I've forgotten what it was but it was probably connected with the Pharaohs. Anyhow it was a major occasion, the Egyptians were very proud and excited and the event was to take place on the river Nile in the centre of Cairo – I gather not far from where we are now. Is that right?"
"Yes"
"How did ordinary Egyptians react to what the President had organised? What did they think about the American influence of Frank Sinatra and one of his wives turning up with singers and dancers and a couple of bands and being asked to be present throughout the four or five days of the festivities? Wasn't it meant to be a serious celebration of your history and culture? And didn't a few film stars also turn up to add to the glamour and glitz of American culture?"

This led to an avalanche of criticism and in some cases a near hatred of Sadat and his government and the way they had cozied up to the Americans. It seemed that this pro-American stance had made him unpopular amongst ordinary citizens but not amongst the military, politicians, business, banking and much of the secular middle-class. The Cold War was still at its height, but from what Samir and various colleagues said, the feelings about Sadat were not brought on by the communists or the extreme left.

"Were you surprised by his assassination in 1981 by Muslim extremists?"
"No"
"Did you support the Muslim extremists?"
"No – although some of us supported the Muslim Brotherhood."

Certainly in Britain most politicians and the media maintained that the assassination had been carried out by the Muslim Brotherhood with little support from the Egyptian people. Soon after returning from Egypt I found myself at the home of a good friend who had recently resigned from the FCO. Friends from the FCO would often visit him and so it was this Sunday morning. I was introduced to a couple of his contemporaries and it was explained I had recently come back from Egypt. The conversation touched on Sadat and what impression I had gleaned about the present government. I had to reply that I had no knowledge or information about Hosni Mubarak. What about Sadat and the assassination? I explained that for my part I didn't know if the Muslim Brotherhood had been taken over by the extremist Wahhabi sect, but I offered them the opinions of Samir, his colleagues and others regarding Sadat. They were aware of reports sent back by the Ambassador and his staff to the FCO which had dismissed the idea that many Egyptians were pleased Sadat had gone. The Ambassador and the staff of an Embassy in a country like Egypt were far more likely to be in direct contact with members of the government, the military, lawyers, bankers, businessmen, senior academics and the upper middle class than ordinary members of the public and citizens like Samir and his colleagues, and I was more than irritated by the certainty with which these two FCO diplomats dismissed out of hand my interpretation of what I had been told. To them only the diplomats within the Embassy could possibly understand the complexity of the politics, yet disturbingly over the past thirty years the Embassy in Cairo has continued to seriously misread the situation on the ground.

Any spare time I had I wandered around the Old City – it was easy to be overwhelmed by the mosques and minarets, the ancient gateways and parts of the original city wall. The mediaeval part was around the Citadel and the vast area covered by the north and east cemeteries. I was surprised to find small mud-brick dwellings built among the old tomb stones and the larger tombs – at least some families had a place to protect them from their miserable poverty. Children were everywhere, washing lines wherever they could be fixed, and in every direction mosques and minarets in varying stages of decay.

Being prepared to walk, I was astonished how much of the city's magnificent architecture didn't in fact require a bus or a taxi. As I meandered through the narrow winding alleys and back streets with their overhanging wooden balconies, I was able to absorb the street scenes and the cacophony of noise produced by the repetitive cries of street vendors, the regular calls to prayer, the blaring horns of the gridlocked traffic and the exhaust fumes hanging over the dirty pavements. Flocks of sheep, bullock-drawn carts and obstinate donkeys also contributed to the gridlock. Periodically the smell of poverty assaulted the nostrils. Traditional Arab dress had for the most part for men and women been replaced by western waistcoats, jackets and dresses, and of course T-shirts and jeans for the younger generation. Everywhere the ubiquitous tea houses were crowded with men puffing away on their hubble-bubbles or chain-smoking American cigarettes; women found refuge in numerous cafés, often elegantly dressed in the latest fashions, probably discussing family matters or the latest bit of gossip or just showing each other what they had bought. The *souks* and markets were always crowded, traders pressing everyone to barter and buy.

From twisting alleys I was often surprised to come across open spaces surrounded by dilapidated houses, most looking uninhabitable, and many boarded-up premises. What an amazing mix of ugliness and beauty, of the ancient, the old and the new, and centuries of tradition alongside the whirl of modern life. Beggars lying in the streets or curled up in doorways – all were part of the timeless existence of the Arab world's most populous city. The whole experience was so exciting: to come across the al Azhar mosque, dating from the tenth century AD, opposite the al Azhar university, the oldest in the Arab world; the massive Ibu Tulan mosque with its striking minaret featuring an outer spiral staircase; the ancient gateway of Bab Zuwayhah and the largest enclosed mosque, Mulayyad Shaykh, with its twin minarets. The list is endless and whichever building I entered they all had two things in common apart from their religious significance or academic traditions. One was the very thick walls and the colonnaded walkways, some with covered inner courtyards providing a blessed coolness from the scorching sun, or welcome protection from the winter rains and cold winds. The other was the extraordinary sense of calm and quietness, as if in every sense far from the madding crowd.

To leave Egypt without mentioning the Pyramids would be like leaving Paris without mentioning the Eiffel Tower, a sort of inverted travel snobbery. The three pyramids at Giza are staggering – first on account of their age, having been built between 2589 and 2530 BC, and second on account of their engineering.

Tourists, that is you and me, are the main problem, and the intrusive tourist guides who refuse to take no for an answer, plus the obligatory camels, donkeys and horses. The Great Pyramid dominates the scene whilst the Sphinx, the mythical figure with the body of a lion and the head of a man, is simply extraordinary.

From Giza I shared a taxi with three Germans to take us to the vast cemetery of Saqqarah dominated by the Step Pyramid of Zozer built a hundred years before Giza. The step design is apparently unique to Egyptian architecture. The pyramid stands on the edge of the desert and is surrounded by a huge area of tombs in various stages of excavation.

I left the Germans and decided to walk on for a couple of miles to the ruins of the ancient city of Memphis that stands close to the Nile Little remains of the city, and the Alabaster Sphinx is the only thing of note. Made of gypsum (used to make plaster of Paris and blackboard chalk) and greatly damaged by rain, this reputedly eighty-ton figure built around 1300BC is worth one visit, but only one.

However, returning to Giza by another route was worth every step; as I walked towards the Nile everything became intensely green and fertile. Every available space was being cultivated and date palms and orange trees completed a scene of plenty. Mud-brick villages and scattered huts were full of children, and the *fellahin* were hard at work with traditional ploughs using one or two bullocks and scythes for harvesting. All transport was by donkey or camel – what a valuable and valued animal the donkey is in these parts. Strangely the only animal that worried me was man's best friend, the dog – all the way back to Giza stray dogs would be snarling and yapping at me, sometimes quite aggressively.

As I walked along the banks of many barely-flowing canals and ditches it was obvious why schistosomiasis is such a health problem – the majority of waterways were literally a paradise for the spread of the disease, reminding me of what I had seen in the Nile delta.

The Step Pyramid of Zozer could be seen through the trees, a more impressive sight from a distance. I was accompanied through this wooded landscape by birds and birdsong – hundreds of swallows sweeping over the water, wagtails, moorhens, pigeons, various doves and egrets and bright-green finch-sized birds which I'd never seen before. I encountered four large wooden wagons, two heavily laden with harvested clover and two with dried camel hides. Two were pulled by camels and two by donkeys. The workers were wearing long blue or white cloaks and baggy trousers with either turbans or woolly hats. Two men were on each wagon managing the animals and the other two were making sure nothing fell off. A picturesque scene of a bygone age. Finally I reached a good tarmac road leading to Giza and from there I headed back to Cairo by bus.

As I was packing up on my last evening I realised how attached I had become to the Windsor; in spite of its dreadful plumbing, if I ever returned to Egypt I would do my best to return to the charm of this delightful traditional hotel – not the least of which was its memorable antique elevator.

Anyone my age will be well aware that the Pyramids and the Sphinx are one of the Seven Wonders of the World. I am surprised when I think how unexcited I had been about actually seeing them. Probably the endless postcards and photographs had made them too familiar. What a confession to make.

25

YEMEN BEFORE SEPARATION

The history of Yemen can be roughly divided into three parts: first, before the arrival of Islam; second, between the acceptance of Islam and the interest of European countries at the beginning of the sixteenth century; third, the last four hundred years.

Mention is made of Yemen in the Old Testament with reference to the Queen of Sheba travelling to meet King Solomon (1 Kings chapter 10 and 2 Chronicles chapter 9), and by the Greek historian Herodotus sometime in the fifth century BC when he wrote that Yemen was the only known country to produce frankincense, myrrh and cinnamon. Later, the Romans always referred to the south-west corner of the Arab peninsular as Arabia Felix – 'happy' – although no one knows why this appellation was chosen. The Christian story of the Wise Men from the East bearing gifts of gold, frankincense and myrrh to the baby Jesus is known to all of us. The incense route from southern shore of Arabia inland to the wild deserts and rugged mountains of the Hadramant has been explored by many travellers, one of whom was Freya Stark who wrote *The Southern Gates of Arabia* in 1936. In fact all the Wise Men had to do was to follow this ancient highway, which was already famous as the main trade route to the north and ultimately the Mediterranean Sea.

Islam reached Yemen immediately after the death of the Prophet around 632AD. Both sects, Sunni and Shii, were represented and have remained in the country ever since.

It wasn't until the early sixteenth century that the Portuguese and Italians became the first Europeans to realise that the entrance/exit to the Red Sea could be controlled by the port of Aden, although it was not until the opening of the Suez Canal in 1869 that the British first fully grasped the strategic importance of the Red Sea for their expanding empire and the passage to India. Previously the Egyptians and Ottomans had fought and argued over this part of Arabia whilst the endless tribal disputes with the Arabs inhabiting the surrounding desert (now part of Saudi Arabia) made certain this part of the peninsular was in constant turmoil.

In 1839 the British occupied Aden and the surrounding land and this was followed in 1873 by the Ottoman and British Empires arbitrarily dividing the country into north and south Yemen. At the time local tribes and sects were bitterly opposed to this action and the effect of the resulting frontier is still in evidence today.

In 1937 Aden became a crown colony of the British Empire and was able to control the southern end of the Red Sea, the Gulf of Aden and onwards to the Indian Ocean. During the Second World War it played a significant role in helping to protect Allied shipping from the German navy patrolling along the west coast of Africa.

Following the Second World War the north was supported by Saudi Arabia and the south by Egypt, but after many years of bickering and instability, and following the death in 1962 of the Imam of Yemen who had ruled the country from Sana'a, a bloody civil war broke out that lasted six years. In 1967 the British decided to make a hasty evacuation and total withdrawal from its by then small military garrison in Aden just in time to avoid the bloody outcome of the civil war. This finally resulted in 1969/70 in the north becoming the Yemen Arab Republic (YAR) and the south the People's Republic of Yemen – the latter being renamed the People's Democratic Republic of Yemen (PDRY) a year later.

Constant friction and frequent fighting persisted between the YAR and the PDRY throughout the '70s and '80s due in part to Moscow's influence in the south that extended across the Bab el Mandeb (entrance to the Red Sea) to Ethiopia, Djibouti and Somalia. Probably of equal importance were the endless disputes between the many different tribes in both the north and the south. The serious arguments between the differing branches of Islam remained largely in the north – the PDRY had long since declared it was to be a secular state.

26

YEMEN ARAB REPUBLIC

My first meeting at the Embassy of the Yemen Arab Republic (YAR) was in December 1982 with the First Secretary Gazen Abdul Kabeq. The meeting took place just before a serious earthquake in North Yemen, so inevitably my request to visit went on the backburner.

My first contact with the People's Democratic Republic of Yemen (PDRY) had been in 1980 and negotiations had progressed slowly until finally my visit had been fixed for February 1986. In January 1986, however, serious civil unrest – in other words, fighting – had been stirred up in Aden by tribes from the YAR, some even claiming to represent the government in Sana'a. As a result my visit had to be cancelled. At this point the Ambassador and his small staff in Aden managed to organise a dramatic and successful evacuation of all British and Commonwealth citizens as well as other nationalities including Soviet citizens and members of their Embassy.

Negotiating and corresponding with two countries at the same time, particularly when they were hostile to each other, was difficult. Neither country was aware I was planning to visit their neighbour as I had come to the conclusion permission would be revoked and negotiations stopped if either found out.

With the two countries almost on a war footing, the contrast between the two embassies couldn't have been more stark. The PDRY put no obstacles in my way either regarding the visit or granting a visa, while the YAR, in spite of bland assurances from the Ambassador that there would be no problems, proved quite different. First, an official invitation was required before a visa could even be considered, and after a year with nothing achieved I was beginning to feel it was as difficult as dealing with the Soviet Union – I couldn't decide if it was bloody-mindedness, inefficiency, political posturing or a combination of all three. Finally a colleague came to my rescue. David Morley, Professor of Tropical Child Health at the University of London, had been working with the British Council in Sana'a and he kindly wrote to the Head of the Council asking if he could bring pressure to bear on Dr Khaled al Sakkat, Director of the International Relations Department in the Ministry of Health. Telexes and telegrams followed and in the end I received a letter enabling me to apply for a visa; ultimately my date of departure was fixed for 14 November 1986.

The flight was somewhat tedious with stops in Paris, Athens and Cairo, but all was soon forgotten with the amazing sunrise as we flew down the Red Sea, finally turning left over green fertile land stretching up and down the Yemeni coastline. Inland, as we flew eastward, a range of barren mountains of between 7 and 8,000 feet, according to the pilot, could be seen. As we prepared to land at Sana'a, which lies at 7,500 feet, the aerial view of the well-known traditional agricultural terracing that dominated the landscape was an unexpected bonus.

I was through immigration, collected my luggage, no problem with customs, exchanged travellers cheques and was out of the airport in less than an hour – quite remarkable, but I suppose there were few passengers on the flight and the place was hardly a centre of activity – the flight before mine had landed over an hour previously and the next one wasn't due for several hours. I shared a taxi into the city, dropping off a young businessman at the five-star Hotel Sheraton built on a hill overlooking the city. We passed several more five-star hotels, none of which would have been out of place in Paris, New York or Tokyo. We drove on to the Dar al-Hamd, a former palace of the family of the late Imam and now a three-star hotel - a splendid choice by the British Council who had obviously listened to my requests. It possessed a marvellous other-world atmosphere with the interior virtually unaltered since the building's construction at the beginning of the twentieth century – substantial external stone walls, low doorways, wide stone stairways and dark, wooden furniture throughout. I decided on the cheapest room without a shower, opting instead for a communal lavatory and shower – a square structure about three feet high made of concrete blocks in the centre of which was a seat with two raised areas for one's feet; clearly one sat down to have a shower.

In the small restaurant one other person was having breakfast, a Palestinian studying philosophy for a PhD. He had strong views and before we had even finished coffee he had outlined the injustice of the Palestinian situation, the role of Britain in helping to create this injustice, and the inevitability of Israel eventually disappearing off the map, or at the least having to agree to live alongside a Palestinian state. Having survived this unexpected outburst I asked him the quickest way into the centre of Sana'a. He obligingly drew a map and warned me it was impossible to buy a street map even in the one and only tourist shop (which proved later to be a small room with a counter and everything piled on the floor). The Palestinian student, who by this time considered himself my friend, explained it was a public holiday to celebrate the Prophet's birthday (this seemed to be a moveable feast), which was very annoying as I had intended going straight to the Ministry of Health. Anyway he was able to take me to the Ministry, and using his hand-drawn map we then went our separate ways.

Medicine and politics were forgotten on this first day: sightseeing was to be my priority. The distinctive architecture of Sana'a still survived in the old city, which was almost completely surrounded by a medieval wall and magnificent traditional gateways. Unlike Cairo and Damascus it was the domestic architecture which stood out rather than grand mosques or ancient universities. The ground floor of almost every dwelling was made of stone that supported the upper storeys of baked-mud brick, five or six floors high. Geometric patterns were formed by protruding bricks, and the upper floors were decorated with lime wash and open tracery on the walls. Windows had a decorated arch over the top, often fitted with coloured glass, and doorways were commonly crowned with a shell-shape design, very similar to our own Queen Anne/Georgian shell hoods. Blind circular or oval windows as well as balconies and verandas completed this wonder of Islamic architecture.

Whether I was wandering through narrow alleyways or crowded *souks*, along shop-lined streets to open squares, or struggling through the gates of the old city wall to the busy street traders beyond, all the time goats, sheep, chickens, donkeys and even camels formed part of the general melee, reminding me I was close to the countryside. Women wore the *sharshaf*, a severe black cape, veil and head covering, or the *sitara*, a brightly-coloured and attractively-patterned cotton garment extending from shoulder to feet. Girls wore multi-coloured frocks and sometimes head scarves. Men wore skull caps of varying colours, turbans, or the traditional 'Yasser Arafat' chequered headdress and sometimes scarves wrapped around their heads. Some were in the customary white gowns, others wore long skirts or European-style jackets and trousers. The younger men and boys sported the ubiquitous jeans and T-shirt. The most noticeable and unique items worn were the daggers or *djambia* – either the J-shaped *asib* or the less curved *thuma* – the latter was seen less often and I gathered they could only be worn by the upper class and senior clerics.

Heading back to the hotel from a different direction I found myself walking across cultivated fields close to the hotel – cabbage, maize, tomatoes and peppers all awaiting the final harvest. In another area the soil was being turned by a bullock and hand-held plough. Glancing up, eight birds of prey were circling overhead.

A truly fascinating day.

My Palestinian friend and a Lebanese Christian working for the United Nations were having supper together, so I joined them. Both men had lost their homes as a result of the conflict in the Middle East and almost before I had sat down they wanted to tell me their story, or what had caused their personal disaster. First, western nations had concentrated on and supported Israel and ignored all Arab countries unless they had oil or gas. Second, the majority of Arab leaders had done a great disservice to the Palestinian cause and to the Arab world by their extravagant and dishonourable lifestyles, plus their insistence on ruling with some form of dictatorship. The Lebanese believed that the emotive and threatening talk of many Arabs such as 'throw all Jews into sea' or 'kill the lot of them' would make any prospect of a settlement impossible. The Palestinian remained silent. As we were preparing to go up to bed I asked them a question: didn't they think there was a paradox in Israel being the only country in the Middle East and Arab world to carry out democratic elections? Surely that was an irony? Neither replied and we all departed to our rooms.

I had been wandering round for over seven hours and as I collapsed into bed I realised that my sightseeing day hadn't been wasted regarding the actual purpose of my visit to Yemen. I had found Abdul Nasser and Jamal Street, Tahir Square, the Ministry of

Health, the Ministry of Foreign Affairs, the University and Medical School, the British Embassy (just in case) and the British Council, and I had been able to work out how long it would take me to walk to the Ministry of Health in the morning.

An armed soldier was on guard at the Ministry of Health; he reluctantly permitted me to enter after I had managed to explain with the help of an interpreter that I had a meeting with Khaled al Sakkaf at 9am. I found his office and waited outside with another man who was either Korean or Chinese. By 9.30 there was no sign of the Director of International Relations so I ventured next door and chanced to find Dr Haj'ar, Director of Health Affairs, one of Professor Morley's contacts whom he had strongly advised me to meet. He of course knew nothing of my visit and said it was very unusual for al Sakkaf to be late, and offered to phone him at his home. He was informed that he wouldn't be coming in that day. My heart sank.

Haj'ar was on his own, so I gave him the letter explaining the reason for my visit, the programme that had been arranged for me and the people I hoped to meet – the Director of MCH ("out of the country"), the Director of EPI ("may be possible"), the Director of Nutrition ("also out of the country"), the Director of the World Bank Project ("uncertain, nobody knows where he is"). I explained I was expecting to visit both urban and rural PHC facilities ("difficult if not impossible").

However, by 1pm I had managed to talk to the Deputy Director of MCH, the Deputy for Nutrition, the Director of PHC and the WHO coordinator of PHC who readily agreed to arrange visits to both urban and rural facilities within the next couple of days. Just as I was leaving, the Director of EPI breezed in and we arranged to meet the following day. Not a bad outcome considering no one even knew of my existence!

Such disorganised organisation was now familiar to me as was the extraordinary way meetings and private discussions were conducted; the YAR proved to be the epitome of this behaviour. The mind boggled at the flexibility of my Arab colleagues who never appeared to have a fixed schedule of their own and if they did were happy to disregard it. If I was to achieve anything at all I had to accept this modus operandi.

As I walked back to the hotel I noticed something that I had overlooked the day before – men sitting alone or in small groups or just lying in the street chewing *qat*. Later I was to hear about private *qat* parties held in people's homes. Bundles of *qat* leaves are collected, inspected for quality and then laid out on the street or any convenient scrubland. The leaves are chewed over and over to obtain their mildly narcotic juices. The *qat* chewers with their bulging cheeks reminded me of my children's hamsters and their large cheek pouches for storing food. Shelagh Weir's book *Qat in Yemen* published in 1985 provides a full history of its consumption and the social effects brought about by the drug – a very interesting read.

Taking advantage of the thermals at the end of the day, the raptors were again slowly circling over the cultivated fields close to the hotel, today in far greater numbers – between thirty and forty. They were to be a regular feature of my stay.

After an interesting experience with the communal shower I was delighted to find the Palestinian in the restaurant. We were both more relaxed by now and didn't mention politics or the Zionists. He admitted his Ph D was only a hobby – in reality he was a businessman (in what, I forget) with offices in Cyprus and Beirut.

All in all it had been an unexpectedly satisfactory day considering its unpromising start. Nevertheless I remained mystified and somewhat irritated by particular differences between the Arabs and the West. For example, the English translation of the Annual Report on Health Statistics had been promised me via the Department of Statistics. This however proved to be impossible as the Director was away in the United States and (difficult to believe) he was the only person with a key to the relevant cupboard in the department. Someone at the World Bank Project then agreed to translate the report, only for the Director to say he was unable to agree to this without first getting permission from the Ministry of Health. Consequently he decided it would be impossible to meet me. Quite by chance an Arab colleague in an adjacent room helpfully arranged for the translation to be carried out. I never did meet the Director.

This other more helpful side of the coin also emerged when Dr

Saied of MCH very obligingly went to his car to get the latest translated report on nutrition after I had mentioned the Department of Nutrition had told me only one copy was available. When it transpired that this was Dr Saied's only English copy that he had hand-written himself I was particularly grateful, especially when he then arranged to have it photocopied for me.

The YAR in the '80s was one of the least developed countries in the world and poorest in the Arab world. By the end of 1986 only 21% of the rural population had a supply of safe drinking water within three to four miles of each household (although in defence of Yemen's slow progress the majority of villages are built on the sides or tops of hills with water found in the surrounding flat land). The claim that 99% of the urban population had piped water within a short distance of their homes was impossible to verify, but it was an unlikely assertion.

Over the previous twenty years a serious problem connected with water had been developing, but was rarely talked about officially. By chance I had the good luck to meet Mr Kozinski, a Pole working in the Ministry of Public Works, who was willing to talk to me provided his name was never mentioned in my report. The water table had been dropping fast and in the previous six years it had fallen 150 feet. The reason for this potential catastrophe was almost entirely due to the unrestricted private drilling and pumping to irrigate the land for growing *qat,* the drilling and pumping increasing exponentially as the consumption and cost of the leaf escalated. These operations were being financed by ex-patriot Yemenis working in Saudi Arabia, the Gulf States and a few western countries. At the time of my visit the government had started drilling and pumping new bore-holes to try and improve the supply of drinking water, but it was proving difficult to train sufficient personnel to work and maintain the equipment. As I write in 2015, the water table has continued to drop to dangerous levels according to the WHO, and the battle between *qat* and drinking water continues.

By 1986, 12-15% of the population had adequate sewage disposal and interestingly, about 60% of traditional housing in both urban and rural areas had some form of latrine. Throughout the world, and the

YAR was no exception, the introduction of water supply is always far ahead of the introduction of sewage disposal, so it was vital that pit latrines were correctly situated and attention turned to health education; villagers were instructed and constantly reminded not to defecate near any water supply.

Governmental responsibility for primary health care was limited. There were A&E departments in some hospitals in major towns, health centres in both urban and rural areas, and health units only in rural areas. Private health care flourished – over 500 clinics as well as an unknown number of private health centres with 20 to 25 beds were functioning throughout the country. According to the most recent figures in 1986, only 35% of the urban and 10% of the rural population had access to government facilities.

The health centre at Ranada on the outskirts of Sana'a was surprisingly impressive and well organised with a young Yemeni doctor in charge, full of enthusiasm. Originally opened in 1962 it moved to its new premises in 1983 under the guidance and with the support of West German advisers and architects. It covered a population of 20-30,000 in Sana'a, and 60,000 in the surrounding countryside along with the supervision of thirteen health units. The centre was staffed by three doctors, four qualified nurses, five assistant nurses, three trained midwives, a laboratory assistant and a pharmacist. On the day of my visit the centre was functioning well and crowds of patients were waiting to be seen – a most unusual sight compared with the rest of the YAR. 85% of births were at home and the fourteen *dyas* were supported by the three midwives.

I was not, however, allowed to visit an A&E department or any other health centre either in Sana'a or elsewhere – this was not due to lack of time or effort on my part, rather I think Ranada was the only health centre the authorities were happy to show foreigners. Nonetheless it was very disappointing and frustrating.

The rural facilities I visited were confined to the Amran Directorate forty-fifty miles or so north and west of Sana'a. To get there we travelled over a vast flat rocky terrain with unexpectedly cultivated fields surrounded by dry-stone walls – most of the crops had already been gathered leaving only maize and the green areas of *qat*. In the distance I could see spectacular barren mountains and nearer hills with visible terracing.

The health centre in the town of Amran had been opened in 1978, again with West German technical cooperation and continuing support. The German technical director met me and showed me round. Even at 9.30am when I arrived there were few patients. The reality was so different from what I had been told to expect at the Department of PHC. According to up-to-date statistics the centre was responsible for seventeen health units, but only four were functioning, thus leaving most of the scattered villages without any medical care. The Yemeni colleague and the official who were accompanying me explained that the thirteen non-functioning health units were to be joined by another thirty-two and all were to be operational by 1989. I asked the German director for his opinion as to whether this was remotely possible or likely; accompanied by a quizzical smile his reply was measured and tactful – No, he didn't think it likely.

Just cloud-cuckoo-land in other words.

We proceeded from Amran to two villages, Amad and Beni-azzubiar a further ten miles on dirt tracks through villages amazingly well built in the traditional style from black stone and mud bricks. Amad was an area with no roads at all, just isolated houses or groups of buildings, some with fortified turrets, all stone and mud brick, some three storeys high. A particular feature were the many dry-stone walls, not marking out roads or tracks because there were none, so serving no purpose that I could see. Donkeys, sheep and goats were everywhere, children were running around and old men were sitting and smoking. An old chap and his friend, both of them sitting or kneeling on the ground, were weaving brightly-coloured lengths of material. They told us they had started at sunrise and would finish at sunset and that such matting sold easily at the local *souk*.

Between Amad and Beni-azzubiar the occasional Toyota pick-up truck or Japanese motorbike careered along the rutted track, but no sign of any UK land rovers. Beni-azzubiar was different; it was built on the side of a bare stony hill, all the houses crowded together in a crazy network of twisting alleyways.

Both health units were isolated and consisted of two rooms and a storage space. Although utterly basic, both were clean and staffed by a male nurse and an untrained traditional birth attendant (TBA). Both units were almost devoid of patients. In Beni-azzubiar, however, a man turned up full of complaints that neither the nurse nor the *dya* had been there the day before and that nobody was ever given enough medicine. Soon after leaving a lorry driver stopped us to ask if there was a doctor nearby. We told him there wasn't but that there was a clinic further up the road. The clinic obviously hadn't met with his approval as he said he had just been there.

I was quickly getting an idea of what health care was like in the countryside. After all, I presumed Amad and Beni-azzubiar had been forewarned of my visit and presumably would have endeavoured to make a good impression.

My driver and interpreter were by now totally fed up with primary care and were really keen I should see some historic sites close by. They were extremely proud of their country, a trait I found in many Yemenis.

We approached Thula along a rutted track over an unremitting rocky desert landscape and in the distance a large isolated hill with an apparently flat summit; as we approached nearer I could make out deep ravines and turrets of rock reaching up to the edge of the summit. The nearer we got the easier it was to see that this rocky fortress town had been built into the side of the hill and was surrounded by an almost intact mud wall. Many of the houses were three or four storeys high, protecting the winding paths from the heat of the sun. Rocky fortifications on the top of the hill had been built to protect the town below and had been part of the country's history since the early sixteenth century. In *Yemen Rediscovered* published in 1983, Michael Jenner writes:

> 'Thula demonstrates the harmony of stone employed in a variety of functions. The roads and homes, being of the same stone, create a strong sense of organic unity. The town is literally part of the mountainside.'

I was interested in an enormous medieval water tank dug deep into the ground at the base of the hill; it was empty, but in the early 1970s drilled bore-holes at the edge of the tank had provided water pipes to many collecting sites throughout the town.

Less than ten miles from Thula are the twin towns of Shiban and Koukaban, both originating from pre-Christian times. Shiban is most famous for its Grand Mosque, second only in age to the Grand Mosque in Sana'a. However, it was the bustle and activity in the main tarmacked street leading down from the market square that enthralled me. The town is situated at the edge of a large fertile plain resulting in piles of fruit and vegetables everywhere. Street vendors, protected from the sun by black umbrellas, were selling anything and everything one could think of. Other traders had fixed stalls to present their goods. Women and children filled the street and struggled with their purchases whilst donkeys and goats were eating whatever they could find. Ducks and hens pecked around in the dirt whilst the geese behaved in their usual threatening and aggressive way. Clapped-out cars, motorbikes and pick-ups honked their way up and down the street, blocking out the sound of the call to prayer.

A thousand feet above Shiban the town of Koukaban could be seen, built as a fortification to defend the town below. Apparently it was possible to climb up an almost vertical narrow path to the fortifications, which were massive and impressive. It would have taken at least a couple of hours to reach the top and we had no time – there was another historic site to be found.

Barely an hour before sunset we reached Kasr al-Hajjara (Castle of the Rock) or Dar al-Hajjara (Palace on the Rock), a spectacular sight from ground level. How I wished I had my binoculars as I'd never seen so many birds of prey, at least half a dozen species all quietly circling in the thermals. There was a road up to the Castle/Palace from where great views spread out across Wadi Dahr. I had expected a wide, barren stony plateau but even at that time of year it was still green and full of many types of fruit, many varieties of grape, and of course the ubiquitous *qat* bushes. It was difficult to believe that the water table in the Wadi Dahr had dropped as much as Mr Kozinski had indicated in the rest of Yemen.

Dr Karl Rudersdof of the West German Volunteer Service had worked in the YAR for a couple of years and I was able to ask him and one of his colleagues about the state of the health service. They were united that the lack of doctors and all other health workers was the fundamental problem, closely followed by poor education and training coupled with the fact that 90% of all nurses were male – a situation they described as a seemingly insurmountable 'Everest'.

In my opinion the lack of trained female midwives was the most serious problem with the inevitable consequence that 95% of all deliveries were carried out by untrained *dyas.*

In 1984 the Ministry of Health had finally and wisely decided to organise the registration of these TBAs, making it possible for them to be integrated into the government service, although interestingly they would continue to be paid by the patient. It was a huge undertaking as the majority of *dyas* were illiterate. The initial four-week training would clearly be inadequate, but at least it was a start and at the end of the month a maternity bag as well as visual reference cards for high-risk problems such as haemorrhage and difficulties in labour had been provided for the *dyas.* By the time of my arrival, 270 *dyas* had attended the registration course. The plan was to repeat the training every three years.

The training of some primary health care workers to become supervisors as they were subsequently called, commenced in 1981. Local communities were given the responsibility for choosing likely candidates who, it was stipulated, could not be recruited until they were eighteen and should have completed primary school education. The Health Manpower Institute was responsible and had organised the original training that had been carried out by eleven health visitors from Sudan. Eight fully-trained female Yemeni nurses had just returned from a WHO training course in Alexandria and were about to take over from the Sudanese.

The Expanded Programme of Immunisation (EPI) had started in 1977 and yet by 1985/86 only 16% of three-year-olds had been immunised against diphtheria, pertussis, tetanus and polio, 19% against measles and 28% against tuberculosis. Women hadn't fared much better with only 25% against tetanus. Yemen, the WHO and UNICEF were well aware of the dreadfully slow progress and I was informed that a mass campaign of immunisation of children under five years was to be undertaken in 1987 or '88. Certainly the WHO and UNICEF representatives were less optimistic about the start and success of the campaign than Dr Saied, the Yemeni Director of the EPI project when I had a meeting with him.

Ex-patriot workers varied considerably in their attitude to the Yemenis, particularly the Americans – sensitivity was not part of their vocabulary. The WHO adviser was American. I remember clearly – he had been helpful to me personally, but his superior and condescending attitude was embarrassing as was his impatience with anything and everything the Yemenis were trying to accomplish. He rarely seemed to comprehend the almost insurmountable difficulties they had to overcome. The American US AID controller was the same; in particular she gave the impression of being detached and of having no empathy with the people or their country – arrogant and ignorant, in fact.

However, the Swedes in charge of the Save The Children Fund, and the West German volunteers and technical advisers couldn't have been more different. The understanding and support given by the British Council was also good to see and their contribution was greatly helped by both Mr Chenery and Mr Hepburn being fluent Arabic speakers.

Mohammad my interpreter had spoken a great deal about hoping to study in the UK and was really eager to tell me about his family – twelve brothers, six sisters, four mothers and one father. He himself was married with four children and one wife and I was interested to learn that all four births had taken place in hospital – this was very very unusual. He asked what he should do about the UK and if I could help him. I thought the British Council would be his best bet and he was greatly encouraged when he discovered both Chenery and Hepburn spoke Arabic. I was due to visit the Council the next day so we arranged to meet and I was able to introduce him so that he could explain his plans for the future. By the time I left he was still chatting away and seemed to be getting on well.

Hepburn had invited me round for a meal in the evening at a simple Yemeni restaurant, then back to his flat for a drink and chat about my visit and his experience of living in the country. During the meal I asked about Mohammad and he was cautiously optimistic they might be able to help, but I never found out whether or not they did. Hepburn told me what a nightmare it was to organise anything and regaled me with many amusing examples of the government's particular style of bureaucracy. At the time he had been endeavouring to organise a concert tour for a well-known English pianist in the coming year; he had quickly discovered that the government was opposed to its citizens having any contact with western culture. He wondered if perhaps a lutenist playing medieval music would have been easier . . . Still, western culture was safe within his flat as he put on LP records of the choir of New College, Oxford, and we enjoyed a tot of whisky.

While we were talking, Hepburn asked if anyone had ever mentioned another agricultural tradition within the town of Sana'a itself, and serving the same purpose as terracing – I had of course seen the traditional terracing system of agriculture in many places. Apparently the cultivated fields like those close to my hotel depended on a centuries-old network of pipes based around suitably sited mosques. After washing hands before prayers, the water was then piped to the appropriate gardens for irrigation. Over recent years many of these cultivated fields, known as 'radish gardens', had disappeared through lack of water. Those remaining still produced maize, cabbage, radishes, leeks, tomatoes, onions, rocket, lettuce and strawberries. I forgot to ask Hepburn whether the problem was a genuine shortage of water or if the number of suitably sited mosques had declined or were no longer in use –perhaps a combination of all three.

My impression of the health services was not good; I could recall only one facility that had impressed me, the health centre at Ranada run by the enthusiastic Yemeni doctor – he was the exception, as the great majority of physicians were involved and interested in nothing else than private practice.

When I consider the countries involved in *People, Politics and Health*, all of them have produced a response from me regarding primary care, whether it be interest, disagreement, support, hope, disappointment, or perhaps often all of those things. The Yemen Arab Republic is the only country where my reaction has been negative.

Nevertheless, the unique stunning beauty of its domestic architecture, the rugged landscape and the noise and smell of the streets were truly unforgettable, especially the colours – white turbans, black garments and every colour of the rainbow in between. One thing did surprise me – I had expected to see many beggars, but they had been displaced by *qat* chewers.

It was difficult to see how the YAR and the PDRY would again unite, but I was proved to be wrong – they reunited in 1990 and became the Republic of Yemen, with Sana'a remaining the capital and Aden becoming the country's commercial centre. Then in the mid-'90s the south was defeated in a brief civil war and since then the maelstrom of independent sheiks and tribes has threatened to boil over once again. In the 21st century everything has been further complicated by jihadists, Muslim fundamentalists and in particular, al-Qaeda, not to mention the use of drones by the United States which has consolidated the Yemenis' dislike, not to say hatred, for the West.

27

PEOPLE'S DEMOCRATIC REPUBLIC of YEMEN

The Embassy of the People's Democratic Republic of Yemen (PDRY) was on the Cromwell Road in a rather run-down part of London that was entirely appropriate for a strongly Marxist country; compared with other embassies of the communist bloc (except Albania which I never visited) it couldn't have been more different. I often wondered as I climbed the rather dirty staircase up to the first floor, which I did quite frequently for some years, whether they were in fact able to settle the rent or pay the telephone and electricity bills. Anyway, Mohammad Almas, the Second Secretary , became a great help to me from my first visit in February 1981 until I arrived in Aden exactly six years later.

Those six years involved endless phone calls, cables, telex messages and letters between the Embassy in London and the Ministry of Health in Aden. They entailed finding out the cheapest flights, then having to alter and cancel and rebook them over and over again, all of which tested my ability to organise and re-organise my NHS work in Wells. The British Embassy in Aden kept in regular contact throughout 1985, trying I think to warn me about the instability of the country.

Originally my visit had been arranged for mid-January 1986, but it was not to be. On 13 January, the day before I had planned to reach Aden, a violent civil war broke out between those who felt the government had strayed from the ideology of the Soviet Union and those who wanted to encourage private enterprise and had already started giving land back to some farmers. Both sides had been seeking the support of various tribes and sheiks and religious leaders. The war lasted ten days of bloody and ruthless fighting – the official death toll was around 4,500 but it was generally believed to have been much higher, even more than the fight for independence two decades earlier. The dead were simply bulldozed off the streets into mass graves.

The Soviet Ambassador had been unable to mediate and quickly organised the evacuation of some of his staff. Other countries did the same, but many foreign individuals including Russians, East Europeans and the remnants of the Soviet Embassy, turned up at the British Embassy in hope and desperation. At the time the Royal Yacht *Britannia* happened to be sailing close by and became involved in the rescue of 450 people; when it came under fire it moved on and was able to collect another 200 or so from farther along the coast. Many dramatic photographs appeared in the world press and everyone agreed the *Britannia* had carried out a remarkable rescue.

Flying Ethiopian Airlines, rather than Aeroflot, via Moscow or Havana, provided the cheapest but rather tedious flight with long waits in Frankfurt and Rome before reaching Addis Ababa; there a change of aircraft and a superb view of the African coastline which was quickly left behind as we crossed the entrance to the Red Sea and saw ahead the southern coast of Yemen as we started the descent into Aden, arriving Friday, 7 February, 1987.

I was met at the airport and taken to the Hotel September 26 (named in commemoration of Revolution Day 1962) and previously known in the colonial era as the Rock Hotel at Steamer Point and still frequently called the same. To get there we passed through the Maalla, a modern district of Aden with a wide main street lined on both sides by grey, dreary, five-storey 1950s Soviet-style apartments, and bare rugged mountains dominating the skyline on one side. Finally we reached Tawahi residential district and Steamer Point.

Between 1839 and 1967 when the south of Yemen gained her independence, the British influence had remained almost entirely in Aden, the rest of the south and the entire north being ruled by innumerable sheiks, sultans, emirs and lesser tribal leaders. Throughout the 1950s constant bickering and often fighting had taken place between the enclosed Arab Protectorate occupied by the British, and the rest of Yemen, supported by Egypt and Syria, and ruled by the royal family in Sana'a. In 1962 the military coup against the Royalists took over the north of the country and founded the Yemen Arab Republic (YAR) and infiltrated much of the south surrounding Aden.

In the late '50s/early '60s, unlike the rest of Yemen, Aden had flourished economically and there was a high level of employment due to the building of an oil refinery in Little Aden, and the employment of many Yemenis by the British military and their families. According to Robin Bidwell in *The Two Yemens*, only London, Liverpool and New York handled more ships, and this, combined with at least a quarter of a million tourists a year who came to buy duty-free cheap goods, provided considerable wealth. In the *souks* the locals were able to outwit the visitors in bargaining and bartering, thus adding to their relative prosperity. Steam Point, with the building of a number of fashionable hotels, had become a special place for ex-pats and tourists.

In spite of the prosperity they had created, anti-British feeling finally erupted in October 1967 and the British troops and their families made a hurried exit. Everything then changed and two rival political parties – the Front for the Liberation of South Yemen (FLOSY) supported by Nasser, and the National Liberation Front (NLF) a left-wing radical organisation supported by the trade unions and the workers in the port of Aden – were left to fight it out. The NLF won and the country became known as the People's Republic of South Yemen, and then, following the Glorious Correction Step in 1969, a new constitution was drawn up and the Democratic Republic of Yemen was born in 1970, later to become the People's Democratic Republic of Yemen (PDRY), strongly supported and now under the direct influence of the Soviet Union. At independence in 1967 medical services were limited to Aden whilst the rest of the five governorates had been ignored. When the British finally left Yemen they had little to be proud of, and two expert political journalists working for many years in the Middle East confirmed this. I was told that in the rural governorates there were no medical facilities, fewer than ten primary schools and no secondary schools.

In *The Arabs* Peter Mansfield wrote:

> 'No newly independent state has started life in less promising circumstances. Before independence the mainstay of the economy had been Port Aden and the income from the British Military base, which was about 11 million pounds per year. Britain had promised to increase this aid to 60 million pounds for the first three years after independence, but this promise had been made

> when Britain had expected to be dealing with a federation of South Arabian sultans under it patronage. To the nationalist and non-aligned Republic of South Yemen, Britain would offer no more than 1.8 million pounds.'

Fred Halliday in *Arabia Without Sultans* wrote:

> 'The People's Republic of Yemen emerged into a world where danger confronted in every direction . . . the insulation of Aden also reflected a political decision by the British to keep tribal areas as unchanged as possible . . . when the British departed (1967) South Yemen had only fourteen tarmaced miles of road outside Aden, three Yemeni doctors and 950 hospital beds. Education facilities hardly existed outside Aden . . . the British betrayal of their aid commitments deprived the state of 60% if its income.'

Hotel September 26 had suffered from twenty-five years of neglect. It was shabby with a dirty entrance and in need of paint both inside and out, had ill-fitting doors and windows, and most corridors were minus light bulbs. My room was spacious, but plaster was coming off the walls and there was just one dim bulb; no plug in the sink or bath; rusty pipes; the lavatory seat broken and falling off, a flush that didn't work and no lavatory paper; the hot tap fixed so it couldn't be used, and the tiles in the bathroom loose and falling off. The air conditioning fan was noisy and when I eventually discovered how to switch it on and off I had to stand on a chair to reach the switch that was out of sight, except when standing at the opposite side of the room, above the pelmet of the threadbare curtain. At least there was a table where I could write and an old-fashioned wicker chair to sit on which really made me feel quite at home, and I had fun trying to imagine what it would have been like in the days of privilege – it was difficult to believe this had once been a fashionable hotel. Equally it would have been amusing, had I felt like laughing, when one evening the yale key of my room snapped in the keyhole and I had to disturb the next door room by using the balcony that connected us – luckily my window was open. It took over twenty-four hours for the hotel to find another key and to remove the broken key from the lock.

I was ready for Abdullah Salim at 8.30am but received the almost inevitable phone call whilst having breakfast – he wouldn't be round till after 9am – in fact he arrived spot on time explaining it was pointless to start earlier as little happened before 9am. Added to which, he knew the Minister of Health was away and nobody knew where he was – perhaps he had gone to one of the governorates and would be back in a couple of days. This was to have been the first scheduled meeting on my programme.

We started instead with a visit to the only Exchange Bank in Aden to see if the rate was any better than the hotel (in fact little difference) and as we left, Salim explained I needed two photographs as I must register with the Ministry of the Interior within forty-eight hours and they were required. It would have been helpful if the FCO or the PDRY Embassy in London had tipped me off.

On finally reaching the Ministry we found the Director of PHC wasn't in his office so I told Salim I would like to visit the Department of International Relations – he was unhappy about this.

"I think you must wait for instructions."

From whom? From *Allah*? However, perhaps Salim was right as three people were already waiting outside the open door of the office, whilst inside a workman was busy painting the room. After a brief discussion I suggested Salim should speak to the other three and we all trouped into the room. The workman was still up a ladder but there was a man sitting behind a large official-looking desk – I'm pretty sure he'd been trying to hide and wouldn't have invited us in, simply departing without acknowledging us if he'd had his way. I thought it best to let the other three finish their business before I spoke to him. He spoke no English, but Salim came to my rescue and by lunch time we had negotiated with the man behind the desk that I should meet the Minister at 9am the next day – not that I believed this would actually happen even though I had been assured the Minister would be back and that the Director of the WHO office would also be ready to see me. As for the rest of the day, the Director of PHC would meet me in the early afternoon. All these meetings were unrelated to my official programme; it was all very much *'in sha Allah':* God willing.

Dr Abdul Latif, the Director of PHC, was a young man, enthusiastic, well-informed, cooperative and conscientious. It was not until the evening that I realised he was the chap with whom the

British Embassy had been in contact in '84 and who had kept the lines of communication open with the Ambassador. It was very unusual in developing countries for officials to remain in the same post for as long as three years. I was surprised, but could well understand why the Ministry would want to keep him for as long as possible.

By chance the Director of PHC for the Lahej governorate and the Director of the Health Manpower Institute could be heard down the corridor. Latif leapt up and brought them along, introduced me, and within half an hour a two-day trip to Lahej (also the name of the capital town) was organised for me to visit rural health facilities and meet rural health workers. I couldn't believe my luck. Perhaps *Allah* was watching over me as everything had been arranged in spite of the workman up the ladder painting, repairing and drilling holes in the wall, and Latif having to give endless advice to a steady flow of colleagues coming in for a chat, and others requesting his signature on bits of paper.

Some of the most valuable discussions took place at the Health Manpower Institute and the Medical Faculty of the University. The disagreements between the Institute and the Medical School were glaringly obvious, especially in regard to primary care. The Institute was oriented towards the community and PHC whereas the Medical School held rigidly traditional views concerning the hospital service.

Following independence, the introduction of primary care faced almost insurmountable obstacles with the government committed to the expansion of hospitals. However, with the increasing influence of Havana, the first two development plans 1971-'74 and '74-'78 concentrated on building facilities in rural areas. Unashamedly I was informed that the Ministry had concentrated on quantity rather than quality. As Abdul Latif said:

> "What else could we have done?"

Finally, with really strong support from the Health Manpower Institute and advisers from Cuba, the Ministry of Health agreed in 1979 to establish a Department of Primary Health Care, and further resources in 1982. It was interesting to find that in planning and teaching, the influence of Cuba was considerable and far more than that of the Soviet Union or Eastern Europe. Perhaps I shouldn't have been surprised as by this time Cuba had become the leading non-aligned nation on health care, and the WHO, as well as many independent experts, believed they had much to teach countries in the advanced industrialised world and paradoxically, their arch-enemy the United States, most of all

One meeting with the Dean of the Medical School and a Cuban paediatrician was memorable. They openly argued and disagreed about almost everything and the Cuban especially refuted the Dean's insistence that both undergraduate and postgraduate teaching reflected a belief in the importance of primary care. Eventually however the Dean had to admit that teaching was almost exclusively carried out in three hospitals and the interest in primary care was non-existent. A further accusation by the Cuban concerned nearly 150 female doctors who had become unemployed because suitable accommodation had not been provided for single women in rural areas, and the women had simply refused to work in these governorates. The Dean denied this and the Cuban became really angry. Much more went on in this vein and it was amazing to witness the freedom of speech. I had gone to the meeting with a list of questions but they were virtually all answered by just listening to the ding dong battle between them.

The World Bank considered both the YAR and the PDRY to be amongst the bottom ten of least developed and poor countries in the world with life expectancy, maternal, infant, and under-five mortality virtually the same for each country. Further investigation however, showed the PDRY's GNP per capita income of 420 US dollars was much less than the YAR's 590 US dollars.

Like the YAR, the PDRY was an arid country with a serious shortage of water, although a significant difference between them soon became apparent; this concerned the use of water in the cultivation and consumption of *qat*. The Marxist government in the south had taken an almost Calvinistic approach by restricting *qat* consumption to Thursday afternoons and all day Friday, the Day of Prayer. In public the law was enforced by the police and only one *qat* market existed in Aden. Although disapproved of by the authorities, *qat* was chewed in private at home. What a contrast with the YAR.

Dr Latif's Department of PMC consisted of three small rooms in a quadrangle of single-storey concrete buildings with flat corrugated iron roofs: typewriters, three desks, three telephones, a number of bookcases and little else except piles and piles of reports and suchlike lying on the floor. This was indicative of the extent of his authority in what was one of the least prestigious and certainly one of the least influential government departments.

Urban facilities consisted of People's and Workers' clinics providing curative care for the adult population and for those in employment. In 1983 the first polyclinic had been built and by the time of my visit a further four were in operation providing curative and preventive work and the follow-up of specific diseases. MCH Centres originally built as separate facilities were now being incorporated within the polyclinics.

I visited a number of facilities in Aden and Crater – two polyclinics, two People's clinics and four MCH centres. Abdul Ali Ahmed, the chief nurse, acted as my guide/interpreter in Aden and Crater – a pleasant, helpful, well-organised man who spoke and understood English pretty well. I very quickly realised that if I could act as a safety-valve and just listen to him I would probably find out a great deal more than by asking questions, and this proved to be the case. His frustration was bubbling over and preventing him from doing his day to day work: so much bureaucracy and unnecessary paperwork; a telephone system that was continually breaking down; and seriously unreliable transport for both patients and health workers, either breaking down with no mechanic available to carry out repairs, or due to a fickle supply of fuel. Sadly he was also very conscious of how poorly he had been trained, yet nobody seemed to care.

The People's Clinic and the MCH centre in Ma'alla were just what I had anticipated would be provided for the poor living in the grim Soviet-style flats as well as the residential districts of Rowda and Sheikh Othman. The two facilities were in need of repair, were unclean, ill-equipped, understaffed and largely empty of patients – they just didn't want to use them. Abdul encouraged the health workers and a few patients to talk and there was no holding back their complaints, everyone interrupting and trying to have their say. I had to rely on Abdul to translate honestly and he ended by saying:

> "The Ministry likes to tell you foreigners about things that don't exist and things that never happen."

The polyclinics at Al-Mansoora and Kharmaksar were a complete contrast. Opened in 1985 both were well staffed including pharmacists, laboratory and x-ray technicians. The population of Kharmaksar was less than 16,000 – three times less than that covered by a standard polyclinic; for the most part they were either Yemeni politicians, wealthy traders and money lenders, or foreign diplomats and people working for international agencies. Clearly this was the most prosperous district in Aden and as Abdul so accurately commented:

> "A population that the Ministry of Health wanted and needed to impress."

In addition eight 'national service' girls had been attached to the polyclinic in order to start two years of nurse training. 'National service' for boys involved two years in the military.

In Crater most of the housing, shops and *souks* were in the main volcanic bowl whilst the poor shanty dwellings and squalid slums were clear to see in the three or four smaller craters. In theory the People's Clinics were open between 8am and 8pm with doctors, medical assistants and practical nurses in attendance. The October 13 People's Clinic covered a population of around 70,000 and the facilities and staff were hopelessly inadequate, as was the nearby MCH centre. Abdul did his best to get some response from the staff; their reaction was largely anger and frustration at the way they and their patients had been let down – 'all the money goes to the hospitals'. A few made comments about their poor training. As for the patients, mothers sat with their babies, quietly whispering and waiting; old men leaned on their sticks, and old women twisted and turned on the uncomfortable couches. A striking feature of both the People's Clinic and the MCH centre was how few patients had turned up considering how many people the clinics were responsible for (I asked to see the register). It was utterly depressing from everyone's point of view.

The two days spent at Lahej governorate did not disappoint, but on the other hand only confirmed what I had already been told at the Department of PHC and the Health Manpower Institute, and later at the Health Services Directorate in Habyleen in the Radfan district of the governorate. Latif and his colleagues in the Health Institute had been completely honest and made certain I realised that coverage was at best variable and in three governorates was totally inadequate. Latif said he couldn't emphasis enough that the data supplied by the Ministry rarely reflected the reality at the coalface.

The usual complaints of not enough money or rather not enough of anything, and the concentration on hospitals, were repetitive and universal, although as much discussion centred on the urgent need for more women to be involved in the rural scene. Both men and women were certain that females would be more likely to remain in an area, were more likely to be interested in health matters (universal throughout the world), and be more conscientious on timekeeping and looking after instruments, dressings and drugs, which were all in short supply. A strong case was certainly made, but an equally important point was highlighted in connection with the extremely low, sometimes non-existent, level of education in the rural population resulting in a complete lack of understanding of the link between faeces, flies, food and poor hygiene with simple diarrhoea and vomiting – the cause of death in so many babies and children under five.

In the rural sector, small villages with populations between 200 and 500 had health guides providing simple first aid and advice on sanitation and the maintenance of clean water. It has also been hoped that mothers would bring their children for immunisation but so far this hadn't happened. Traditional Birth Assistants (TBAs) were available if wanted. In the early '80s in the Lahej governorate health guides had started to receive further training, whilst *giddas* were being used in managing childbirth – a *gidda* literally means a grandmother or woman in the close family circle who traditionally was far more involved than the TBAs. Reliable data did not exist, but it was accepted that at least 80% of deliveries were dealt with by *giddas,* about 18% by TBAs and only 2% by trained midwives.

Rural health units provided care for villages with populations between 3,000 and 8,000 – again just simple curative care plus the usual *gidda*/TBA work. In addition there would be a small locked dispensary with some prescription drugs.

By the time of my arrival two types of health centres had been established. Type 1 was just an upgraded rural health unit and type 2 was a rural hospital with up to 20 or 30 beds for medical and obstetric work, a dispensary, a simple laboratory and sometimes an x-ray unit for chest, skull and limb x-rays.

I managed visits to two health units and two health centres, journeys that took some time as they were on unmade roads and tracks. The PHC Directorate and the Health Manpower Institute in Al Hotta as well as the Health Services Directorate in Habeelin completed my first day and it was in these organisations that a strong case was made against women doctors. It was alleged they were no different from their male colleagues in being reluctant to work in rural areas and often didn't turn up for work. Female medical assistants rather than doctors were acceptable as they were more likely to live locally, and the continuity of care they provided might encourage mothers not only to turn up themselves but at the same time bring their children along for immunisation.

Everyone working in the health units and health centres agreed that more supervision and regular checking of facilities was needed – this would raise standards and greatly improve morale. Finally, regular clinics conducted by visiting paediatricians and obstetricians and/or gynaecologists should be introduced, and there was united agreement that the specialists should be female. The problem was to persuade hospital specialists to work in the community.

Lahej governorate, in spite of being adjacent to Aden, was quite different. I had not anticipated the amount of fertile land enclosed within the dark barren rocky hills. I recall clearly the sudden appearance as if from nowhere of two gardens filled with flowers of the most wondrous and breathtaking colours, to be followed by desolate *wadis* mostly of scrub and flattened eucalyptus trees resembling inverted umbrellas, and then the occasional undulating waves of golden sand. Army camps were a regular feature and we passed through three military checkpoints – all very tedious with the officers cross-questioning my companions and pointing at me while young soldiers surrounded the car and proudly showed off their kalashnikovs.

On that first day we had only been driving for about an hour when we arrived at a small village with a busy market on both sides of the road. I asked if we could stop and wander. There was a profusion of fruit, vegetables and salad as well as a mind-boggling display of anything you could think of – piles of empty bottles, paraffin in large metal containers, hairbrushes and combs, old car and bicycle wheels and tyres, ladies' necessities and bottles of perfume, half-used biros, a few pencils and pencil sharpeners, rusty scissors and knives and an endless selection of china and metal plates. There were replacement parts for cars and lorries, and broken-down donkey carts could be repaired on the spot. Children's clothing was neatly laid out along the road with bundles of well-worn sandals and shoes and much else beside. Everyone was shouting and bargaining – something Arabs love to do.

On returning to the car I found my colleagues talking to the Director of Health Services for the Radfan district, which lay north-east of the village. He had been travelling in the opposite direction to us but turned round to follow us instead. Presumably the meeting he had been due to attend came to nothing – a perfect example of the Arab way of doing things.

Our destination was the health unit at the small village of Al Habeelin, and about a mile before the village we stopped to pass the time of day with two male medical assistants and their donkeys, which were used for transport. We all arrived at the unit, including the Director, and chatted for a while, but I could see the medical assistants were keen to show me something in the village. It turned out to be the nearby water supply which was having to be pulled from the well by hand as the pump had broken three years ago and the promised replacement had never arrived. I brought this to the attention of the Director, but whether a replacement ever arrived I never found out. My enquiries about sanitation caused embarrassment as, even though official pits had been dug, the population ignored the pits and defecated almost anywhere.

The health unit we visited the next day in a small village was much the same as that at Al Habeelin. However, the health centre in a large village had an attached MCH unit with a delivery room and a few beds for both pregnant mothers and medical problems. It was a surprise to find most homes had piped water, and the majority of them had also recently been connected to electricity. Sanitation remained the same – the clearing of sewage from the pits was virtually non-existent, so not surprisingly people preferred to defecate at the edge of the village rather than in fly-infested pits.

As we drove towards the frontier with the YAR a really noticeable change was taking place. First of all it became more mountainous with a dramatic, stark, inhospitable backdrop and second, the majority of buildings took on the distinctive unique character of the memorable architecture of its northern neighbour.

On occasions I felt embarrassed by the efforts that had been made on my behalf and the way I had been welcomed and the friendly behaviour of everyone I met. For thousands of years or more Yemen had been isolated and difficult to reach, but for the past four to five hundred years reports from European travellers had one constant, unchanging observation on the warmth of their greetings, however rich or poor they might be. I could certainly confirm this.

It was noticeable how much less I heard the *muezzin* on its call five times a day to prayer: a great difference compared with other countries I had visited. It would seem that the Marxist ideology of Soviet socialism had had a considerable effect on day to day life.

For Muslims, Friday, the holy day of prayer, is more like a public holiday in the PDRY, so I was determined to make use of the day off, and not by attending midday prayer. The distance between my hotel and Crater was about two and half miles. It was about 80° F when I set off and I decided not to stop and explore but make my way to Crater as quickly as possible. I had climbed up through Ma'alla and was just able to see the road leading up a steep incline through a gap in the barren hills. Two young policemen stopped me and asked if I was Russian or East German, finally asking to see my passport – in fact I had been asked on a number of occasions if I was Russian. They spoke a little English and asked where I was going. When I replied I was heading for Crater, to my astonishment they hailed a taxi and insisted on paying the fare. I was puzzled and nervous – what were they expecting from me and was the taxi driver involved? It was all very strange but nothing untoward happened and the taxi driver didn't ask for more money. As I left the two policemen all I could say was:

"Shukran, shukran, salaam aleikum"

"Thank you, thank you, peace be with you."

Only a few buildings remained from earlier times but evidence of British influence was everywhere with little attempt to change old imperial connections – the buildings still bore an eclectic mix of names such as Wellington, Kew, Dorset, Isis, Stevenage, Cumbria and others I have forgotten. Red PO boxes were still standing and on an outcrop of land on the edge of the town was an Anglican Gothic Revival church built at the end of the nineteenth century, now closed and falling down. No one stopped me entering the mosque Sayyid Abdullah al Aidrus, originally built in the fourteenth century and rebuilt in the nineteenth. It had a quiet calm interior with a few men sleeping and a couple of crows gently rotating on a fan hanging down from the ceiling. There was no religious service happening or even any evidence the mosque was still used.

In the middle of the town a dirty white minaret still stood, but the mosque was no more. The *souks* that sold gold and silver were not easy to find, but the market and the *souk* selling *qat* were crowded, and tempting smells lured me to the main market selling fruit, vegetables, herbs and all manner of spices and incense. Most of the goods came from the Lahej governorate. Children were everywhere; the most popular games seemed to be hopscotch and football. Old men played dominoes and chess and while most played chess at the usual leisurely pace small groups were playing at breakneck speed – fascinating to watch but I never discovered why nor have I ever seen the like since.

I hadn't found the most famous site in Crater, the Tanks, or more accurately I hadn't been looking as I'd decided to leave them for the following Friday. As I walked back to my hotel the grimness of Ma'alla really sank in; the street was about a half mile long with quite a steep gradient which was obviously hard work for the women as the shops were inconveniently spread about. Keeping control of the many children was also pretty testing. On reflection, though, running tap water and flush lavatories probably compensated for almost anything so perhaps their lives were not as difficult as I imagined.

A hundred yards or so beyond the end of the flats I came across a large Christian cemetery surrounded by high metal fencing. How I hadn't spotted it earlier God knows. It didn't appear to be part of the Imperial War Graves Commission. The graves were mostly for men and boys in their late teens to middle thirties, a number of women who had died in childbirth, and babies and children succumbing to illnesses of the Victorian/Edwardian eras as a result of the lack of immunisation and living in an age before the advent of antibiotics. Most of the men had been in the army or the navy and I could well imagine very few would have had any idea where Yemen was, no idea why they were there or who they were fighting. Two graves in particular interested me – 2nd Lt W J Stephen, and Lt Starkey from Rosscarbery in County Cork, a small village in the Republic of Ireland which my family and I know very well.

As I left the cemetery groups of Soviet sailors were coming up from the harbour. Their battle cruisers had docked a couple of days earlier, which had created a feeling of reassurance as it was only a year before that the bloody uprising had led to the difficult evacuation of foreigners. If some internal unrest were suddenly to arise at least the Soviet navy might be able to rescue me and other foreigners. Nothing happened, of course – perhaps I had been unsettled by the episode on the causeway (more of this later). The sailors looked so young, barely out of school, and like the dead young men in the cemetery I felt certain they had little idea where they were or why.

Before this, however, as I was leaving Crater and had just reached the roundabout where the Yemen policemen had been so helpful, I could see many Soviet sailors wandering all over the place. A small group approached me, obviously thinking I was Russian, two of them shaming me by speaking a little English. They wanted to know how to get to Aden. They didn't want to catch a bus and anyway hadn't realised they had to buy a ticket before they could get on, so I managed to persuade them to walk rather than take a taxi, and they set off cheerfully. They seemed such open friendly lads, none of them drunk or rowdy, and I could well imagine their officers giving them strict instructions before they disembarked about how they should behave. It was difficult to accept they were my 'Cold War' enemy.

My second 'Holy Friday' enabled me to climb *Jabal* Shamsan, the mountain dominating Aden. Having no map I was advised to start at Gold Mohur beach, much used by the locals. The taxi driver wasn't keen to take me and hailed a couple of locals. They were united in their advice – 'no it's only for the military' – and I had to agree there were rather a lot of armed soldiers about. There was no alternative other than to walk further round the coast to the next beach which was crowded with Russians of every shape and size, just as I imagined the Black Sea might be.

Fortunately it was cloudy otherwise I think the heat plus the extra walking might have deterred me. The first half mile or so was over barren rocky terrain with a few stunted trees. The track then became steeper but still presented no real difficulties except for areas of scree which were quite dangerous – the ground was so dry that even quite large rocks were easily dislodged. Temporarily losing my way I had to retrace my steps to get round a gully so as to reach the ridge. All was deserted and silent except for a Russian sailor who gave me a wave, some interesting birds with distinctive calls and spectacular colours, a few little birds similar to rock pipits, and a variety of raptors.

It had taken just over two and a half hours to reach the main ridge and what a view awaited me although I was still not at the actual summit. Luck was with me when I spotted a track coming up from the Crater area – two Yemenis appeared climbing slowly up, so I followed them to the summit.

In spite of a heat haze I was able to identify Gold Mohur beach, Little Aden, Steamer Point, the Clock Tower and Tawahi district, the Christian cemetery, the flats of Ma'alla, the dreaded causeway, Kharmaksar, the beach from where the evacuation to the Royal Yacht *Britannia* had taken place, and finally Crater. By the time I had taken in the wonderful panoramic view the two Yemenis had disappeared.

The walk down to Crater was easy and the Tawilla or Aden Tanks quickly came into view; they had been dug into the mountain to conserve any rain as it poured down from *Jabal* Shamsan. On the highest slopes eighteen tanks of varying size had been cut out of solid rock. The upper tanks obviously filled up first and overflowed into the lower ones, finally ending up with the largest at ground level. Nobody is certain, but the consensus is that they were originally constructed about 400BC. The British can take credit for the careful repairs carried out over the first half of the twentieth century, a truly amazing engineering achievement, and the beautiful gardens surrounding the lower tanks added something quite special. The best view of course is from above.

What was the 'dreaded causeway'? I had been in the country for three days and a meeting had been arranged at the last moment in connection with the Expanded Programme of Immunisation (EPI). I decided to catch a bus to the Kharmaksar area, sit and have some lunch in the colourful shaded gardens and then walk along the causeway to the Ministry of Health – the sea on one side and a muddy lagoon on the other full of many birds – I managed to identify flamingo, black and grey heron, redshank and dunlin, but without binoculars a number of ducks and waders remained a mystery.

I had noticed military aircraft coming in to land and flying over the causeway, but had thought no more about it and started taking photographs in the hope I might later be able to identify some of the birds – a stupid idea in itself as I only had a small instamatic camera that was not at all up to the job. At the end of the causeway a small number of military vehicles had gathered. Again I thought no more about it and continued bird watching. The noise of one of the army trucks made me suddenly look up. It was speeding towards me and stopped in a dramatic fashion. Two soldiers jumped out and ran towards me, indicating with their kalashnikovs to move towards the truck. A couple of officers arrived and we stood looking at each other, unable to communicate. Very soon a police van screeched to a halt and I was driven to a small concrete pillbox near the Aden hotel, which still showed bullet holes and damage from the fighting the previous year. With no windows and just a small doorway, after the best part of an hour it was getting extremely hot and I was becoming very anxious as my passport, camera and other papers had been taken. No one spoke. Eventually a couple of air force officers arrived and took me to the main police station in Kharmaksar. Upstairs in the main office a portrait of Lenin hung on the wall and a metal bust stood on the table. Still no one spoke but at least I was given a chair so I could sit down. An interpreter then arrived and explained we were waiting for someone else, but he refused to say who it was.

A further forty minutes passed before a man in civilian clothes came in and started to question me about almost anything, and I was made to write down my replies. He asked aggressively:

> "Don't you know you have been in a forbidden military zone and photographing a military airport?"

He didn't believe I didn't know and continued:

> "How long have you been in the army? Are you allowed to take photographs in the UK? Are you free to go into a bookshop? What do you know about the PDRY? How many photographs have you taken in Aden already? Do you have a wife and children? Where do your parents live?"

And so he went on with a bored expression on his face, his questions becoming more and more bizarre and seemingly pointless.

After some argument I was allowed to try and phone Dr Badr at the Ministry of Health, but without success as he was still away from Aden; at least the Ministry knew why I hadn't turned up for the EPI meeting. Nearly five hours after my arrest I was driven back to my hotel – minus passport, documents and camera and – later as I was to discover – my airline tickets. Looking back I've no idea why I didn't contact the British Embassy sooner as by now I was really quite worried.

In the morning I phoned them and was instructed to contact them again if all my possessions hadn't been returned within twenty-four hours. It was interesting to find out where the Ministry of Health came in the pecking order of influence and importance in the eyes of the Ministry of the Interior – almost at the bottom, so my Yemeni colleagues informed me, probably on a par with Education. It transpired that the Deputy Minister had contacted the Ministry of the Interior on two occasions, but to no avail. It was only when Dr Badr finally arrived back in Aden that I was promised my passport, camera and tickets would be handed over the next day.

The presence and commitment of UNICEF, the WHO and the World Bank, seemed as strong here as in the YAR, and even though there were differences, the overall strategies were similar. However, the medical input from outside countries was quite different. Only Sweden was represented in both countries with their Save The Children Fund projects related to MCH, to the training of midwives and TBAs and family planning – their commitment was impressive.

But neither East nor West Germany nor France were present and US Aid was also absent as was the British Council. Without any doubt the country with the greatest presence and most influence was Cuba – financially, the Soviet Union.

For my final day two meetings had been organised. The first one was at the Ministry of Health with Dr Badr, the Minister. We had briefly met in Kuwait at a meeting of the Council of Arab Ministers of Health in September 1986 when he had renewed my invitation after my initial visit had been cancelled on account of the revolution. He was genuinely apologetic about my 'arrest' and we parted on good terms. At the Department of PHC a long chat lasting most of the morning with Abdul Latif confirmed my initial impression that he was a decent, hard-working, conscientious and intelligent man. Our conversation meandered and at one point he 'confessed' that when he had visited Europe he was frequently ashamed of being an Arab because of the behaviour of many from Saudi Arabia and the Gulf States. He was anxious for me to understand that he and his family might be poor but they knew how to behave – his parents were believing Muslims. He was certain that if the PDRY had similar wealth to Saudi and the Gulf States the money would be spent more wisely and certainly in a more socially responsible manner. I regret we never met again.

The Embassy in Aden had been most helpful and had supported me over the years in negotiating with the Ministry of Health and keeping up the pressure on contacts within the Ministry. Mr Marshall, the present Ambassador, who had been closely involved in the evacuation of hundreds of people to the *Britannia*, had suggested it would be best, certainly more useful to him, if we could meet at the end of my visit. He could then listen to my assessment of health care and ask his own questions.

We duly met at the Embassy the day before my departure. Mr Marshall was on his final posting. Unpretentious and easy to talk to, it soon became clear he was genuinely interested in getting appropriate aid and support to the PDRY. Over the past months, in fact since the uprising the previous year, he had been in regular contact with the

Ministry of Overseas Development in London over a number of suggestions he had made, including some that related to health. He had been deeply frustrated and annoyed at receiving no response. He asked me what I thought. This enabled me to talk about one of my bête-noires regarding health – the Ministry of Overseas Development! In my experience their plans were either hospital-dominated or focused on the supply of hi-tech equipment – making money out of exports was their primary interest rather than becoming involved in giving appropriate advice or endeavouring to focus on the needs of the country concerned. To me the Ministry of Overseas Development in relation to health matters gave the most inappropriate type of aid – mostly useless and even harmful to the poorer countries of the world.

We retired to his residence for drinks in the garden before lunch, all very civilised. David Spencer the First Secretary, who had also helped me, accompanied by his awful wife from Newcastle, another couple whose name I have forgotten, and the Ambassador's Indian wife who was also his secretary, made up the lunch party. The awful wife must have been a great embarrassment to him, seemingly unaware of her ignorance about the Arabs and even more where Russians were concerned.

After a very pleasant couple of hours I decided, to everyone's surprise, to walk back to my hotel – admittedly it was a couple of miles. It transpired none of them had ever used the public bus service and even the Ambassador had no idea how or where you bought a ticket – he mistakenly thought the ticket was bought on the bus, just as I had thought on my first trip to Crater.

The final *'blick'* from this faraway land was at the mini-bar in the small departure area of its tiny international airport. I was using up my local currency on a glass of mango juice and a cup of black coffee. I then asked for orange juice and waited for departure. Unexpectedly the girl at the bar came over with a cup of black coffee as well, which naturally I offered to pay for. She simply refused to accept any money, a circumstance very similar to the young boy when I first ventured on a bus only to find I couldn't buy a ticket on the bus – in the confusion he came over, gave me a ticket and refused any payment. And I mustn't forget the two young policemen and the taxi . . .

What a fascinating but almost unfathomable country.

28

ARABIAN/PERSIAN GULF

Britain's influence over the small sheikhdoms and villages along the coast of the Arabian/Persian Gulf began at the beginning of the nineteenth century. Starting with Bahrain in 1816, then Abu Dhabi, Dubai, Sharjah, Ras al-Khaimah, Ajman, Umm al-Qaiwan and Fujairah, they became known as the Trucial States, so called because of a special treaty of relationship with Britain following the signing of a maritime truce in 1836. These seven sheikhdoms, all being little more than fishing villages with populations of around 2,000, experienced regular attacks by pirates and the Truce put them under British protection.

After the Second World War oil and gas exploration in the Trucial States were initially ignored as discoveries had already been made in Kuwait and Qatar and of course Saudi Arabia. Oil was not in fact discovered in Abu Dhabi until the late 1950s. Eventually the seven states united in 1971 to form a federation that became known as the United Arab Emirates (UAE). Qatar had been part of the Ottoman Empire throughout the nineteenth century and didn't become a British Protectorate until the middle of the First World War, remaining so until 1971 when it became a sovereign independent state. Both Bahrain and Qatar were approached to join the UAE but declined.

Kuwait had been an independent and autonomous Arab sheikhdom under the rule of an Amir from the eighteenth century although the British had established a protectorate from 1897 until independence in 1961. At no time had the Amir of Kuwait shown any interest in joining the Trucial States or later the UAE. Two neighbouring countries, Saudi Arabia and Oman, did not become involved with the UAE, the former because of its size and its oil and gas reserves and the latter because of its strategic position at the Strait of Hormuz.

*

Had I been visiting a hundred years ago all these villages and settlements would have been indistinguishable except for their size: small harbours surrounded by mud-brick houses amongst narrow twisting alleyways, probably with a central market. There was sufficient ground water from wells to support the small populations and enough to allow for the growing of some fruit and vegetables. Beyond these settlements lay the inhospitable empty desert.

The Ottoman Empire and Persia (Iran) had always been significant powers in the region and the language and culture of these two countries as well as their politics have left their mark, and both Turkish and Iranian are still spoken. During the nineteenth century Tsarist Russia began to view the Gulf with a predatory eye although no more than Britain and France.

Diving for the most exquisite pearls, trading with the East, fishing, traditional *dhow* boat building and weaving were the main sources of employment whilst the safe harbours provided some protection against marauding pirates. However, in the 1930s the introduction of high quality artificial pearls from Japan caused a serious downturn in income – the artificial pearls were so much cheaper than the natural pearls, however beautiful. And so the Trucial States soldiered on in comparative poverty until the discovery of oil and gas changed everything for these isolated desert people.

Religion, especially over the last eighty to ninety years, has unfortunately not succeeded in creating peace and harmony. Islam is the official religion of the region although small Jewish and Christian minorities have been permitted. 80% of the indigenous population are Sunni and the remaining 20% are Shii who have been marginalised and ignored and have largely remained what they have always been – poor. A significant group of Islamic puritans known as *Wahhabis,* originating in Saudi Arabia and Qatar, believe many Muslims have fallen away from the strict true orthodoxy and discipline of Mohammad. Shii in particular and many Sunnis as well totally reject the *Wahhabis'* teaching and the historical basis of their claims.

In political terms whether these countries, in fact the entire Middle East, are described as autocracies, oligarchs, plutocracies, royal dynasties or military dictatorships matters little – all pretend to be governing with some form of democracy, yet nothing could be farther from the truth and whether they call themselves amirs or kings or presidents, all refuse to relinquish power.

Gerald Butt, the BBC's Middle East correspondent during the 1980s wrote in his book *The Arab World* about the region I am attempting to describe (but he does it so much better):

> 'Scattered pin pricks of orange flame in the blackness far below. An occasional cluster of white lights, the fingers of light marking the jetties stretching out into the blackening sea and further out the splodges of light where tankers are unloading. It's a view from an airliner at night which is familiar to hundreds and thousands of foreigners who have flown into the Gulf countries drawn by the magnet of work and high wages which accompanied the oil boom. That view from the plane tells you a lot about the region – the oil wells on and off shore with gas being flared off, the lonely dots of civilisation in vast tracts of emptiness which by day amount to seemingly endless miles of khaki-brown sand broken occasionally by the needle line of an oil pipe or a cross-desert road.'

Is there anything to add to Gerald Butt? Not much really. In essence it is just a vast empty land mass, very sparsely populated along the coast with the miniscule population living in barely a dozen towns.

As a first-time visitor to this part of the world I immediately wondered how the culture and traditions of the locals would cope with the prodigious wealth provided by oil and gas. Writing now, twenty-five years later, I believe my unease was not misplaced – I felt even then that contemporary architecture was overtaking the UAE and this was only a prelude of what was to come. It was not that traditional buildings and markets and *souks* had been destroyed or allowed to fall down or disappear, rather it was that tradition had been totally overshadowed by ostentatious excess with every chain of banks or financial centres or hotels or government buildings vying with each other to become the tallest or biggest or most spectacular structure in the world. Qatar, Abu Dhabi and Dubai are regularly seen on our television screens and we can all see what money and technology and an obsessive need to demonstrate they are now part of the modern world, has done to society. Wealth is displayed in an unashamedly up-front, almost vulgar manner: how many more buildings of even greater height can be constructed? The urban skyline of America, Japan, China, Brazil, in fact anywhere in the world, has now been equalled and will be overtaken. But what has this technology of steel and glass done for the locals' way of living?

29

THE STATE of KUWAIT

Kuwait occupies the north-west corner of the Persian Gulf: the kingdom of Saudi Arabia lies to the south and west, the Republic of Iraq to the north and west, and 160 miles of coastline lies to the east. Its landmass is flat stony desert and scrubland, remote, undisturbed and involved mainly with camel trading and the building of *dhows* for use in the Gulf, along the east coast of Africa and beyond as far as Indonesia. Everything changed in the early 1930s with the discovery and subsequent drilling of oil.

Soon after the publication of *An Analysis of Primary Medical Care* in 1979 I wrote to my editor at the Cambridge University Press floating the idea of a similar study of the Arab world – at the time no publication either in English or Arabic had been attempted on the subject of primary health care. Soon after this my editor was transferred to New York and he passed on my suggestion to his successor, who responded by saying she was definitely interested but my proposal would not be at the top of her current plans. She didn't think this would create any problems for either of us as it was going to take me some years to complete the study and the travelling involved. Some three or four years later she wrote to ask if I was getting impatient and suggested that if I wanted an immediate contract I should perhaps look elsewhere than the CUP. I asked her advice, the MacMillan Press was proposed and they agreed to publish.

Obviously the more support and interest I could garner the better, so I made contact with the WHO Director for the East Mediterranean Region in Alexandria and the chairman of the Arab Board of Health Ministers with it headquarters in Damascus. It was finally agreed I should meet members of the Arab Board and representatives of the WHO at their Regional Conference in Kuwait in October 1986 – I hoped that I could combine this with my study of primary care in Kuwait. I arrived at Kuwait on Friday, 3 October, 1986, about six weeks before my visit to the YAR.

On my first morning, promptly at 9am my driver Abdullah Mobarak, whom I got to know well in a very short time, turned up at the Sheraton hotel to take me to the Ministry of Health. Dr Ali al-Said, chairman of the Arab Board of Health Ministers was to meet me at the WHO conference at the Regency hotel, which seemed reasonable enough; al Said's secretary suggested I should go straight over there. I was delayed by an almighty traffic jam caused by the Amir and his entourage who were just departing from the opening ceremony of the Conference, and it was after 11am by the time I managed to get into the hotel. In the foyer a pleasant young doctor collared me and asked if I was Dr Stephen – apparently I should have met him at the Qadesiya Health Clinic at 9.30 for the start of my programme on primary care. We both shrugged shoulders but inwardly I was furious at this cock-up.

Dr Sami Matar, the Director of PHC, introduced me to the Director of Clinics and to the Director of MCH and we set about discussing the programme for my visit. From the primary care point of view it was fine, but no time had been allocated for a meeting with the Board of Health Ministers, which was essential if the book was to be written. There was no reason why Matar should understand the importance to me of meeting the health ministers; as far as he was concerned I was just writing a report on Kuwait. He did his best to reassure me:

> "No problem for you as there's a dinner tonight for the Ministers when you can meet them. Everyone will be there. I will arrange your invitation."

It was an extraordinary evening with the dinner being held in one of the city's most exclusive restaurants, and clearly I was meant to be impressed – comfortable surroundings, mountains of food and plenty to drink, starting with champagne. It was difficult to accept that the Arab ministers and delegates of the WHO were here to discuss the problems facing the health services in the region, and not least to focus on the issue of widespread poverty in most of the countries in the Middle East. The inappropriateness of the great majority of delegates stuffing themselves with food and drink appeared to cause no embarrassment to anyone. The final absurdity were the toilets with scented lavatory paper.

As I tried to talk about my book to His Excellency the Minister of Health of Kuwait, it was impossible for him to listen to me at the same time as shaking hands with a long queue of delegates, which was exactly what I had predicted. Still, to give him his due, he suggested I meet with him and his colleagues the next day. Who knows, it might even happen! One delegate seemed to know as few people as I did and he turned out to be most interesting and extremely talkative, mostly about politics and poverty and the problems for the Palestinians. Eventually I discovered he was the representative for the Palestinian Liberation Organisation (PLO).

The next morning Abdullah drove me to the PHC Office even though it was only two minutes walk from the hotel. Dr Matar had no idea why I was there, and as I had no idea either he immediately suggested I should go to see Mrs Amal, the Minister's secretary, whom I had previously met as she had been responsible for arranging my programme.

"Which hotel are you staying in?"
"The Sheraton"
"Oh my god, I especially arranged the Regency for you – that's where the WHO conference is being held. Did you go to the Qadesiya clinic yesterday morning?"
"No, because I didn't get the programme in time."
"Oh my god, I do all this work and it's just a waste of time."

I felt really sorry for this poor lady but didn't have the nerve to agree with her. However, after a couple of cups of sweet tea she recovered and set about re-arranging my meetings. I owed a lot to her.

After thanking Mrs Amal I met His Excellency, as had been suggested, and all his colleagues on the Board. A fortuitous meeting with the Minister from the PDRY was a real bonus as I was able to tell him about my intended visit to Aden the following year. A final meeting with the Board before they all departed was agreed, so I felt reasonably satisfied.

I was undecided about sitting through the final two-hour session but when I learned that Halfdan Mahler, the Director General of the WHO, was to speak I needed no persuasion. He was the man who had changed people's thinking about health care and had been responsible for the International Conference in Alma Ata in 1978; it was from this conference that the slogan 'Health For All by the Year

2000' had emerged. He had highlighted the necessity of concentrating on primary care if any progress was to be made. Writing today in 2015, he remains the most distinguished and influential thinker at the WHO since its inception in 1948. He spoke clearly and briefly and without doubt was in a class of his own. How he was able to tolerate spending so much time listening to what he already knew and to people who had nothing fresh to say, was the penalty I suppose for being in charge of an international bureaucracy.

One person I had particularly hoped to meet was Dr Ali al-Said, the Director of the East Mediterranean Region, but he had been delegated to escorting Halfdan Mahler to the airport. Anyway, I was told not to worry as it was being arranged that I should attend the final dinner that evening.

The evening was as lavish as the previous night, no holding back, no thought of restraint, as extravagant and excessive as the sumptuous entrance hall and the grand staircase, a sort of Arab rococo. Indescribable, really. The get-together and the food were outside beside a pool where three young women played a piano, violin and cello – Palm Court music mixed with classical and pop and occasional outbursts of organ music, from where I couldn't decide except that it seemed to emanate from the darkness of the beach. Again no one was concerned about the extravagant provision of food and drink, except for the PLO chap and a delightful representative from Afghanistan, Dr Sayed Ahmed who, like the PLO representative, felt isolated, lonely and had nothing in common with anyone – very much a poor relation, and in fact his government could barely afford to send him, unlike the four or five delegates from most of the other countries represented there. It is certainly a small world – it transpired he had studied for his Diploma in Public Health in Bristol in 1971. He was complimentary about the Department of Public Health/ Community Medicine, valued his studies in the UK and considered his training to have been thorough. I found it really refreshing talking to him, as if we were from the same planet. En passant I found he had visited Wells.

International organisations certainly know how to look after themselves and spare no expense, but inevitably they become remote from the people they are meant to be helping.

Endeavouring to combine a study of primary care with organising meetings with the WHO and the Board of Arab Health Ministers was proving difficult and frustrating, and looking back it was probably rather an ill-advised idea. Changes from day to day, often hour to hour, was like a game of Snakes and Ladders – just as I thought everything was fine the crucial person or essential document would go missing. Or like a jigsaw when, about to put in the final piece, I would find two others had been removed.

At the time of my visit 63 phc facilities were operational – 49 Type 1 centres (originally called dispensaries) and 14 Type 2 centres (previously called Combined Centres or polyclinics). Type 1 provided basic care and was slowly including care of children. Type 2 provided MCH services as well as visiting specialists carrying out regular weekly out-patient sessions. Seven of the Type 2 centres had 15-30 beds plus one or two labour rooms for normal confinements, staffed by trained midwives.

The idea of general practice had been superficially discussed in the '60s but nothing happened until the Ministry of Health and the Royal College of General Practitioners in the UK met for the first time in the late '70s. At this point the Ministry agreed that family practice was to be the corner-stone of primary care and would require post-graduate training culminating in an exam for the Diploma of Family Practice. In 1984 the first doctors started their training (carried out under the supervision of the College of GPs in the UK), and gained the Diploma in 1987.

The training was based in two Type 2 centres at two districts in Kuwait City – Medan Hawalli and Qadesiya – where I was able to see trainers and trainees at work. Dr Mansour Sarkhol was a splendid, enthusiastic, intelligent and well-organised young man – his official titles were Director, Family Medicine Training Unit and Chairman, Faculty of Family Medicine at the Institute of Medical Specialisation. He was not remotely surprised about my disorganised time and was confident that had my programme been handed over to him by Mrs Amal everything would have run smoothly. Naturally I passed no comment but thought he was probably right. Anyhow, I enjoyed listening to the keen and interested group of trainers he was supervising – it seemed to bode well for the future.

Modern medicine had been introduced to Kuwait by an American missionary group about the same time the Amir had formed a government under a British Protectorate. The first government clinic for women was set up by the American missionaries in 1917 but it wasn't until 1939 that the first primary care dispensary was opened, and a further ten years before the first hospital was established.

Public health had progressed steadily as Kuwait's new-found wealth had been used wisely. By 1986 clean piped water had reached the majority of the population, over 80% of houses were connected to a piped sewage system and rubbish was regularly collected from the streets. Electricity and air-conditioning followed, reaching most homes in the main urban areas. State education was free as was the health service, demonstrating again the judicious use of wealth. The status and attitude towards women and girls was astonishing; 95% of boys and 92% of girls attended primary school while 86% of boys and 79% of girls were enrolled in secondary school. Within the state health service 300 Kuwaiti male and 335 female doctors were employed. Compared with the rest of the Arab world the position of women was remarkable and something that took me by surprise.

Under-utilisation of primary care facilities was common throughout the Arab world due to the filthy, unhygienic conditions for both patients and health personnel alongside the serious lack of female health professionals. None of this applied to Kuwait.

The socio-economic situation, which had improved dramatically since the Second World War, had clearly improved the mortality and morbidity statistics regarding mothers, babies and children. But could everything really be quite as rosy as it seemed? Two things enabled me to get a better perspective and a more realistic feel of how people I would never meet might be living. The first was through my driver Abdullah Mobarak, and the second through not having a car and being able to walk wherever I wanted.

The day after the evening reception given by the WHO, Abdullah had asked me how things had turned out and what was it like. I told him, he asked me some questions and finally said:

> "You can't build a culture with money, you can only build buildings and they're always being changed."

We talked a little about his family and friends and how they lived.

They had no air-conditioning for at least four months in the year and it was really grim without it. He knew a number of ex-pat men working in the construction industry and told me how little they were paid and how their passports had been confiscated, some even stolen. His wife knew a number of women, mainly from Indonesia, India and Pakistan who had confided to her many of their troubles. Abdullah was adamant that construction workers spoke with one voice – 'of course the pay is poor, what else can a foreigner expect?' and all were angry about their passports – 'we are prisoners'. Abdullah and his wife and people like them were rarely heard and I suspect never listened to.

I asked him what he could suggest for me to do during my short stay in his country and how I might get a more accurate impression of the place:

"Just walk around and look."

At every opportunity I did just that. I had an excellent map and Abdullah gave me suggestions about where I should go. It was interesting, and not just from a medical point of view. Many houses and buildings were in a dilapidated state and the inhabitants were obviously poor. I don't remember seeing any real slum conditions which in part was due to there being little overcrowding in the more recently built houses. Superficially I saw no serious malnutrition and all the small shops were full of locals, as were the vegetable markets.

People from the Indian sub-continent dominated the main streets with the women wearing the most beautiful dresses, gowns and saris in every colour and shade. One Sunday I was standing in the large open space in front of a Roman Catholic church. It was simply heaving with people as they left the church and it was noticeable that there were many more people here than I'd seen at the main mosque on the previous Friday's midday call to prayer, where of course there were only men to be seen. I needed to remind myself that those from the Indian sub-continent gave a misleading impression; they tended to be the entrepreneurs, were mostly wealthy and were certainly not employed in the construction industry or in sweeping roads or in domestic service – no, it was not easy to find the poor, who were mostly indigenous Kuwaitis and females from Indonesia brought in primarily for domestic service.

Britain and Kuwait have had an entangled relationship and the only reminders I found of our presence there were two red double-decker buses and two Rolls Royce cars (surrounded by wealthy Arabs and Indians).

About eighteen months after talking to Abdullah and listening to his wife, a symposium was held at the University of Kuwait's Department of Educational Psychology. The conclusion at the end of the meeting was that Kuwait's society was being seriously undermined by the absence of proper parenting, which was directly related to misuse of domestic servants – parents had in many cases virtually opted out and servants had been forced to accept responsibility for the children. When a child was ill it was the servant who took them to see a doctor or a nurse in spite of the fact they rarely spoke or understood Arabic. A study in 1986 had shown that when domestics (mainly Indonesian) had been enticed or otherwise persuaded to come to Kuwait, no mention was ever made that they could be fully in charge of the children – permanent baby-sitters in fact. Poor pay, often no pay at all, as well as the confiscation of their passports completed the story.

Article 10 of the Constitution of the State of Kuwait states:

> 'The State provides care to the youth and protects them from exploitation and from moral, physical and spiritual neglect.'

Grand words, but it was now clear that the culture of affluence and greed was changing society. Anxieties were surfacing concerning the impact many aspects of western culture were having on traditional Arab societies. I recall meeting two Kuwaiti doctors, one a trained psychiatrist, and both were adamant that the increasing tensions within families were leading to the breakdown of society as well as an increase in psychiatric illness. This symposium had certainly highlighted what I had been told by Abdullah and his wife.

At the final meeting of the Arab Board of Health Ministers, Professor Khageli, Dean of the newly-founded Gulf University centred in Bahrain, had been invited to join us. He had been given an impossible task at the very last minute – just twenty-four hours to read the Introduction and four completed chapters of my book. He was quite complimentary and supportive and expressed his belief that there was a need for such a book. So far so good.

I was nervous that five years' work was in the balance – how much support and interest could I really expect? A member of the Board explained they had no executive power to purchase a specified number of copies, but the Board seemed quite optimistic, particularly if the book was marketed well and published in both Arabic and English. Then came the proviso I had been dreading and half expecting – regarding the Persian Gulf I had only included Kuwait, and unless Bahrain, Qatar and the United Arab Emirates were also included this would prove to be an insurmountable obstacle and support would be withdrawn. I enquired about Saudi Arabia and Oman who also hadn't been included, explaining I had been refused visas by both countries. Inexplicably neither the absence of Saudi or Oman proved to be a stumbling block – I never understood the reason.

The years rolled on and almost exactly four years after meeting the Arab Board of Health Ministers in June 1990, David Grist, senior editor at MacMillan, Dr Curtis Rhodes, the Director of Mediterranean Medical & Health Care Resources working at the time in Cyprus, and an Arab publisher from Lebanon, all met at my home in Wells to discuss the final layout of the book, its production, publication and sales. We all agreed how vital it was to publish in both English and Arabic. Everything seemed to be heading towards a satisfactory conclusion.

Unfortunately the world-wide economy at this time was in dire straits and MacMillan UK was taken over by MacMillan USA ten days after our meeting in Wells. David Grist was informed that a North American publisher had to be found specifically to organise sales in the USA; he was given three months to sort this out. Contact was made with a number of university presses – John Hopkins, Harvard, Washington, Yale, Seattle, Chicago, Stanford and others. Not surprisingly it was impossible to organise anything within such a short timeframe; it seemed to me a way in which MacMillan USA could divest itself of a book it had no interest in. Within a couple of months David Grist contacted me to say he had been sacked. I felt genuinely sorry for him – I might not have my book but at least I hadn't lost my job.

Subsequently *Primary Health Care in the Arab World* was produced locally by Somerset House in Wells, by a friend, before he retired from publishing.

30

THE STATE of BAHRAIN

Bahrain lies just off the east coast of Saudi Arabia in a bay formed by the Qatar peninsular, and is made up of an archipelago of thirty-three islands, the largest being the island of Bahrain itself. The refining and export of oil is the main component of its economy and comes in a pipeline from Saudi Arabia to the terminals and refineries on Muharraq and Sitia islands, which are joined by separate causeways to Bahrain island. Two years before my visit, the construction of a fifteen-mile-long causeway linking the eastern province of Saudi with Bahrain island had commenced and was due to be opened at the end of 1988.

Occupied first by the Portuguese and then the Persians in the nineteenth century, Bahrain, like Kuwait, was involved in endless treaties with the British, finally becoming a British Protectorate at the end of the First World War. Oil was discovered in the 1930s and in fact Bahrain was the first Arab country to export oil. Soon, however, it became evident that the oil reserves were small, so the country changed course and took on extensive construction projects, at the same time expanding into banking and finance. In many ways Bahrain mirrored Kuwait but didn't gain independence until 1971, ten years after Kuwait.

Following independence, the National Assembly was set up by the Amir, but in 1975 it was dissolved, thus giving the Amir the freedom to appoint his own cabinet. Since then he and his extended family have retained complete control with little intention of developing anything resembling a democratic society, and over the last forty years the Amir has introduced only the most primitive elements of democracy, and always as a result of the demands of the poor who were and remain predominantly Shii, the Amir and his entourage being Sunni.

*

My flight, direct from Heathrow, arrived in Bahrain around 2am on Saturday, 6 February 1988. I was met and steered through passport control and customs efficiently and easily. The airport was sparklingly clean. As I was dropped off at a hotel, the driver told me I'd be picked up around 9.45am for a meeting with Dr Rashid Fulayfil, the Under-Secretary at the Ministry of Health, in fact the person I had been corresponding with over the last couple of years.

The meeting started promptly at 10am and it was the first time in any Arab country that the door was firmly closed and the office was not treated like a public thoroughfare. Nobody interrupted us – British influence perhaps?

Fulayfil was in his late fifties, knowledgeable and helpful, but over and above that he was organised and efficient. No time was wasted on tea or coffee, we just discussed the programme he had arranged. At one stage the Director of the College of Health Services joined us to confirm our meeting the following day, whilst the meeting at the Directorate of Health Centres was confirmed by phone. As the meeting came to an end, Fulayfil gave me the most up-to-date report on primary health care – it had been sitting on his desk so no need to ask his secretary to search for it. It was an impressive document with every aspect of primary care analysed.

The next meeting, with the Dean of the Medical School at the Gulf University, was not for a couple of hours so a driver was instructed to take me to the Old *Souk* and central market in Manamah (the *souk* was hardly old, being mostly built in the past twenty years). My impression of Manamah was of space and cleanliness, the buildings a dazzling white and the majority of roads lined by pavements – perhaps another legacy of the British. The skyline was of the usual tower blocks of banks, financial centres, luxury hotels and government buildings, all of which could be found anywhere in the world – traditional Arab architecture was rarely to be seen.

Gardens and parks and trees were a pleasant surprise, reminding me that Bahrain had never been short of water until quite recently. This valuable asset, almost unique in the Gulf region, was provided by artesian wells, many *ains* or natural springs, and sources of fresh water found in the shallows surrounding Bahrain island. Then, in the late 1970s, as the increasing population began to exceed the capacity of the natural supply of water, the first very costly desalination plants were built. By 1985 desalination provided the main supply of water.

My driver, who seemed happy to talk about the government, explained it was hell-bent on two policies – to reclaim as much land as possible and to build new towns. Large areas along the coast had already been reclaimed and it was to be an ongoing project. We drove quickly to Medinat Hamad, a new town which was near completion despite construction having started only two years previously, all the buildings, shops and the almost-finished mosque dramatic in their startling whiteness. The majority of labourers were from Pakistan or South Korea.

We had no time to linger if I was to see the Saudi causeway, which was near completion. Opinions were definitely divided about the benefits of this massive roadway for the ordinary citizens of Bahrain. Amongst the poor it was seen as just a means by which the Saudis could come to enjoy the fleshpots of Bahrain including the drugs and sex trade involving young women, girls and boys; little wonder there was anger amongst the mainly Shii population. A great number of the Wahhabi sect were in cahoots with the Amir and his extended family, and with wealthy financiers, businessmen and the officer corps of the army. As selling alcohol, gambling, frequenting night-clubs, and even playing music was and still is strictly forbidden in Saudi Arabia, unsurprisingly they were despised for their hypocritical behaviour.

Constant tension between the Amir and most of the population has led to endless riots and periodic fighting. The Shii represent 65% of the population and the Sunni ruling class the rest. Probably the grim sight of Saudi troops with tanks and armoured vehicles crossing the causeway in response to the Amir's request for help with serious unrest, had been a perfect example of the Amir's attitude towards his people. A number of western countries, with Britain to the fore, supplied and continue to supply military equipment to both countries.

A recent episode that showed how little understanding there was, concerned the holding of the 2014 Formula One Bahrain Grand Prix whilst the Amir's military police were killing rioters who were protesting against the unlawful imprisonment of intellectuals and of doctors who were treating those injured in the riots.

*

We arrived at the Medical School on time, but then the first hiccup occurred; the Dean was at another meeting, so Fulayfil arranged another meeting for the following day. The Director of Health Centres was happy to see me at short notice, explained about the organisation of primary care and provided me with a lot of data. Basically there were three types of health centres in operation. Type A covered populations of 20-30,000 and provided adult care, MCH and dental departments, and eight out of the ten centres had simple x-ray departments (chest, skull and limbs) and laboratories for basic procedures. Type B covered populations of 10-20,000 and provided the same services as Type A except there was no x-ray department. Type C with populations of 5-10,000 provided only a basic curative service. MCH services were provided by a visiting trained midwife and doctor, but this was in theory rather than fact.

It had been arranged I would visit four areas – al Maim, al Razin, al Hura and A'Ali. In spite of being the most basic Type C health centre A'Ali proved to be the most interesting. The building of this new town began in 1965 and was completed in roughly four years. By this time a basic dispensary was in operation and over the years it expanded until in 1983 it was upgraded to Type B. At the time of my visit A'Ali had become a suburb of Manamah and its population had risen to around 12,000.

The chief doctor was Egyptian and to start with she detailed the social conditions of her patients; all had clean piped water and electricity and most also had air-conditioning. Sewage disposal was less satisfactory due basically to the pipes rusting as they came out of the houses to connect with the main pipes in the road. Houses and flats were small, but she assured me they weren't overcrowded and offered to take me to look for myself (I had obviously been sceptical about this claim) but irritatingly I was told there was no time. She spoke English well and as she showed me round she was happy to answer questions and to admit to the problems she encountered. Family planning was now carried out by female doctors (mainly the oral contraceptive pill) and she was keen for me to understand that an ante-natal clinic had been included in the past year staffed by a female doctor, a trained midwife, and a female community nurse similar to a health visitor in the UK. All attended once a week. I wasn't able to verify if the addition of MCH services to Type C clinics had spread throughout the country.

In 1979 an interesting idea had been introduced into Type A and B clinics – the concept of the Family Physician, initiated by the American University in Beirut. As yet no training had begun in Bahrain but there was much talk about the 'Family Folder' which was to be kept in Type A and B clinics. When I asked my Egyptian colleague about this project and when it was likely to start, she replied with a smile and without hesitation:

"It's only a vision for the future."

Dr Ali Mohammad Matar, Dean of the Medical School at the Gulf University, was able to give me a history of this unique project. It had been founded in 1984 although the first students had already carried out two years' pre-clinical studies, which was to be followed by five years' clinical training with graduation in 1989, and then a year's internship. The initial intake of forty students had risen to sixty-five in 1988; originally a quota system had been in operation with preference given to the three countries without medical schools – Qatar, United Arab Emirates and Oman, but in 1987 things became complicated when Qatar and UAE opened their own medical schools. The setting up of the original medical school in Bahrain had been political in an attempt to convince the world that cooperation in the Gulf States was possible. There was even talk that cooperation might extend beyond medicine. Perhaps the main reason was that until 1984 all Bahraini doctors had had to be trained abroad, mainly in Egypt, Lebanon, the USA and the UK – and recently in Saudi Arabia.

The curriculum was to involve a new approach to medical education in which the focus would be to concentrate on the community; for this part of the world the concept was thought to be innovative, even futuristic. As I discussed this with the Dean and some of his colleagues it seemed to me it was going to be almost impossible to impose community participation in the health service when none existed in society itself. In simple terms, unless radical changes in the structure of society were to take place, primary care would remain the poor relation for the foreseeable future.

The Family Practice Residency Programme (FPRP) had in fact been introduced in 1978, as said earlier, under the supervision of the American University in Beirut; by 1987 thirty-three physicians – nineteen Bahrainis and fourteen from elsewhere – had finished the three-year course and been certified as Family Practice Trained. If all primary care physicians were to be trained as family doctors then it seemed to me great benefits could follow if Bahrain decided to cooperate with the Family Practice course in Kuwait rather than with the American University in Beirut. This would avoid the likelihood of conflict between the two supervisors – the American University in Beirut and the Royal College of General Practitioners in the UK.

Like the other countries in the Gulf, Bahrain had a significant expatriate population estimated in 1986 to be roughly 35% of the total population of 351,228, approximately 60% being male and 40% female. No information at all was available regarding their level of education, or how many were manual labourers or domestic servants.

With regard to the health service there was one physician per 800 population – at first glance this was a remarkable statistic but it was concealing two fundamental problems. The first was that three times as many doctors and six times as many nurses were employed in hospitals as in primary care. The second was that the number of doctors and nurses employed in primary care was almost equal, thus highlighting the serious shortage of nurses. The majority of non-Bahrainis working in hospitals were Indian and those in primary care were Egyptian. This in fact was a positive feature as it meant that the majority of doctors working in health centres were Arab speaking, and furthermore 50% of doctors both Bahraini and ex-pat were female.

The excellent maps of Bahrain and Manamah and the archipelago of surrounding islands, which had been produced in association with the Oxford University Press, provided a cultural imprint from the UK. Looking from the road that ran along some of the reclaimed land on the edge of Manamah, I was able to see Muharraq island and the well-known *Qalaat* (fort) Arad, other less well preserved *qalaats,* and the dhows and fishing boats in Muharraq harbour.

Three pieces of modern sculpture have been erected in the centre of Manamah: the stone model of two dhow sails on the Shaikh

Hamad Causeway, standing in a small ornamental garden – I think to commemorate independence; the monument of six curved white beams meeting at the top to hold and enclose a white sphere or pearl, representing the six nations of the Gulf, situated on a roundabout on the Manamah-Muharraq Causeway (known as the King Faisal Highway when I was there); and the large metal *dalla* or coffee pot to celebrate Bahrain's coffee-drinking tradition. The making of such pots had been a speciality for hundreds of years or more. Sadly this expertise has now disappeared, further indicating how the traditions and culture of the Gulf states are in danger of being swallowed up by different values.

The government is, however, aware of such dangers and has decided to try and preserve as many interesting and historic sites as possible, in particular the unique wind towers built in the traditional Gulf style – they were in use prior to the advent of air-conditioning and were surprisingly effective. A particular feature was how quiet they were in operation and many of the older generation preferred the peace and silence of the wind towers to the noise of air-conditioning. As I wandered around I was especially taken by the beauty of the carved wooden balconies on many private houses.

My experience was clearly limited, but I'm pretty sure that if I were an Arab I would resent the invasion of my culture by foreigners – in fact as a westerner I was at times embarrassed by their behaviour. One lunch time Fulayfil and the Minister's secretary took me to the Holiday Inn. It was surrounded by colourful gardens, an enchanting spot where the locals walked quietly about and family groups sat picnicking on the grass, their children playing around them. Inside the Inn all was bedlam and as the foreigners staggered out many were shouting and swearing and quite a few were drunk – the women were worse than the men – and it was still only early afternoon. It was an unqualified display of ostentatious vulgarity and bad taste.

Next stop Qatar, and little did I realise as I moved down the Gulf that I was going to find how Arab culture and customs were again being uprooted and replaced . . . .

31

THE STATE of QATAR

It should have been no surprise that the plane was preparing to land in Doha almost as soon as it took off from Manamah, since a number of the small islands that make up the archipelago of Bahrain lie less than two miles off the west coast of Qatar.

Saudi Arabia and Qatar are joined by salt flats; across this unmarked and unguarded frontier, nomads, Bedouins and others have journeyed to and fro for hundreds, probably thousands of years.

Qatar's royal family came from Central Arabia, now Saudia Arabia, and are directly related to the present Saudi royal family. Most of the Qatari population are Sunni, belonging to the Wahhabi sect, a strictly orthodox and puritanical movement originating in the eighteenth century. The royal family of Bahrain is also connected to this sect.

Qatar, like the other Gulf states, had unreliable data regarding demography, particularly in relation to the Qataris and the ex-patriates. According to a British estimate at the outbreak of the Second World War, the total population was around 28,000 in Doha and a few coastal villages – the central desert area with many nomads was ignored. By 1970 another British guess was that the population had risen to just over 100,000. In 1986 the first Qatari census found the figure had reached 396,079.

The census also revealed that 65-70% were non-Qatari. Of the total population 66% were male and only 34% were female – this extraordinary difference was due to the preponderance of males in the ex-pat workforce from the Indian sub-continent and Iran – curious, as the majority of Iranians are Shii. The oil/gas and construction industries, followed later by banking and the financial sector, accounted for the steady increase in ex-pats. 84% of the population lived in Doha and the industrial town of Umm Sa'id close by.

The Sheraton hotel was situated at the far end of the promenade on the tree-lined shore of the Gulf, and was the most expensive hotel in the country. The Ministry of Health had arranged my accommodation and my heart sank even though the Ministry had agreed to pay half the cost. Throughout all my visits to the Gulf states, the authorities had found it impossible to accept that I was paying my own expenses and wasn't connected to a university medical school or the department of health or some academic organisation.

The interior was lavish and extravagant with a large indoor fountain, a sumptuous lounge and endless music from a spacious entertainment area. Waiters were rushing everywhere. Before settling into my luxurious bedroom I stood on the balcony with a by now chilly breeze coming off the sea and viewed the twinkling lights around the Bay of Doha – and wondered about tomorrow.

I managed to walk to the Ministry by 8am to meet Dr Ahmed Dajani, the Director of Primary Health Care. He was Pakistani by birth but had trained in the United States and had been working in Qatar for six years. At the start of our meeting he was keen for me to understand how much had been accomplished since independence in 1971. Even before this, whilst still under a British Mandate, the Ministry of Public Health had been established in 1951, a Directorate of Preventive Medicine in '61, a Department of Hospital Services in '64, and at the time of independence, on the advice of the WHO, the Ministry of Public Health was reorganised into two separate Directorates – Hospital Services and Public Health & Preventive Medicine. Following the Declaration of Alma Ata in 1978 the Department of Primary Health Care was set up as the third Directorate.

In the early '50s, the Amir had decided that all treatment both in hospitals and in the community would be free – I wondered if this decision had in any way been influenced by the recent introduction of the NHS in Britain, where treatment was free at the time of use. Since 1982 *all* children, at least in theory, had been attending primary school starting at the age of six. The figures for secondary school were 79% for boys and 92% for girls. The adult literacy rate (sixteen years and over) was 78% for males and 91% for females. These statistics, even if perhaps exaggerated, are remarkable, and so different from anywhere else in the developing world.

All doctors and nurses employed by the Ministry of Health,

whether in hospital or primary care, were forbidden to work in the private sector, but this was not to say that private practice wasn't flourishing. However, there were no private hospitals, and private patients requiring hospital treatment were transferred to Saudi Arabia or the United Arab Emirates.

Until the Declaration of Alma Ata in '78, the health service had concentrated on building hospitals – in '57 the 120-bed Rumaila hospital and in '59 a 120-bed women's hospital. This emphasis on hospitals continued for the next nineteen years although by 1988 there were 23 government-run health centres functioning, thus providing competition to the private clinics, which had been active for many years.

I had the great good fortune to have Pauline Keena, Head of Nursing in the Department of Primary Care, to accompany me throughout my stay. She had been working in Qatar for a number of years and understood the country well. She came from southern Ireland and had the charm of the Irish as well as being well informed about the health service in Qatar. Unfortunately, like most ex-pats she spoke little Arabic, but a bi-lingual colleague always accompanied us.

The drive north out of Doha to Khor was on a good tarmac road through gently undulating, rather monotonous, unremarkable stony desert traversed by many dry *wadis* interspersed with shrubs, bushes and stunted trees. Isolated settlements and herds of goats completed the scene except for glimpses of nomadic tribesmen and their camels in the middle distance. Since first coming to Qatar, Pauline had noticed a marked decline in the numbers of camels:

"Today's Bedouins prefer Japanese pick-up trucks to camels."

Khor was a large village with a population of around 16,000 and had been built around a natural harbour. Many dhows were pulled up on the sandy beach as the locals continued to fish. I was surprised by the size of some of the dhows and it signified that fishing was still taking place some distance out into the Gulf. The harbour, and its immediate neighbourhood of traditional housing, was picturesque, evocative of another age. Alas the days of pearl diving were long gone, victim to the cultured pearl industry that had emerged in Japan.

The health centre was open from 7am until midnight and was staffed by six male and two female doctors, a senior nurse, ten trained nurses with some midwifery experience, plus a couple of pharmacists and laboratory and x-ray technicians. The x-ray department was modern but greatly under-used as it had not occurred to anyone to suggest that a radiologist from Doha might visit every fortnight, or as required.

I have mentioned many times that patient usage of phc facilities is closely related to the cleanliness and standard of hygiene of the staff; in Qatar great importance had been placed on these two points. Khor was an excellent example of what could be achieved and a survey carried out a few months prior to my visit showed that on average at least one person per household had visited a health centre five times a year. Furthermore, only 40% of the population lived more than one hour's walk away.

The centres were staffed almost entirely by Arabic-speaking females, either Qatari or Egyptian, and males who were mostly Indian or Pakistani who didn't speak Arabic. Pauline was convinced the nationality of the health worker was not an issue, what mattered was the ability to speak and understand Arabic. In hospitals the majority of all health workers were non-Qatari and mostly from India, Pakistan, the Philippines and Indonesia, plus a small number from the western industrialised world who were exclusively employed in high-tech tertiary departments – virtually none of these workers spoke Arabic.

A decision had been made that doctors working in health centres should be trained as family doctors à la Kuwait and Bahrain, but not surprisingly, without a medical school, it had proved to be impossible. The reluctance to use the Gulf University medical school in Bahrain was an added obstacle. Pauline considered the idea of a family doctor to be sound in principle and we both came to the conclusion that, if a family doctor was not possible, it would be preferable to have a general physician for adults, and paediatricians (all of whom should be female) to provide MCH services; all of course should speak Arabic.

The continuing poor communications and feedback between secondary and primary care was a great concern to Pauline; she was also convinced that hospital specialists needed to be better informed about the needs of patients living in the community and to understand how different their problems were from those in hospital. In a nutshell, their training and education needed to be re-thought. She was frustrated too that most mothers didn't understand how important it was to attend health centres even if their child was well – for immunisation and development checks, for example. However, she accepted that health education was going to be a long uphill battle that would require constant coverage via tv and radio, and most important of all, on every visit a mother made to a centre.

Medinal Khalifa, originally a small suburb on the northern edge of Doha, had been developed into a new town with a new health centre; again, it was clean, the staff being aware of the need for strict hygiene. Three paediatricians for developmental screening and carrying out the immunisation programme, three paediatricians for sick children, six physicians for the care of adults, and a female gynaecologist, comprised the staff. Although 99% of births took place in hospital, health centres were only just starting to be given information about mother and baby and the date of their discharge, hence it was impossible to work out which mothers needed post-natal visiting and follow-up. As has already been said, the lines of communication between primary and secondary care left a lot to be desired.

I came across a new law that had recently been passed that strangely Pauline had not mentioned – home visits had now been forbidden, even by female doctors and nurses. The reason and purpose of this insane new law were truly beyond comprehension, and equally incomprehensible was the acceptance of it. I could only assume that Wahhabi bigotry must have been responsible.

In 1960 infant mortality was 145 per 1,000 births. Under five years mortality was 239, both statistics mirroring the situation in the poorest countries of the developing world. Twenty-eight years later the figures had dropped to 30 and 37 per thousand live births. Maternal mortality had not been recorded in 1960, but between 1985 and '88 there hadn't been one death. This dramatic improvement in maternal and child health was really impressive.

I tried to find evidence that everything was not as satisfactory as the Ministry of Health and the Department of PHC maintained, but for the most part it was all good. In Doha virtually 100% of the population had a piped sewage system with a sewage treatment centre on the edge of town. From what Pauline had told me and what I had seen, in rural areas septic tanks were the rule and were regularly emptied by suction trucks. The streets were free of garbage, although in Doha and places like Khor, dust, rubble and sand lay everywhere on account of the enormous amount of building work taking place.

Clean drinking water reached nearly 100% of the population, a statistic that had been accepted as accurate by the WHO and UNICEF. In remote areas water tankers made regular distribution runs, which I had seen on my way to Khor. But an unexpected report had been released soon after my return to the UK, although whilst I was in Qatar the subject had never been mentioned or even whispered about:

> 'Qatar has one of the largest per capita rates of water usage; a typical household uses three times as much as a European household. Government officials blame air-conditioning and garden watering for these excessive levels . . . irrigation and private farms have also caused water engineers headaches. Legislation exists to protect water resources but it is difficult to enforce and the flow remains largely unchecked.'

Certainly private farms were continuing to sink water pumps and, judging by the beauty of the promenade and the wonderfully coloured flower gardens and parks, the authorities were also guilty of excessive water consumption. (Water was not used for the cultivation of *qat).* Water produced by desalination cost at the time 25% more to produce than pumped water from a depth of 180 feet. During my stay nobody ever posed a question about running out of this most precious resource, but when the water table finally disappears how long will desalination be affordable for a steadily increasing population? What will the situation be in twenty-five years time?

There was electricity in nearly every home and for those in the middle of nowhere generators and fuel were provided completely free. Nutrition was certainly adequate judging by the fact that in 1986 almost 95% of new-born babies had birth weights of at least 5lbs 8ozs. Education and literacy were improving, and most importantly girls were being encouraged and were often out-performing boys at every level.

My endeavour to find evidence that everything was not as successful as I had been told had not been confirmed. Peter

Mansfield writing in *The Arabs* in 1985 had stated:

> 'Qatar, the smallest of the independent Arab states, has developed against powerful odds into a flourishing and well-ordered city state with a distinctive identity.'

Everything pointed to the Amir spending his wealth wisely and to the benefit of his people. But hidden away, or at least never openly discussed by government officials or the Amir's supporters, were nuggets of doubt. The profligate use of water, the potential danger of Wahhabism, the attitude and behaviour of the upper echelons of society towards migrant domestic servants, and the absurd new law against home visits by health professionals, are just a few examples. At a meeting of the Ministry of Education to discuss problems within the School Health Service, it was only on getting back to the hotel and reading a report, 1984-87, that I found information hidden away in an appendix in small print – venereal disease, particularly gonorrhoea, had been steadily rising among boys as young as fourteen. Nobody at the meeting mentioned this. There was no reference either to the other cloud on everyone's horizon – HIV. There was no mention that it even existed or that, if the facts about venereal disease were accurate, HIV would initially spread like wildfire through the male community. Perhaps after all the Amir's utopia was not quite all it professed to be.

My first impression of Doha was of cranes and construction sites and four, wide, well-built semi-circular ring roads, the outer one separating the town from the edge of a barren stony desert. The other side of Doha extended along the semi-circular, tree-lined promenade on the coast of the Persian Gulf. Across the bay I could see a number of buildings from my hotel; first there was a dazzlingly white building close to some sort of tower, and beyond this another impressive building, again whiter than white in the sunshine – perhaps another palace. Obviously the town needed exploring on foot.

It was enchanting to walk through the attractive and peaceful gardens and trees of the promenade with the sea lapping on my left. Suddenly I had a glimpse of contrasting cultures: the earnest western joggers pounding the ground, looking out for their next stop so they could check their watches to see if they were achieving their goal –

red-faced, earnest, sweating and anxious; then the Indian and Pakistani families strolling about, many of the women in colourful saris or long dresses and the men (mostly overweight) in European suits, the girls laughing and giggling and the boys with cricket bats and balls trying to persuade their families to stop so they could start a game. The Arabs were mostly picnicking on the grass with a wonderful display of food and drink, the older men often sitting quietly on the concrete slabs of the promenade in groups of twos or threes, always smoking, as does most of the Indian sub-continent. Nobody was drinking alcohol and no one was causing any trouble.

I watched a number of young men and boys fishing with a simple rod and line, and like fishermen the world over who find excuses when few fish have been caught, their excuse on this occasion was the water was too cold. However, the cormorants flying close to the shoreline, at almost every dive came up with a decent-sized fish in their beak!

The first building I had seen across the bay was one of the original Amir palaces, quite breath-taking in size, which had been renovated and converted into the National Theatre. Nearby was the Clock Tower, apparently one of Doha's most famous sights, and close by, too, the Grand Mosque and Minaret. A little wander round this more traditional area took me to a small, well-restored Ottoman fort which had been used by the Turks in the First World War. Large areas of rubble disfigured the locale, with its variety of *souks* and markets and many simple single-storey houses with flat corrugated iron roofs. They had all seen better days and reminded me that despite the overall impression of immense wealth, it was well to remember 'the poor you have always with you'.

The final building I had seen from the hotel proved to be another palace belonging to another member of the royal family, which had been carefully restored, almost rebuilt, to become the National Museum of Qatar. Beyond the museum up a slight incline Doha harbour came into view – and opened up another world. There they were – the Doha Club, the Beach Club, the Gulf Oasis luxury hotel, all proudly offering swimming pools, motor yachts, tennis, squash and bowling and much else I have forgotten. They were the domain almost exclusively of ex-patriate westerners, instantly recognisable by their lobster-coloured skin and clothing more suited to Hawaii or the beaches of Australia. It was noticeable that ex-pats from the Indian sub-continent, Indonesia and the Philippines were absent.

Supper at the Sheraton on my final evening: West Indians playing calypso music or jazz; Americans, Australians and Europeans consuming mountains of food and booze served by Korean waiters. What on earth must the ordinary Qatari think of us as we steadily take over and seem to rob them of their own culture and traditions?

After breakfast in my room and before being taken to the airport, a last look from my balcony. A spectacular scene met my eyes – thousands, yes thousands of birds migrating from north to south across the Persian Gulf, filling the sky in truly breathtaking fashion. And then, looking down at the hotel swimming pool, at the trees and shrubs that surrounded it, small birds of every possible colour flitting from branch to branch through the dappled sunlight, put the finishing touch to this perfect picture.

32

UNITED ARAB EMIRATES

Out of the blue, in response to a telex sent to Dubai from Doha notifying them of my time of arrival, a return message from Dr Ghaffor, Director of PHC Dubai, with whom I had been in frequent correspondence over the last two or three months, informed me he would be unable to meet me and I would have to arrange another visit. Obviously this would be a total disaster for me as I would have to return to the UK and there would be no way I could re-organise a further visit. My primary responsibility had to be with my practice in Wells, and anyway I couldn't afford a return visit. Furthermore I would be forced to renege on the promise I had made to the Arab Board of Health Ministers with the result they would withdraw their support for *Primary Health Care in the Arab World.* In all honesty, too, I was beginning to lose interest in what I was doing.

Shortly after receiving the news from Dubai, I had a meeting with the Under-Secretary of State, who wasn't interested in helping. Then quite by chance a young Qatari doctor, whom I had never met, who had somehow heard of my quandary, offered to phone Dubai for me to see if he could do anything. Within an hour he had managed to contact Ghaffor and had persuaded him to change his mind and continue with our original arrangement. Apparently Ghaffor's rather lame excuse was that he thought I was going to Oman before visiting Dubai. I was so grateful to that young Qatari doctor and am certain he had no idea how much he had helped me; to my genuine sadness he just disappeared and I never saw him again – I didn't even know his name. How I wished I could have thanked him properly.

The flight was delayed for an hour or so, giving me time to think about Qatar. I had experienced almost universal cooperation and that young man was a wonderful example of help way beyond anything I could have expected.

Coming in to land at Dubai gave me a perfect view of the Creek and the coastline of Abu Dhabi, and then the smaller Emirates spreading out along the coast to the Strait of Hormuz. Passport and customs posed no problems and, as I half-expected, no one was there to meet me. I decided to take a taxi to the Ministry of Health, not that I expected it to be open as it was a Friday, but at least I would know where it was. Having located the Ministry I asked to be taken to the cheapest hotel nearest to it; I could then estimate how long it would take me to walk there the following morning – taxis were expensive and money was running out. I smiled as I was dumped at the Claridge's hotel and as I waited at reception for nobody to appear I couldn't avoid a comparison with its illustrious namesake in London. Eventually a man turned up:

> "Yes, we have a single room with a basin and water but no air conditioning and no breakfast."

I now had a free day but as yet I hadn't come across the excellent map of the UAE, again produced by the Oxford University Press, which I had been told I must get. What to do next? I walked to the Ministry and reckoned it would take me a half hour in the morning. The taxi ride had given me a vague idea of the direction of the famous Creek so I set off. What immediately caught my eye was that cricket was being played on every spare bit of open ground – usually a small group of men and boys knocking a ball about, the stumps represented by the nearest oil can or wooden box or wall that could be marked out. Spin bowlers were much in evidence, certainly more than the speed merchants that were in fashion at the time. Only Indians and Pakistanis were involved, the Sikhs standing out on account of their colourful turbans. But no West Indians.

When I eventually reached a large open sandy area close to the edge of the Creek, I found two matches being played. The batsmen and wicket keepers at the match I watched were wearing pads, and there were proper stumps at both ends. Spectators sat around the uncertain boundary, a mixed bunch consisting mainly of women and small children with a few Arab men squatting and talking together and largely ignoring the game. I imagine they were probably totally mystified by the strange spectacle.

The Dubai side of the Creek was a fascinating mix of old houses, many wind towers, as in Bahrain, a variety of small *souks* and numerous old dhows stretching up the Creek. The 180-year-old Al

Fahid fort had been well restored as had the Grand Mosque nearby.

Looking across to the Deira side there was just an expanse of modern commercial buildings indistinguishable from anywhere else in the world. Nevertheless I decided to take a water-taxi, or *abras*, and on landing I found a busy scene; dhows were moored for about a hundred yards up and down the quay, which was piled high with goods waiting to be loaded or had recently been unloaded. Trade was mainly with Somalia, Iran and places up and down the Arab side of the Gulf coast and beyond the Strait of Hormuz along the coast of East Africa. It was a truly atmospheric, colourful sight, with not a single non-smoker amongst the not-very-energetic dockers!

As I meandered around I found an alleyway quite by chance leading almost secretively away from the quay to the famous Gold *souk* – that was indeed a sight to behold.

To the Ministry by 8am and straight to the Department of PHC. It turned out Dr Ghaffor was at a conference, but then a voice hailed me from another room – Dr Abdul Wahab al Muhaideb, the Assistant Under-Secretary for Health, who proved to be a great help. First he provided the recent Ministry of Health Annual Report which I had requested, and second he endeavoured to reassure me that a programme of work would indeed be organised, so at least Ghaffor must have spoken to him.

Al Muhaideb explained he was going to Abu Dhabi the next day, that I was to accompany him and we would be staying for a couple of days. I was to meet him at the Hilton hotel in the morning; for the life of me I couldn't understand why he couldn't pick me up from Claridge's, but I was in no position to quibble.

As part of the programme a visit to a health centre in Deira had been arranged for the afternoon. I waited in vain, but nobody turned up – fortunately I had become used to the unreliability and unpredictability of the Arab world so I shrugged my shoulders and accepted the inevitable. In any case the Annual Report provided plenty of work when I got back to the hotel.

al Muhaideb arrived at the Hilton in a large Mercedes equipped with a large mobile phone – very modern for those days – plus a radio-cassette with speakers. He was a large man and climbed out of the car with some difficulty, hampered by his *dishdasha* (a long white cotton robe). I noticed he was also wearing *serwals* (cotton pyjama trousers) under his *thobe* (full-length dress), and to complete his outfit he had on the traditional headdress, Yasser Arafat style. He showed me how complicated it was to put on: first a *ghahfeyah* (crocheted cap) was worn under a *ghetral* (large triangular scarf), all kept in position by the *agaal* (black woollen headband). In both Dubai and Abu Dhabi the majority of physicians wore traditional dress.

It was noticeable that in the UAE both sexes wore traditional dress more often than in Kuwait, Bahrain and Qatar. The *abbaya* (black covering over a woman's dress or jeans and her head) was worn less often than the *nigah* (a black veil that covered the whole of the face except the eyes). Girls seemed to be introduced first to a headscarf and then in their mid-teens to a simple veil – but not the *nigah* until they were older.

al Muhaideb spoke and understood English and had visited the UK – or to be more accurate, London – on a couple of occasions. The purpose of both visits had been to try and buy a property or properties, and the property market and visiting estate agents appeared to be his main interest, not medicine – although this might be doing him an injustice as in fact he managed to arrange an excellent couple of days for me.

The drive took a couple of hours over an endlessly flat stony landscape with an occasional small oasis and the sudden appearance of brightly coloured flowers. It was a well-tarmacked carriageway that passed through small settlements, indicating easily available natural water. Throughout the journey I was quizzed about the most expensive and fashionable parts of London, which towns and cities were popular, how Cambridge compared with Birmingham, or Oxford with Manchester. He wanted to know if it was true that living in the country was often many people's dream. And so it went on. I'm certain I wasn't much help.

My immediate impression of Abu Dhabi was a feeling of space: wide roads, clean streets, much greenery and a few beautiful parks and gardens, but rather spoilt by the forest of tall buildings – some quite ridiculously high – demonstrating the ingenuity and expertise of architects and engineers working with glass and steel. I discovered that old buildings, people's homes and even mosques were being flattened to make way for I know not what – almost certainly endless shopping malls and luxury hotels, whilst banks, business and commerce and the financial world competed to become the most prestigious exemplar of modern architecture. Abu Dhabi provided and has continued to provide what the Emir and his extended family, the wealthy, and the majority of tourists, want. However the multi-storey apartments for ordinary citizens at least provided air-conditioning rather than the old wind towers, which had been demolished, so on reflection I mustn't be too harsh.

The Ministry of Health had arranged my programme: a meeting with the Director and Technical Coordinator of EPI; next a meeting at the UNICEF Regional office to discuss the strategy for PHC which had been produced by the WHO, UNICEF and the Ministry of Health in 1986, and a discussion on the UNICEF Gulf Area Annual Report of 1987. Both meetings were excellent. Then on to the School of Nursing to finish a good morning's work.

In the afternoon a young Lebanese doctor, Dr Karim Hashish, accompanied me while I visited two primary care facilities. She was feeling sad, having just returned from her father's funeral, and was very distressed by the situation in Beirut. She had left Lebanon eleven years ago and had lived in the Emirates ever since, returning regularly to visit her family, but this time on going back for the funeral she had found Beirut unrecognisable. Extremists had taken over and she felt totally alienated from her own country. In the streets she felt unsafe, never knowing if she was going to be stopped and asked for her passport and other documents or asked questions about who she was, where she was staying, or where she was going. She felt she could easily have been taken hostage.

Al Nahyan MCH centre had been open for fifteen years and provided ante-natal care, children's curative and preventive care, and health education for mothers. The Rodha health centre had originally been opened as a dispensary but in 1985 had been upgraded to a health centre with an attached MCH unit which was finally installed in a small dispensary storeroom that proved to be too small for health education, so this could only take place when the patients' waiting area wasn't in use. Planners love planning and what interests them most is to have plans in their office so they can proudly demonstrate the improvements in their facilities. Nobody seemed remotely concerned whether they were patient-friendly. Karim agreed with my criticism and was convinced that PHC still remained at the bottom of health service priorities.

The ruling classes and the upper echelons of society perceived health almost exclusively in terms of secondary and tertiary care. Politicians by and large were not interested in primary care, looking upon it as second-class care or just an irritation and certainly not of concern to them. Anecdotal stories had a ring of truth about them and I remember hearing about the number of MRI and CAT scanners and other high-tech equipment that had been installed in the UAE, yet MCH centres often had no baby scales, thermometers, or pregnancy-testing equipment. Likewise health education projects could not be established on account of lack of transport to bring in the mothers, and the project already established at Al Nahyan and Rodha could not be expanded. Lack of money was surely not the reason; rather it was a complete lack of interest.

We both needed some fresh air and decided to walk along the promenade. Seemingly hundreds of gardeners toiled over the fabulous gardens, working on their hands and knees as they meticulously cleared every inch of ground and pavement and trimmed the edges of the grass as if done by scissors. Karim pointed out the full extent of land reclamation (similar to Bahrain) with ten-lane highways filling up the space. The shops bulged with food and consumer goods – everything you could possibly want but little you really needed. Shopping was the only thing to do, reminding me a little of Japan.

Karim remarked about modern Abu Dhabi, how she disliked the atmosphere of consumerism and missed very much the everyday street life of an ordinary Arab town or village. The Gulf states had become the mecca of a different culture, and just as she had felt an alien in her homeland of Lebanon, so here too she felt herself a stranger in her adopted country, though for different reasons. It was reassuring to know that she felt as I, and I'm sure others, did.

Like the rest of the Emirates as well as Bahrain and Qatar, Abu Dhabi and Dubai had initially found it difficult to collect accurate data on population, basic health and education statistics, as well as information about clean drinking water and sewage disposal. It was very refreshing though to find that the poor quality of data and the inaccuracy of many surveys was openly admitted.

The UAE had undertaken three national population censuses, the most recent being in 1980. Its main shortcomings were the composition of the population by nationality, which limited meaningful interpretation of the results since immigrants probably constituted about 70% of the total population. According to the WHO, even the recent 1987 vital statistics were virtually non-existent, whilst demographic and socio-economic surveys didn't exist at all.

Access to clean drinking water in both urban and rural areas had definitely improved over the past twenty-five years, but I found it impossible to discover the situation regarding ground water – broad generalisations or straightforward obfuscation was the order of the day; honesty was no part of the vocabulary. Few disputed that fresh water was scarce and most agreed that 80% of drinking water was supplied by desalination. Water engineers, economists and desalination experts all agreed in a variety of reports that desalination was expensive, but nobody was prepared to give figures about the drop in the level of ground water. Worst of all I never once heard anyone mention the obvious – that desalination depended on money, or in other words, the continuing production of oil and gas.

Health services were provided by the individual countries of the UAE but were under the supervision of the Federal Ministry of Health in Dubai. Primary care was organised through a network of health centres with no difference between urban and rural services. Facilities were provided on population numbers – up to 5,000, from 5-15,000, and over 15,000. All centres had a pharmacy and only the smallest didn't have a simple laboratory. Rural hospitals were operational in six of the emirates. The health of immigrant workers, as in the neighbouring Gulf states, was likely to remain ignored and unchanged for years to come.

The University of the UAE had been established in 1977 in Al-

Ain, an oasis town in the foothills of the Hafit mountains on the Oman border, more or less equidistant from Abu Dhabi and Dubai. In 1984 a steering committee had been appointed to start planning for a new medical school and two years later, in consultation with the WHO, a Dean was appointed, and the first workshop on medical education followed later in the year. Visits were made to medical schools and institutions throughout the world; this led to an imaginative curriculum being agreed on. There was to be strong emphasis on community health, the safety of the environment, epidemiology and medical/health economics. The focus on economics was very unusual at that time and was real forward-thinking. It was therefore a curious irony that the study of health economics had failed to point out the folly of the continued emphasis on hospitals and high-tech medicine rather than the need to concentrate on a strong primary care sector. The training of medical students was to foster a problem-based approach rather than passive learning, and in addition it was intended that most teaching would take place in health centres, which by then would have adapted to the primary care philosophy.

The opportunity to visit Al-Ain was too good to be true. I was picked up around 8am; it had been raining heavily all night and many roads were half-flooded, and it wasn't until we reached the main road to Al-Ain that the flooding disappeared. The three-lane highway with a central reservation and motorway-style overhead electric lighting extended for at least two-thirds of the hundred-mile journey. The central reservation was mainly grass, shrubs, hedges, trees and clumps of flowers. On either side of the road were strips of date palms about a hundred yards long, and, alongside, some form of agricultural activity. Beyond that lay the desert and endless rolling waves of sand extending as far as the eye could see; the nearer we got to Al-Ain the more striking the sand – white, yellow, orange, and even red. As we neared our destination I could see the town was dominated by the Jebel Hafit mountain range with large areas of thriving agriculture surrounding the rest. We were soon hooting our way through cars, goats, bikes and camels to the university. Al-Ain seemed to be a town of shaded parks and gardens – a real blaze of colour. This was a great surprise as I'd never realised an oasis town could be so beautiful. Jebel

Hafit was the source of the water producing this Garden of Eden.

We went straight to the Faculty of Medicine and Health Services to meet members of staff, one of whom gave me a resumé of the short history of the medical school. The course was for seven years – two years' pre-clinical study and five years' clinical training, with students working and being taught, it was hoped, as much in health centres as hospital wards and clinics. Graduation would be followed by a one-year internship before being allowed to practise – the course so far, then, almost identical to that in the western world. Finding enough teachers would undoubtedly be a problem, at least in the short term, as well as the self-evident fact that new health centres would need to be built, and in the right locations.

I was able to talk to quite a few of the staff, both Arab and Indian, and it was clear both nationalities were not convinced that primary care was the correct approach. It was difficult to know how much the steering committee were aware of this opposition or were just pretending it didn't exist. Teaching in all its aspects was going to pose a number of problems. In 1986/87 thirty-three students had been accepted, twenty-one female and twelve male, and it was intended they should begin their clinical training in '88, around the time of my visit. Two hospitals and sixteen health centres – eight in Al-Ain and eight in the surrounding desert – were the responsibility of the medical school.

My initial impression was that much study and thought had gone into this potentially first-class project, but on reflection everything was happening too quickly, almost before the groundwork was in place. Perhaps this had been recognised as no students had been admitted in 1987/'88. Whether the impatience was due to the UAE believing they had been left behind by the creation of the Gulf Medical School in Bahrain, I don't know.

On my way back to Abu Dhabi it was suggested we should make a detour, but not before the cattle/camel market had been visited – utterly fascinating, with sheep from Australia and goats from Iraq, but mostly it was camels – strange, smelly creatures. The market was crowded with men who were as interesting as the animals, and judging by the number plates of their trucks, most of the buying and selling involved Oman. The adjacent vegetable market was spread over all the available ground and stacked high with every vegetable and fruit I could think of – except Brussels sprouts! For the first time since I had arrived in the Gulf I felt I was in Arabia.

The reason for the detour was another oasis town, Buraimi, about ten miles from Al-Ain – in fact it was in Oman, but nobody took any notice or cared on this unmarked desert frontier. It was a most attractive small oasis full of date palms, markets and gardens, and small mud-brick single-storey houses. I saw no poverty and the inhabitants looked healthy. It had a well-preserved stone fort – I think Ottoman – with four small crenellated towers joined by a high wall. But the real interest was the running water, its source twenty-five miles away in the mountains. It was explained to me (although I still didn't fully understand) that underground channels (*falaj*) carried the water from the source half way up the mountains, the water finally surfacing in Buraimi. Here it was diverted on rotation either for agricultural irrigation or to the numerous gardens. It reminded me of the constant flow of water in Wells, coming from the Mendip hills, that is diverted daily down alternate sides of the High Street. The water was clear and sparkling with small brightly-coloured birds continually dipping in for a drink, while children played at the edge. An enchanting place and so unexpected to see the running water.

al Muhaideb suggested I should book in at the Excelsior Hotel instead of Claridge's, and on returning to Dubai I was somewhat dismayed to find it was on the outskirts of Deira. However, it cost less. In Abu Dhabi I had been treated well with reduced rates in the hotel – this had been arranged by the Ministry in Dubai and it turned out at my final meeting I had been overcharged, so I was given 60 *dirhams* to compensate. Everything helped as I had banked my last travellers cheques – plastic cards had yet to arrive!

An extraordinary storm brewed up and continued all night, and to my astonishment, in the morning the hotel was surrounded by flooded streets and abandoned cars with water lapping over the tops of the wheels. The foyer too was flooded, mainly due to a leaking roof, and three men spent most of the day sweeping the water down the steps of the main entrance. The deluge lasted most of the day with severe winds and lightning in the afternoon. To say the British are the only people to talk about the weather is simply not true! The town soon looked as drab and dreary as anywhere in Britain on a wet and windy day – all the brilliant whiteness had disappeared and gloom had descended. I was mystified as to why the roads flooded so quickly as drain covers were visible on all but the smallest roads. There was no mystery; the drains were not connected to any pipes so the water soaked straight into the sand. I wished I had my gumboots with me but I knew I wouldn't be able to buy anything as practical or useful as that in this paradise of consumerism – I know because I asked.

Anyway, at midday, my shoes having been filled with sandy water on a couple of occasions, the Director of PHC collected me. Dr Mohammad Fahmy was Egyptian, spoke English well and a little Russian – he had studied and trained in the Soviet Union in the '70s. A reliable and conscientious man, he seemed determined I should see and discuss as much as possible and explained he had been embarrassed by the disorganisation that had greeted me on my arrival. Clearly he wanted to make amends and was as good as his word.

Al Rashidiya health centre in Deira, the Al Mankhool health centre in Dubai, and the Satura peripheral clinic also in Dubai had all followed a similar pattern of development since independence. The two health centres were clean and had been kept in a good state of repair, but both experienced the usual difficulties – the main complaints from patients concerned the rapid turnover of staff, both medical and nursing. The peripheral clinic had been set up long before independence and in the beginning only carried out simple tasks, but in 1982 ante-natal care (ANC) was introduced and quickly followed by MCH services, the ANC being carried out by two female doctors visiting once a week. The chief doctor was a Palestinian who had been working there for fourteen years and it was his enthusiasm and the continuity he provided that was the main reason for its success. The number of patients attending the clinic had been steadily rising over the years and by the time of my visit around 450 patients attended every day. This was by far the greatest number I had encountered in any Arab country I had visited. Seven doctors including two paediatricians covered this considerable workload – I don't recall the number of trained or assistant nurses.

Fahmy again pulled out all the stops on the following day. Al

Ghesus health centre had opened in 1983 and had been quickly upgraded to include MCH care. As in Abu Dhabi, separate MCH centres had been the norm until 1983, but since then it had been integrated into all health centres. We were able to spend time talking to three members of staff and a really worthwhile discussion highlighted several issues – the lack of nurses; the need for but the difficulty in getting specialists to provide regular out-patient clinics; and the problems posed by the number of languages, apart from Arabic, spoken by patients – Parsee, Iranian, Somali, Bengali, Indian sub-continent and various south-east Asian languages.

The school health service had been in operation since 1968 and strangely, as in Abu Dhabi, was organised and supervised from Kuwait, which was also in charge of the Department of Education. Again I never understood why or how this arrangement functioned. Anyway, by the time of independence, twenty schools each with a small attached health clinic had been opened, and by '81 a further sixty schools plus their attached health clinic were operational. During the next seven years two-thirds of schools had regular input from a full-time nurse who had responsibility for five or six schools, carrying out development check-ups, immunisations, and referrals to a newly opened School Health Service Polyclinic. The method of referral (ie whether the nurse could refer directly) had not been settled, and everyone agreed it was going to take at least five years to see how successful the polyclinic project would be.

The day ended rather quietly at the Nursing Institute attached to Rashid hospital where two courses had been running for some years – the training was three years for a full qualification and eighteen months for assistant nurses. It was all very low key and I was given the usual list of problems, but no ideas about any solutions. I felt sympathy for Fahmy; he had remained enthusiastic and helpful, and for the day to end so tamely was a big disappointment for him. As we said goodbye I think he knew how grateful I was – I hope so.

Certainly the UAE was full of strange paradoxes.

What were my final impressions of Kuwait, Bahrain, Qatar and the United Arab Emirates? Certainly a strong feeling that their history, culture and way of life was in danger of disappearing. Who is responsible and why it is happening is difficult to answer. The decision to follow the western industrialised world and the underlying imperative to outdo the US, Japan and western Europe, had been displayed superficially by the skyline of these countries, but how had they come to believe that their success depended on supplying foreigners with whatever they wanted, even if this involved accepting some of the crudeness, vulgarity and excess of western culture?

Such behaviour is contrary to the revelation of the 114 *Suras* (chapters) communicated to the prophet Muhammad in the Sacred Book of Islam, the Koran. Such behaviour is also just as alien to the culture and tradition of secular Arabs. Or is it that rulers and dictators are simply ambitious and want influence and power at any cost?

Unfortunately it is more than this, and in particular over the last twenty years Qatar appears to have been leading the way in corruption and bribery so that it has become the accepted way to live. The fiasco of allegations of corruption by FIFA, the International Federation of Association Football, in awarding Qatar the 2022 World Cup tournament, and the – repeatedly denied – allegations that the Gulf state bought votes, will have resounding consequences far into the future. Qatar's moral corruption, draconian medieval laws and human rights record were apparently overlooked.

However, it is not only Qatar but each country from Kuwait to the UAE that is guilty of treating foreign labour with absolute contempt – the female domestics almost slaves within the family and the men in construction having to work in dangerous conditions with no regard for health and safety, often unpaid for months and with inadequate food and housing. Both men and women have their passports taken from them and so are unable to leave the country.

The shortage of water throughout the Gulf is obvious, yet the UAE has shamefully managed to lead the way, almost to the point of lunacy, by using water to provide superb golf courses, two large stadiums for Test cricket and much else besides. Only rarely is the voice of caution or reason heard, and never amongst sportsmen and women, supporters, journalists and sponsors. In fifty to a hundred years how will the southern shore of the Arabian/Persian Gulf look when oil and gas have run out and the expensive desalination of water is no longer affordable?

These small countries need to remember they have literally been built on sand, that they depend on the restrained and sensible use of water, and that everything is ultimately supported by the continuing flow of gas and oil.

As we look at life today, surely none of us must forget the warning of the poet Shelley as he travelled the Middle East early in the nineteenth century. Rulers come and go: empires fall into ruin: power is transient. Does no one think of the past, or the future, or is the present all that matters? Let the Gulf states ponder over his poem:

Ozymandias

I met a traveller from an antique land
Who said: two vast and trunkless legs of stone
Stand in the desert . . . near them on the sand
Half sunk, a shattered visage lies, whose frown,
And wrinkled lip, and sneer of cold command,
Tell that its sculptor well those passions read
Which yet survive, stamped on these lifeless things.
The hand that mocked them, and the heart that fed:
And on the pedestal these words appear:
'My name is Ozymandias King of Kings:
Look on my works, ye Mighty, and despair!'
Nothing beside remains. Round the decay
Of that colossal wreck, boundless and bare
The lone and level sand stretch far away.

33

FINAL THOUGHTS

Looking back, what do I think about the countries visited in this book?

I think I can safely say that it is not really the countries I remember but the people. I realise how immensely fortunate I have been to travel as a physician, where possession of a stethoscope gave me immediate access to ordinary people and to their homes, however poor they might be. This nearness to a family is a privilege granted to very few and something I experienced in every country. To be asked to lay your hands on a little boy's tummy or auscultate a young girl's chest or support a worried mother in her anxiety about a long-standing nappy rash, or listen to the trials and tribulations of being old, is indeed a special honour.

To have experienced such proximity to people in spite of being totally unknown to them, is almost beyond belief. To have found such folk throughout the world has been wonderfully reassuring and confirms what I suspect we already know – it is not those whose sole interest is power and politics who are needed, it is the 'common man', ordinary mortals of the human race.

Printed by: Copytech (UK) Limited trading as Printondemand-worldwide, 9 Culley Court,
Bakewell Road, Orton Southgate, Peterborough, PE2 6XD